RARE DISEASES

Dr. Sheeana Gangadoo

ALLIED
HEALTH
PRESS

Rare Diseases

Author: **Dr. Sheeana Gangadoo**

Allied Health Press
4164 Lakeshore Road
Burlington ON L7L 1A4
Canada
www.alliedhealthpress.com
Email: orders@arclereducation.com

ISBN: 978-1-77956-270-8

ABOUT THE AUTHOR

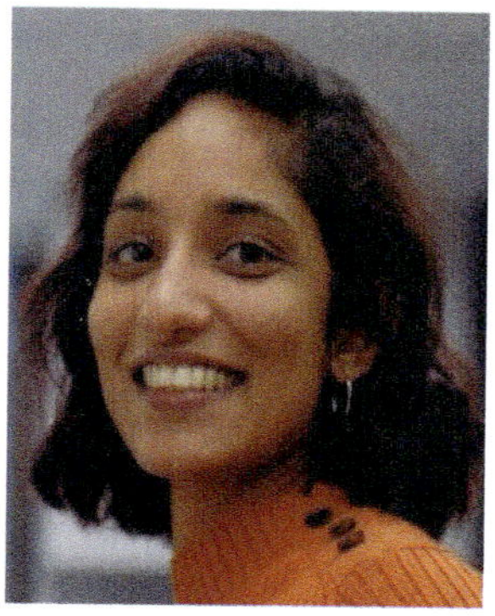

Dr. Sheeana Gangadoo was awarded her PhD in Microbiology and Agricultural Sciences, where her work focused on the influence of nanoparticles to improve the gut microbiota and overall health of broiler chickens. As a postdoctoral researcher, she focused on the investigation of antimicrobial materials to reduce the spread of antibiotic resistant microbes and was trained on various spectroscopic and microscopy techniques. She was later employed as a microbiologist in collaboration with Australian biotechnology company, Biomebank, and successfully optimised a novel anaerobic bioreactor for the production of probiotics in treating gut diseases.

Word Roots, Prefixes, and Suffixes by Chapter

Chapter 1 Introduction to Rare Disease

-itis: Inflammation (e.g., arthritis refers to inflammation of the joints).

-osis: Condition or disease (e.g., fibrosis refers to the thickening and scarring of connective tissue).

-opathy: Disease or disorder (e.g., neuropathy refers to nerve disorders).

-genic: Originating from or produced by (e.g., pathogenic refers to disease-causing agents).

Chapter 2 Chronic Respiratory Diseases

-itis: inflammation (e.g., bronchitis)

-osis: condition, usually abnormal (e.g., fibrosis)

-opathy: disease (e.g., cardiomyopathy)

-spasm: involuntary contraction (e.g., bronchospasm)

-ectomy: surgical removal (e.g., lobectomy)

Chapter 3 Pneumonia

-itis: Inflammation (e.g., pneumonia, meaning inflammation of the lungs).

-osis: Abnormal condition (e.g., pneumoconiosis, a lung disease caused by inhaling dust).

-pathy: Disease or disorder (e.g., pneumopathy, referring to any disease of the lung).

Chapter 4 Infant Leukemia

-emia: Referring to a blood condition.

-cytosis: Indicating an increase in cells.

-blast: Referring to an immature or precursor cell.

-genesis: Denoting the formation or development of something.

-pathy: Indicating a disease or disorder.

Chapter 5 Rare Tumors of the Colon and Rectum

-itis: inflammation

-plasty: surgical repair

-scopy: viewing or examination

-genic: producing or originating

-sarcoma: malignant tumor of connective tissue

-carcinoma: malignant tumor of epithelial origin

Chapter 6 Cystic Fibrosis

-osis: Condition or disease.

-pathy: Disease or disorder.

-itis: Inflammation.

-genic: Causing or producing.

Chapter 7 Tuberculosis

-osis: A condition or disease, used in terms like "tuberculosis" to indicate the disease caused by the bacteria.

-itis: Inflammation, sometimes seen in related conditions like "pneumonitis" when the lungs are inflamed due to tuberculosis.

-genic: Producing or causing, as in "tuberculogenic," which refers to the production of tuberculosis.

Chapter 8 Human Immunodeficiency Virus Infection

-itis: Inflammation, used in contexts like HIV-associated conditions (e.g., lymphadenitis)

-osis: Abnormal condition or disease, as in immuno-compromised status

-pathy: Disease or disorder, often seen in discussions about HIV-related illnesses (e.g., neuropathy)

Table of Contents

LIST OF FIGURES

LIST OF TABLES

PREFACE

Rare diseases, while individually uncommon, can collectively have a significant impact on the population and affect around 5–8% of people globally, with 7.9% of that population under 25 years of age. There are approximately 6,000 rare diseases worldwide which affect 300 million individuals and share common features. They are often difficult to diagnose promptly, tend to be chronic and debilitating, are largely genetic, and have limited treatment options. These diseases can have severe impacts on individuals' health and quality of life, as well as caregivers' lives, and lead to a high morbidity rate. Some examples of rare diseases include Hemophilia, Thalassemia, Sickle-cell Anemia, Cystic Fibrosis in India. The World Health Organization (WHO) defines a rare disease as one with a prevalence of 1 or less per 1,000 population. However, different countries may have their own definitions based on the prevalence, severity, and availability of treatment options for these diseases.

Research on rare diseases is accompanied by a unique set of challenges, including 1) conducting large-scale clinical trials and studies due to their low prevalence, 2) limited understanding of the underlying mechanisms of these diseases, further hindering the development of effective treatments, and 3) lack of awareness and expertise among healthcare professionals as a small number of individuals are typically affected, leading to delays in diagnosis and treatment.

Research on rare diseases is therefore crucial for improving outcomes for affected individuals. Advances in genetic and molecular research have led to the development of targeted therapies for some rare diseases, offering hope for improved treatments in the future. Additionally, increased awareness and collaboration among researchers, healthcare professionals, and patient advocacy groups are essential for advancing research and improving the lives of those affected by rare diseases.

Despite their low prevalence, rare diseases collectively affect a significant portion of the global population, making them a substantial public health concern. This book seeks to explore cutting-edge research and innovative approaches aimed at improving the lives of those affected by these conditions. For example, recent advancements in therapies targeting specific genetic mutations and gene therapies have shown promise in improving lung function in cystic fibrosis and conditions such as spinal muscular atrophy. These developments not only offer hope for better treatment but also highlight the importance of continued research and support for individuals with rare diseases.

This textbook aims to provide a comprehensive overview of these often-overlooked conditions, aiming to educate and inform healthcare professionals, researchers, students, and caregivers alike. Through detailed exploration of the diverse landscape of rare diseases, including their epidemiology, pathophysiology, diagnosis, and management, the textbook bridges the gap in understanding and fosters interdisciplinary collaboration in the field. By highlighting the unique challenges faced by individuals living with rare diseases and their families, the book aims to raise awareness and promote advocacy for improved access to specialized care and innovative therapies. Furthermore, by showcasing the latest research developments and therapeutic advancements, the textbook endeavors to inspire readers to contribute to the ongoing efforts to address the unmet needs of this vulnerable population. The overarching goal of this textbook is to empower readers with the knowledge and tools necessary to make meaningful contributions to the field of rare diseases, ultimately enhancing the quality of life for those affected by these conditions.

Chapter

INTRODUCTION TO RARE DISEASE

1

Contents

Introduction

Rare diseases are a group of diseases that only affect a very small number of people. Definitions vary, but in general, a disease is considered rare if it affects fewer than 1–5 people per 10,000 people in the general population. Most people suffering from rare diseases have limited treatment options for their disease, and in many countries, there are no plans, policies, or laws in place to advance rare disease research and improve the management of these numerous diseases. The awareness and understanding of rare diseases are often minimal, and many patients struggle to find adequate information about their afflictions related to their rare diseases. As a result, patients can feel isolated, overwhelmed, and unsupported after diagnosis, and the emotional, psychological, and financial impact of diagnosis and living with a rare disease is significant. Traditionally, research and development of therapies for rare diseases have been neglected in favor of more common diseases. Over the last 20 years, however, concerted policy efforts have led to a significant improvement in the understanding of many rare diseases and the availability of effective treatments. Rare diseases pose a particular challenge for research and clinical development. This is due to the small number of patients, the limited epidemiological data on the natural history of many rare diseases, and the fact that all phases of research and development are more difficult and protracted than for more common diseases. In general, patients struggle to access quality care and support. Even when treatments are available, patients can wait several years for a correct diagnosis, and many patients are unable to receive them as they are often not reimbursed by their national healthcare system or are simply not available in their country. Rare diseases must be considered a policy priority in all healthcare systems, and patients should have the same right to treatment and care as patients with more common diseases. Improving care for rare disease patients should therefore be seen as a priority by national governments around the world (Abbas et al., 2021).

Orientation and Directional Terms

Term	Definition	Illustration
Rare Disease	A rare disease is a condition that affects a small percentage of the population, typically fewer than 200,000 people in the U.S. or 1 in 2,000 in the EU.	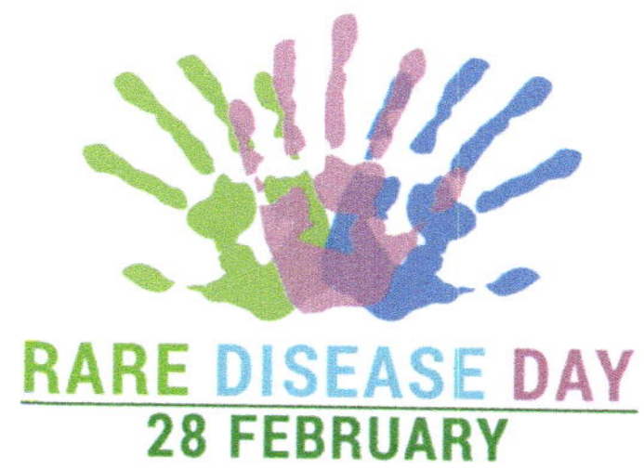
Clinical Trials	Clinical trials are research studies that test new medical interventions, treatments, or drugs in human volunteers to assess their safety and efficacy.	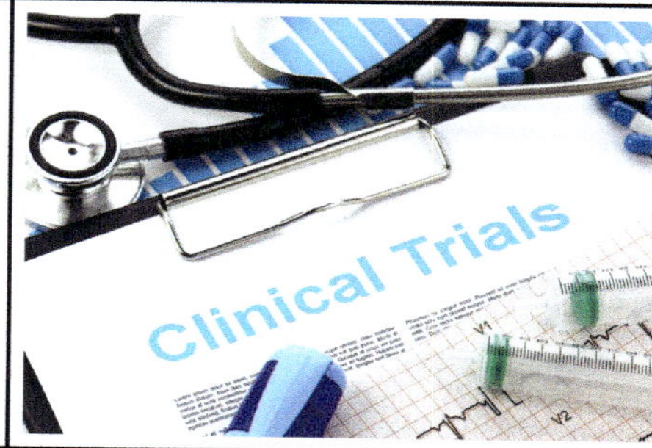
Public Health	Public health refers to the science and practice of preventing disease, prolonging life, and promoting health through organized efforts and informed choices of society.	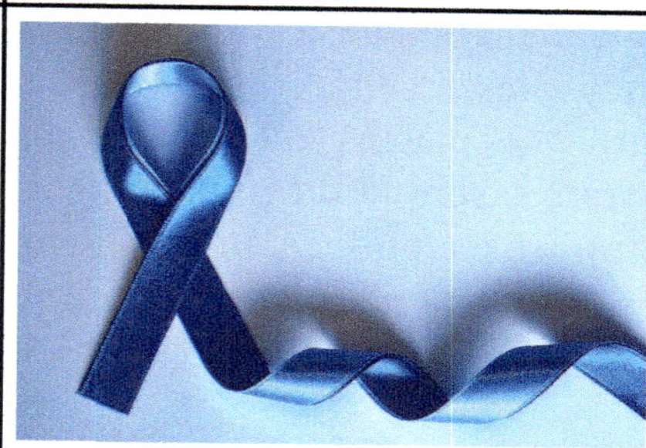
Genetic Disease	A genetic disorder is a disease caused in whole or in part by a change in the DNA sequence away from the normal sequence.	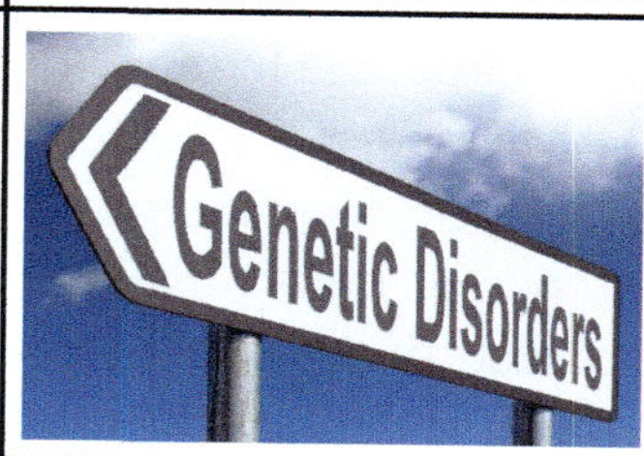
Health Workforce	The health workforce consists of all people engaged in actions whose primary intent is to enhance health, including doctors, nurses, and other health professionals.	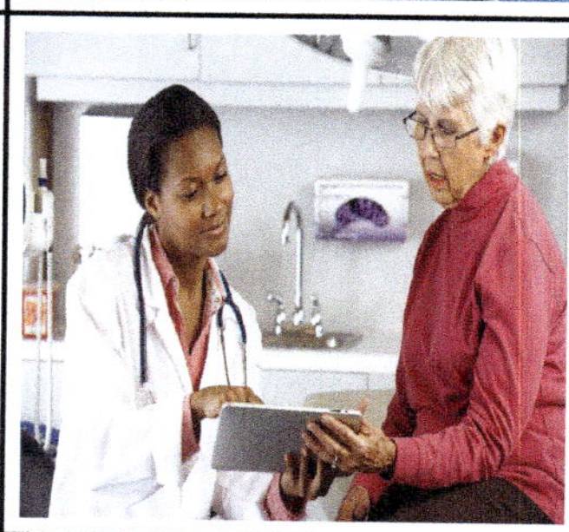

1.1. An Overview of Rare Disease

Rare diseases, also known as orphan diseases, are a group of diseases that affect only a small percentage of the population and usually occur in early childhood but can also be observed in a chronic phase in adulthood. These diseases are often progressive, disabling, and life-threatening, where approximately 30% of affected children die by the age of 5 years. Rare diseases not only have a severe psychological and financial impact on patients and families but also place an enormous burden on communities/societies and countries. It is estimated that there are around 7,000–8,000 different rare diseases. Most rare diseases are genetic in etiology and pathology, with clinical phenotypes varying widely. The Global Genes Project estimates that types of rare solid cancers, and hematologic malignancies (liquid cancers), such as myelodysplasia syndrome (MDS) and myeloproliferative neoplasms (MPNs) including polycythemia vera, essential thrombocythemia, primary myelofibrosis and chronic myeloid leukemia, affect approximately 300 million people worldwide (Adeniran et al., 1993).

Although some definitions of rare diseases are based on the number of people living with a disease and depend on various factors, such as the availability of appropriate treatments or the severity of the disease, there is unfortunately no single, universally accepted definition for rare diseases. The most widely accepted definition is that no disease is rare if it affects someone you love.

Nowadays the treatment of infectious and nutritional disorders has been well established. In contrast, pediatric onset genetic disorders and cancer in children constitute a substantial load in pediatric clinics, and rare diseases are the major clinical load (Figure 1.1).

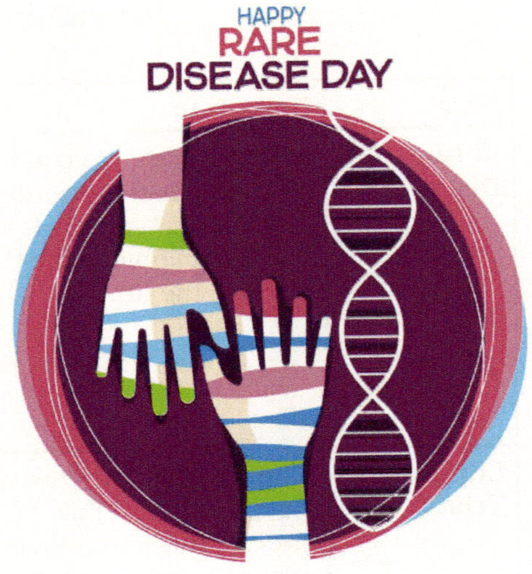

Figure 1.1. *Illustration of rare disease.*

Source: Getty Images, Creative commons license.

1.1.1. What Are Rare Diseases?

Rare diseases are a diverse group of diseases that are generally characterized by the fact that very few people are affected by them compared to more common diseases such as diabetes or heart disease. Rare diseases are usually severe, chronic conditions that are often progressive, debilitating, and life-threatening. For example, 30% of patients with rare diseases die before the age of five (Agarwal et al., 1999). There is no universal definition for rare diseases, and countries set different thresholds for classifying a disease as "rare."

1.1.2. Definitions of Rare Diseases Around the World

The threshold for the definition of rare diseases varies from country to country as shown in Table 1.1. In many countries, there is no official definition, although there are often proposed thresholds. Because of the complexity of rare diseases, it is important that each country or region develops a definition in the context of its unique population, culture, resources, and healthcare system. In addition to prevalence, there may be other situations that apply to rare diseases. In Japan, for example, rare diseases are mainly defined as diseases that are chronic and require a high level of care for the patient and their family.

Table 1.1. *Prevalence of Rare Diseases in Different Countries*

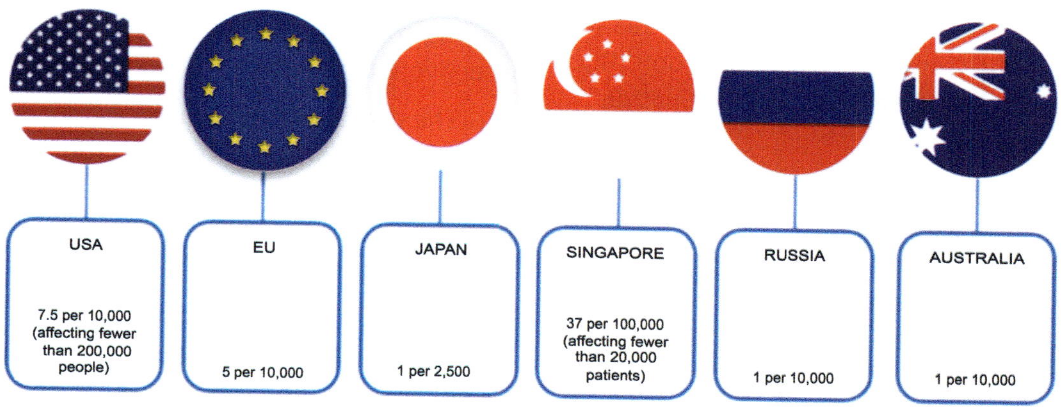

1.2. Advances in the Diagnosis and Treatment of Rare Diseases

In the past, before the age of Genomics, the diagnosis of rare diseases was challenging, and the detection rate was very low due to the lack of diagnostic techniques. Therefore, delayed or incorrect diagnoses were not uncommon, causing stress, frustration, and worry among patients and their families.

Studies have shown that only 36% of rare patients/individuals were diagnosed at an early stage; of those, about 25% received a different diagnosis, 15% sought a second opinion and 5% were treated and cared for unnecessarily (Al-Hassani et al., 2017).

Over the past two decades, rare disease research has been the hallmark of the genetic era in medicine, which has moved from the clinical-symptomatic to the pathologic-etiologic phase with the development of new technologies. With advances in genomics, the rate of discovery of genetic rare diseases has increased dramatically.

The applications of next-generation sequencing (NGS) technology will primarily benefit rare disease patients. Excitingly, the concept and practice of rare diseases have changed dramatically in recent decades.

For approximately 50% of the estimated 7,000 rare diseases, the responsible genes have been identified to determine their molecular etiology, and it is predicted that the remaining 50% of genes will be identified by 2020, which will be accelerated by NGS technology.

To guide the treatment of rare diseases and accelerate progress in rare disease research through international cooperation and collaboration, the International Rare Disease Research Consortium (IRDiRC) was established in 2011, and strategies and guidelines were documented in 2013.

Over the past 10 years, major efforts have been consolidated to increase the knowledge about the epidemiology of rare diseases, including recognizing the specificity of rare diseases; developing information for patients; educating health professionals and the general public about their diseases;

training health professionals to better recognize rare diseases; organizing screening and access to diagnostic tests; improving access to treatment and the quality of patient care; continuing efforts to promote rare disease medicines; addressing the special accompanying needs of people suffering from rare diseases; promoting research on rare diseases; and building national and international partnerships.

A nationally coordinated and collaborative approach involving data collection and utilization, coordinated care, equitable access to services, equitable access to diagnosis and treatment, and nationally coordinated research for both malignant and non-malignant phenotypes has been established (Ambur et al., 2022).

Great progress has been made internationally in the care and treatment of rare diseases. The last day of February each year is recognized as Rare Disease Day. In 2015 and 2016, the Food and Drug Administration (FDA) approved 47% of new drug medications for the treatment of rare diseases. The goal is to develop 200 new therapies for rare diseases by 2020.

1.3. Advances in Rare Disease Research

In the past, rare diseases have been under-researched in many ways and have been hampered by the lack of population-based epidemiology, studies of disease-related etiologic mechanisms, clinical treatment trials, diagnostic tools, health services research, and family/community and social research.

In recent years, studies on the genetic and environmental causes of disease and their interactions with rare diseases have become a key area of medical research. It is believed that such studies hold the key to overcoming human diseases. Rare disease studies have gone from being side stream to the mainstream in pediatric research (Aydin et al., 2007).

High-throughput sequencing techniques (whole genome sequencing and whole exome sequencing) have revolutionized research, leading to accurate and specific diagnosis and effective treatment.

The discovery of disease-causing genes, the identification of inherited mutations, and the detection of genetic variations have brought great benefits to patients and families with rare diseases.

The knowledge and experience gained from rare disease studies have not only improved our understanding of phenotype-genotype relationships but have also informed other medical fields, particularly personalized medicine. These research findings have been reflected in the development of therapies.

Rare disease studies have provided exciting opportunities for identifying genes that cause disease in humans, for understanding common diseases, and for translating genetic findings into clinical practice.

Fanconi anemia (FA) is the most classic, representative rare disease and the best example with the greatest success. FA is a rare hereditary disease associated with developmental disorders, progressive bone marrow failure, and a tendency to develop cancerous cells, often manifesting as acute myeloid leukemia (AML). It was first described and named by the Swiss pediatrician Guido Fanconi in 1927.

FA has several synonyms such as Fanconi pancytopenia, hereditary aplastic anemia, hereditary pancytopenia, constitutional aplastic anemia, hereditary bone marrow failure syndrome, premalignant disorder, chromosome splitting syndrome, and DNA repair disorder. The incidence is 1:160,000 in the general population, but 1:20,000 in some ethnic groups.

So far, 23 responsible genes have been identified, and interestingly, several of them are genes that are also associated with other cancers, including the breast cancer genes BRCA 1 and BRCA 2.

It was the first successful example of umbilical cord blood stem cell transplantation in 1988, so the FA study has been called a paradigm for understanding cancer and aging.

1.4. Factors That May Encourage Rare Diseases

1.4.1. Technology and Occupation

As knowledge grows, it acts synergistically with technology, and recent advances in the field of environmental environment and health are a gateway to health hazards, risks, and vulnerabilities. Technological advances have brought more people together, and improved production processes, but have inadvertently led to increased consumption, and associated wastes (gaseous emissions, solid, and liquid waste), exacerbating human health via degradation of the aquatic ecosystem, pressure on water resources, deforestation, and increase in agrochemicals. Human occupational exposure/contact through inhalation, ingestion, and skin contact have led to the disruption of hormonal enzymes, inhibition of fetal growth, and the trigger of DNA damage. A hallmark of technology is found in industrial emissions, transportation such as roads and airplanes, radiation from telecommunications and military armaments activities that trigger climate change imprint. Air pollution occasioned by dust particles, vehicular emissions, soot, nitrates, NH_3 and nitrogenous gaseous oxides (NOx), sulfur oxides, aerosols, CH_3, PM2.5, and PM10 activate biomarkers (ceruloplasmin, orosomucoid, C3, and alpha-1-antitrypsin), may be a pointer that can indicate high risk even at moderate exposure levels, and can significantly and positively increase the risk of cardiovascular disease through chronic systemic inflammation (Barros et al., 2017). The aforementioned effect also exacerbates and promotes the progression of atherosclerosis and the increase in cardiovascular events, including regularity of the incidence of non-communicable respiratory diseases (NCRDs) with asthma, chronic bronchitis, obstructive respiratory disease, and allergic rhinitis. Human diseases such as cancer, renal kidney problems, cognitive impairment, bronchitis, and neurological disorders have been attributed to environmental toxins such as heavy metals (Cd, Ni, Cr, Pb, Hg, As).

Human factors that may exacerbate the incidence of rare diseases may include low attention emission from the pharmaceutical industry, inadequate government policies and lack of public health advocacy groups, low monitoring and surveillance, and inadequate reporting by the global health research community. Occupational exposure plays an important role in the occurrence of rare diseases. Hexavalent chromium (Cr+6) is carcinogenic, attacks the skin, and causes the denaturation and precipitation of tissue proteins. Occupational exposure to chromium usually occurs through inhalation, but the gastrointestinal (GI) tract and skin can also be affected, making the respiratory tract the primary target organ for Cr+6 and its compounds. Nickel is absorbed through the lungs, GI tract, and skin but is excreted in the urine. The artisanal effect, respiratory abnormalities, and industrial occupation take up a large aspect of the rare disease that may be undocumented and show that it may be of public health importance through occupational exposure, showing that individuals exposed to heavy metals in a paint factory and spraying automotive paints may have impaired health.

1.5. Climate Change and Rare Disease Occurrence

The history of the occurrence of infectious diseases is geographically determined and occurs mainly in places with hot and humid weather. Diseases are expected to continue to spread with global warming, as the latter plays a role in the widespread emergence, re-emergence, and redistribution of infectious diseases. Most commonly, insect-borne diseases are highly sensitive to climate variability. This category includes vector–borne diseases such as dengue, malaria, hantavirus, and cholera; others include salmonellosis, cholera, and giardiasis. Temperature fluctuations are likely to lead to changes in the life cycle of pathogens as they can cause pathogen death, where increased temperatures have been shown to affect the fecundity and sporogony of microorganisms. Changes in climate parameters such as humidity, amount, volume, and duration of rainfall can influence the spread of waterborne pathogens, which are particularly prevalent during the rainy season. At extremely high temperatures, which can lead to drought, water resources in a particular location tend to decrease and concentrate, and run-off waterborne pathogens increase in quantity and impact (Broesby-Olsen et al., 2008). Infectious diseases are also affected by atmospheric water vapor (humidity), a well-known example being the transmission and survival rate of the influenza virus. An important fact about the effects of climate change on infectious diseases is that they cannot be generalized, as the effects in one environment may differ from those in another, as climatic factors change. Microclimate can have profound effects on the hosts harboring pathogens, but also on the host.

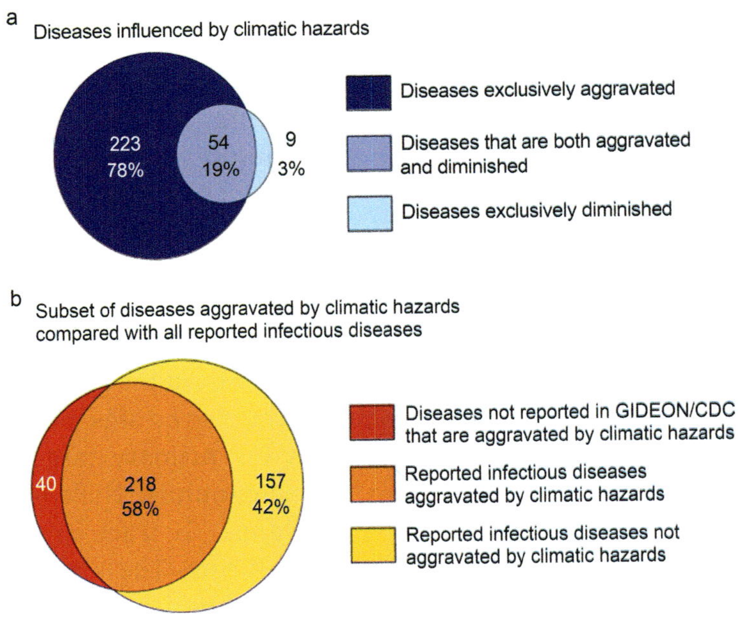

Figure 1.2. *Over half of known human pathogenic diseases can be aggravated by climate change.*

Source: https://media.springernature.com/lw685/springer-static/image/art%3A10.1038%2Fs41558-022-01426-1/MediaObjects/41558_2022_1426_Fig4_HTML.png.

The pattern of changes in population and geographic location affects the insect vector, which is closely linked to the pattern and variation of climate. The small-scale environment (microenvironment) can serve as a shield to contain the disease vector/host because the variation in microclimate is insignificant, but at the large-scale level, climate differences may differ across the regional impact scenario. In a localized extreme heat environment, heat rash, heat edema, heat syncope, cramps, exhaustion, life-threatening heat stroke and other related diseases may occur in the population (Chu et al., 2003) (Figure 1.2).

1.6. Issues in Clinical Development and Access to Treatment and Care

The drug development and approval process is costly and time-consuming and poses a particular challenge for rare diseases, which ultimately affects patients' access to new treatments. The development of therapies for these diseases is also difficult because different countries have different definitions of rare diseases (Cimen et al., 2007). To encourage pharmaceutical companies to conduct research and develop drugs for rare diseases, drugs to treat rare diseases have been classified as "orphan drugs" – with corresponding legislation. However, not all rare disease medicines are designated as orphan drugs. Orphan drug legislation has significantly changed the number of treatments available for rare diseases. For example, prior to the adoption of the Orphan Drug Regulation, only 8 orphan medicinal products were authorized in the European Union, whereas since the entry into force of the Orphan Drug Regulation, over 125 products have been authorized. However, treatments are still only available for around 5% of rare diseases and many challenges still remain.

1.6.1. Discovery and Early Phase Research

A better scientific understanding of rare diseases is crucial as it will lead to the development of new drugs and treatments for rare diseases. As mentioned above, insufficient knowledge and understanding of the causes and clinical course of rare diseases can make it difficult to determine the best strategy for treating a particular disease. Also, research efforts are often scattered and poorly organized across groups, which can lead to duplication of research efforts. This in turn can slow down research efforts and potentially the development of new drugs for rare diseases (Consigli et al., 2000).

1.6.2. Clinical Trials

Clinical trials are designed to test whether a new drug is effective and safe for use in humans. Clinical trials for rare diseases face particular challenges: Small patient populations make it difficult to recruit a sufficient number of participants, making it difficult to achieve statistically significant results. Patients can be spread over large geographical regions, making trials expensive and complex to conduct. A large proportion of rare diseases affect children, often in very small numbers, and therefore require special consideration in clinical trials. In some cases, there are no other treatment options for a rare disease. Additionally, the use of a placebo as a comparator in a clinical trial can raise ethical issues if the new product is very effective. This is also a challenge with other diseases but is much more common with rare diseases.

1.6.3. Registration and Marketing Authorization

To place new medicinal products on the market, a registration or marketing authorization must be obtained in each country. Approval procedures vary considerably from country to country, which means that the time in which potentially life-saving medicines are available to patients varies greatly. Existing regulatory procedures are often poorly suited to rare diseases. For example, regulatory authorities and their advisors often lack expertise in certain rare diseases, leading to significant delays in the approval process (Dominiak et al., 2016). In addition, in some countries, there are no laws that promote the registration and approval of drugs for rare diseases, and patients are therefore forced to access medicines by other means.

1.6.4. Access to High-Quality, Safe, and Effective Treatment

Even if a new drug is approved, it is not necessarily immediately available to patients, as the decision to fund or reimburse a medicine can be a lengthy process and is not generalized across the globe. The delays in accessing these new treatments can depend on the ones responsible for paying – governments, private insurers, or patients. In some countries, these decisions are made at a regional level, which can further delay the time it takes for new treatments to reach patients. Furthermore, existing procedures for accessing new therapies are often not adapted to the particular challenges of rare diseases and orphan drugs, leaving patients to pay for new therapies out of pocket, often with devastating financial consequences. As there are rarely comprehensive and structured reimbursement or authorization procedures, especially in low- and middle-income countries, many patients do not have access to treatment, and in some countries, such as Brazil and India, the only way to access treatment is through litigation and court cases.

1.6.5. General Access to High-Quality Care

Even when medicines are available, it can be difficult for patients to receive quality and timely diagnosis, care, and support due to a lack of specialized services. Few rare diseases have clinical guidelines for best practice, making it difficult to provide optimal care to patients. Even with the existence of guidelines, healthcare professionals may not be expertly fit or trained in the etiology of rare diseases. Due to the often-complex nature of their condition, it is recommended that patients with rare diseases are cared for by a multidisciplinary team. However, in many instances this is not the case, which then leads to poorer outcomes for patients (Federica et al., 2022).

1.7. Policy Priorities for Rare Diseases

In light of the above challenges, there is a clear need for continued political commitment to improve care for rare disease patients (Feldman & Maize, 2007). The key policy priorities for rare diseases are listed in the table below and described in more detail in the following section (Figure 1.3):

- Ensure that rare diseases are a public health priority by raising awareness of rare diseases among policymakers, health professionals, and the public,
- Promote continued research and development, strengthen political commitment to support research, innovation and strategies for rare diseases, and increase collaborative research efforts to improve scientific understanding of all rare diseases,
- Empower patients and their communities to enable better disease management and give patients more influence on the decisions that affect them,
- Ensuring sustainable access to diagnosis, treatment, and care, improving the rare disease workforce and infrastructure, and developing and strengthening legislation that improves access to essential medications, specialized care, and financial support for individuals with rare diseases are critical steps in addressing the challenges faced by this population.

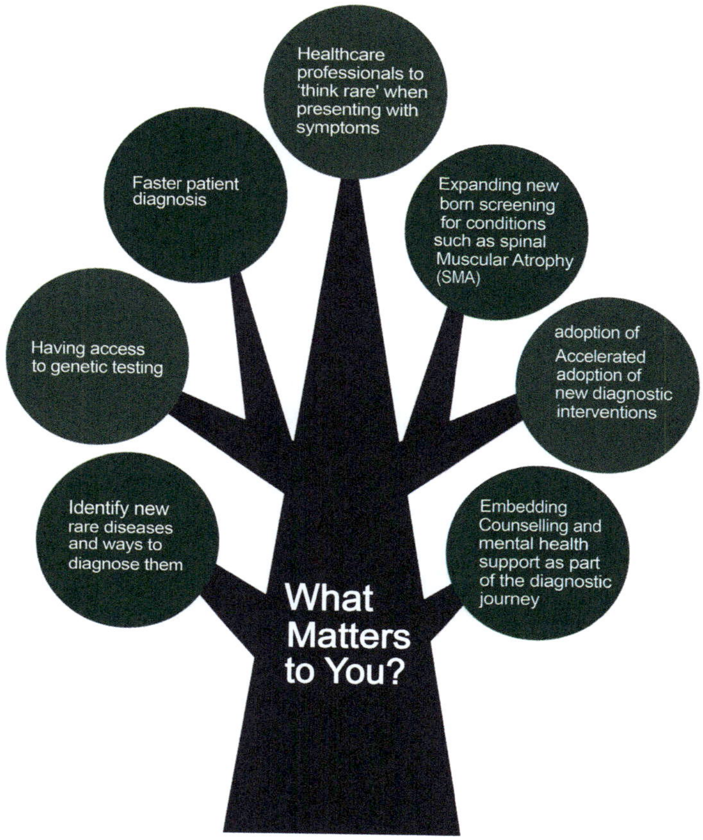
Healthcare professionals to 'think rare' when presenting with symptoms
Faster patient diagnosis
Expanding new born screening for conditions such as spinal Muscular Atrophy (SMA)
Having access to genetic testing
adoption of Accelerated adoption of new diagnostic interventions
Identify new rare diseases and ways to diagnose them
Embedding Counselling and mental health support as part of the diagnostic journey
What Matters to You?

Figure 1.3. *Implementing rare disease framework.*

Source: https://www.gov.scot/binaries/content/gallery/publications/strategy-plan/2022/12/rare-disease-action-plan/SCT11223736061_g01.png.

1.7.1. Ensure Rare Diseases Are a Public Health Priority

Due to limited support and information, patients, and caregivers, often need to become experts and advocates for their own rare diseases. Patients should therefore be empowered and given more support to engage with and shape the policies and systems that affect them. Patients and caregivers have unique insights and perspectives that should be especially considered in research and development, regulatory processes, campaigns, and policy development. Efforts such as the establishment of more patient groups, either in person or via social media, and the development of educational materials and supportive policies across all sectors will be central to better empower patients to drive change (Feldmeyer et al., 2016).

1.7.2. Promote Continued Research and Development for Rare Diseases

To advance research and improve care, greater collaboration is needed at all levels. Close collaboration between scientists, policy, and decision-makers, physicians, and patients is essential to advance research and improve care. International research groups, such as the International Rare Diseases

Research Consortium (IRDiRC), are at the forefront of research. However, there is still no treatment for the vast majority of rare diseases, and further prioritization of research and collaboration is essential to provide treatment options for all rare disease patients and improve care (Foxton & Delaney, 2011).

1.7.3. Ensure Sustainable Access to Diagnosis, Treatment, and Care

Efforts to reduce inequalities in access to care and treatment, which are often limited to those who can afford to pay for their care or who can travel to seek expert advice, require strong political will in the face of limited resources. Such inequalities are regularly observed both within a country and between different countries, due to the limited availability of specialists and different regulatory and reimbursement procedures (Goudie, 2020).

1.7.4. Legislation Is Required to Continue to Increase Access to Orphan Drugs

It is important to develop orphan drug and rare disease legislation in countries where such a framework does not exist, and to strengthen and improve existing regulatory procedures – especially as our understanding of rare diseases increases. The Orphan Drug Act of 1983 in the United States of America was the first law to recognize the lack of treatments for patients with rare diseases and the urgent need to prioritize these diseases in drug development. A number of countries have then followed suit, creating laws and incentives that have led to a significant improvement in treatment options for patients with rare diseases (Havenith et al., 2021).

1.7.5. Investment in the Health Workforce and Infrastructure for Rare Diseases Is Needed

The lack of expertise and infrastructure for the diagnosis and treatment of rare diseases is a constant challenge for rare disease patients. To reduce inequalities in access to treatment, it is essential to invest in the health workforce and promote specialization in rare diseases and genetics in every country. Improving material resources for the diagnosis and treatment of rare diseases, such as genetic testing, newborn screening and pathology, can also improve the diagnosis and prevention of rare diseases (Karampinis et al., 2023).

1.8. The Way Forward

There have been significant advances in the understanding and treatment of rare diseases in recent years, and patient advocacy has been central to these developments. Despite these advances, much remains to be done to reduce the unmet needs of patients, their families, and caregivers. Many policymakers are unaware of the various challenges patients face in obtaining a diagnosis or appropriate treatment (Khaddour et al., 2020). Awareness-raising activities are essential to ensure that rare diseases are considered a top public health priority. The limited access to treatment remains a key issue for rare disease patients worldwide, and stakeholders must work together to establish rare diseases as a global priority on the health agenda and improve equitable access to treatment and care. The existing knowledge and understanding of rare diseases must be shared, and collaboration between all stakeholders is crucial to make the best use of existing knowledge and avoid duplication. Patients' unique expertise and insights should inform research and policy so that patients can help shape the decisions and policies that meet their specific needs. Additionally, legislation to facilitate the development of and access to medicines for rare diseases must continue, and regulatory processes should be further improved with efforts concentrated on reducing inequalities in access to treatment and all aspects of care. Rare diseases are a key health challenge that should not be ignored. A supportive global, regional, and national policy environment is essential to ensure that patients receive the high-quality specialized diagnosis, care, and support that is essential to manage their disease – and to offer the 95% of patients who do not yet have treatment options a chance for better outcomes and a higher quality of life (Litaiem et al., 2022).

A Closer Look at Public Health

Public health is a multifaceted discipline focused on protecting and improving the health of populations through education, promotion of healthy lifestyles, and research into disease and injury prevention. It encompasses a wide range of activities, including epidemiology, biostatistics, health services, environmental health, and social and behavioral sciences. The World Health Organization (WHO) emphasizes that public health is about "promoting and protecting the health of people," highlighting its crucial role in enhancing community well-being and quality of life. For instance, a study by Marmot et al. (2008) illustrates how social determinants of health, such as income and education, significantly influence health outcomes, underlining the importance of addressing these factors within public health initiatives.

Epidemiology, a cornerstone of public health, involves the study of the distribution and determinants of health-related states or events in specific populations. This field has been pivotal in identifying risk factors for diseases and guiding interventions. A landmark study published in the *New England Journal of Medicine* (Doll & Peto, 1981) established the link between smoking and lung cancer, fundamentally transforming public health policy and leading to widespread anti-smoking campaigns. Furthermore, modern epidemiological studies continue to evolve, incorporating advanced statistical methods and data analytics to address complex health issues, including the impact of environmental pollutants on respiratory diseases, as explored by Wang et al. (2019).

Public health also emphasizes the importance of vaccination and disease prevention programs. The success of immunization programs has been a defining achievement in public health, significantly reducing the incidence of preventable diseases such as measles and polio. Research by Andre et al. (2012) indicates that vaccination programs prevent an estimated 2-3 million deaths annually. However, vaccine hesitancy poses a significant challenge, as seen during the COVID-19 pandemic, where misinformation led to decreased vaccination rates. Studies by Roozenbeek et al. (2020) reveal that targeted communication strategies can effectively combat vaccine misinformation and enhance public trust in vaccination programs.

The COVID-19 pandemic underscored the critical role of public health systems in managing health crises. The rapid response of public health agencies to track and contain the virus showcased the importance of surveillance, data collection, and community engagement. Research by Paltiel and Zheng (2021) discusses the lessons learned from the pandemic, emphasizing the need for robust public health infrastructure and interdisciplinary collaboration to better prepare for future health emergencies. This experience reinforces the need for sustained investment in public health, ensuring that systems are equipped to respond swiftly and effectively to emerging health threats.

Summary

- Rare diseases, also known as orphan diseases, are conditions that affect a small number of people compared to the general population. In the United States, a disease is considered rare if it affects fewer than 200,000 people. While each rare disease is uncommon, collectively they affect millions of people worldwide and can be a result of genetic, environmental, or infectious influence, and typically manifest early in life.
- Due to their low prevalence, rare diseases pose significant challenges for patients, healthcare providers, and researchers. Diagnosing rare diseases can be difficult due to their unfamiliarity, leading to delays in treatment and management. Additionally, the lack of awareness and understanding of rare diseases can result in social isolation and limited access to appropriate healthcare services for patients.
- Treatment options for rare diseases are often limited, with many lacking approved therapies, which can lead to a heavy burden on patients and their families, both emotionally and financially. However, advancements in medical research, particularly in genomics and personalized medicine, are providing new hope for rare disease patients. These developments are leading to a better understanding of the underlying causes of rare diseases and the development of targeted therapies.
- Despite these challenges, the rare disease community is strong and resilient. Advocacy groups, patient organizations, and researchers are working tirelessly to raise awareness, improve diagnosis and treatment, and support those affected by rare diseases. Through collaboration and innovation, progress is being made to improve the lives of people with rare diseases and their families.

References

1. Abbas, M. N., Tan, W. S., & Kichenadasse, G. (2021). Sorafenib-related generalized eruptive keratoacanthomas (Grzybowski syndrome): A case report. *Journal of Medical Case Reports, 15*, 481. https://doi.org/10.1186/s13256-021-03044-4.
2. Adeniran, A., Townsend, P. L. G., & Peachey, R. D. G. (1993). Incontinentia pigmenti (Bloch-Sulzberger syndrome) manifesting as painful periungual and subungual tumors. *Journal of Hand Surgery, 18*, 667–669. https://doi.org/10.1016/0266-7681(93)90194-y.
3. Agarwal, M., Chander, R., Karmakar, S., & Walia, R. (1999). Multiple familial keratoacanthoma of Witten and Zak—A report of three siblings. *Dermatology, 198*, 396–399. https://doi.org/10.1159/000018168.
4. Al-Hassani, F., Davies, J., Pang, C., & Knight, S. (2017). Local subungual excision and graft use in patients with incontinentia pigmenti: A case report and review of the literature. *JPRAS Open, 11*, 33–36. https://doi.org/10.1016/j.jpra.2016.09.004.
5. Ambur, A., Clark, A., & Nathoo, R. (2022). An updated review of the therapeutic management of keratoacanthomas. *Journal of Clinical and Aesthetic Dermatology, 15*, S16–S22.
6. Aydin, F., Senturk, N., Sabanciler, E., Canturk, M. T., & Turanli, A. Y. (2007). A case of Ferguson–Smith type multiple keratoacanthomas associated with keratoacanthoma centrifugum

marginatum: Response to oral acitretin. *Clinical and Experimental Dermatology, 32*, 683–686. https://doi.org/10.1111/j.1365-2230.2007.02529.x.

7. Barros, B., Helm, K., Zaenglein, A., & Seiverling, E. (2017). Keratoacanthoma-like growths of incontinentia pigmenti successfully treated with intralesional methotrexate. *Pediatric Dermatology, 34*, e203–e204. https://doi.org/10.1111/pde.13159.
8. Broesby-Olsen, S., Bygum, A., Gerdes, A., & Brandrup, F. (2008). Multiple self-healing squamous epithelioma of Ferguson-Smith: Observations in a Danish family covering four generations. *Acta Dermato-Venereologica, 88*, 52–56. https://doi.org/10.2340/00015555-0368.
9. Chu, D. H., Hale, E. K., & Robins, P. (2003). Generalized eruptive keratoacanthomas. *Dermatology Online Journal, 9*, 36.
10. Cimen, S., Aslan, G., Lebe, B., Tuna, B., Secil, M., Demir, O., Pabuccuoglu, U., & Yorukoglu, K. (2007). Penile keratoacanthoma associated with urothelial carcinoma of the bladder in Muir-Torre syndrome. *Urologic Oncology: Seminars and Original Investigations, 25*, 326–328. https://doi.org/10.1016/j.urolonc.2006.12.014.
11. Consigli, J. E., GonzÁlez, M. E., Morsino, R., Guidi, A., Chappuis, J. M., Papa, M., & Maldonado, S. (2000). Generalized eruptive keratoacanthoma (Grzybowski variant). *British Journal of Dermatology, 142*, 800–803. https://doi.org/10.1046/j.1365-2133.2000.03471.x.
12. Dominiak, N., Hayes, B., Swick, J., Leach, B., Maize, J., & Ralston, J. (2016). Keratoacanthoma centrifugum marginatum: A diagnostic and therapeutic challenge. *JAAD Case Reports, 2*, 206–208. https://doi.org/10.1016/j.jdcr.2016.04.013.
13. Federica, F., Carpanese, M. A., Sacchelli, L., Loi, C., Chessa, M. A., & Bardazzi, F. (2022). Two birds with one stone: Successful treatment with methotrexate in a patient with generalized eruptive keratoacanthoma of Grzybowski and rheumatoid arthritis. *Dermatologic Therapy, 35*, e15787. https://doi.org/10.1111/dth.15787.
14. Feldman, R. J., & Maize, J. C. (2007). Multiple keratoacanthomas in a young woman: Report of a case emphasizing medical management and a review of the spectrum of multiple keratoacanthomas. *International Journal of Dermatology, 46*, 77–79. https://doi.org/10.1111/j.1365-4632.2007.03190.x.
15. Feldmeyer, L., Szeverényi, I., Mandallaz, M., Lane, E. B., & Hohl, D. (2016). Late-onset multiple self-healing squamous epithelioma Ferguson-Smith recurrence induced by radiotherapy. *Case Reports in Dermatology, 8*, 344–349. https://doi.org/10.1159/000451097.
16. Foxton, G., & Delaney, T. (2011). Eruptive keratoacanthoma and squamous cell carcinoma complicating imiquimod therapy: Response to oral acitretin. *Australasian Journal of Dermatology, 52*, 66–69. https://doi.org/10.1111/j.1440-0960.2010.00739.x.
17. Goudie, D. (2020). Multiple self-healing squamous epithelioma (MSSE): A digenic trait associated with loss of function mutations in TGFBR1 and variants at a second linked locus on the long arm of chromosome 9. *Genes, 11*, 1410. https://doi.org/10.3390/genes11121410.
18. Havenith, R., de Vos, L., Fröhlich, A., Braegelmann, C., Sirokay, J., Landsberg, J., Wenzel, J., Bieber, T., & Niebel, D. (2021). Grzybowski's generalized eruptive keratoacanthomas in a patient with terminal kidney disease—An unmet medical need equally ameliorated by topical imiquimod cream and lapacho tea wraps: A case report. *Dermatologic Therapy, 11*, 625–638. https://doi.org/10.1007/s13555-021-00479-x.

19. Karampinis, E., Lallas, A., Lazaridou, E., Errichetti, E., & Apalla, Z. (2023). Race-specific and skin of color dermatoscopic characteristics of skin cancer: A literature review. *Dermatology Practical & Conceptual, 13*, e2023311S. https://doi.org/10.5826/dpc.1301a311s.

20. Khaddour, K., Fields, R. C., Ansstas, M., Rosman, I. S., & Ansstas, G. (2020). Metachronous cutaneous squamous cell carcinoma in a young patient as the only presenting symptom to uncover Lynch syndrome with MLH1 germline mutation. *Hered Cancer in Clinical Practice, 18*, 23. https://doi.org/10.1186/s13053-020-00148-4.

21. Litaiem, N., Khammouma, F., Mrad, M., Bacha, T., Belhadj Kacem, L., & Zeglaoui, F. (2022). Multiple keratoacanthomas of Ferguson-Smith type. *Clinical Case Reports, 10*, e06429. https://doi.org/10.1002/ccr3.6429.

22. Mascitti, H., De Masson, A., Brunet-Possenti, F., Bouaziz, J. D., Laly, P., Mourad, N., Garrigues, J. M., Laurent-Roussel, S., Cavelier-Balloy, B., & Moulonguet, I. (2019). Successful treatment of generalized eruptive keratoacanthoma of Grzybowski with acitretin. *Dermatologic Therapy, 9*, 383–388. https://doi.org/10.1007/s13555-019-00304-9.

23. Miao, Y., Kolb, F., Tomasic, G., Lupu, J., Routier, E., & Robert, C. (2022). Keratoacanthoma or cutaneous squamous cell carcinoma revealing a DNA mismatch repair default (Muir-Torre syndrome). *Journal of the European Academy of Dermatology and Venereology, 36*(1), 74–76.

24. Mlacker, S., Kaw, U., & Maytin, E. V. (2017). Use of photodynamic therapy and acitretin in generalized eruptive keratoacanthoma of Grzybowski. *JAAD Case Reports, 3*(5), 457–459.

25. Nishizawa, A., Nakanishi, Y., Sasajima, Y., Yamazaki, N., & Yamamoto, A. (2006). Muir-Torre syndrome with intriguing squamous lesions. *American Journal of Dermatopathology, 28*(1), 56–59.

26. Nofal, A., Assaf, M., Ghonemy, S., Nofal, E., & Yosef, A. (2015). Generalized eruptive keratoacanthoma: A diagnostic and therapeutic challenge. *International Journal of Dermatology, 54*(2), 160–167.

27. Oakley, A., & Ng, S. (2005). Grzybowski's generalized eruptive keratoacanthoma: Remission with cyclophosphamide. *Australasian Journal of Dermatology, 46*(2), 118–123.

28. Pancholi, A., Collins, D., Lindley, R., & Gandhi, P. (2008). Muir–Torre syndrome: A case report and screening recommendations. *Annals of the Royal College of Surgeons of England, 90*(1), 9–10.

29. Pham, F., Buiret, G., Bonnet-Dupeyron, M. N., Beschet, I., & Skowron, F. (2021). Multiple and aggressive keratoacanthomas associated with Ferguson-Smith syndrome, successfully treated by cetuximab and cisplatin. *European Journal of Dermatology, 31*(3), 271–272.

30. Poligone, B., Hayden, M. S., Chen, L., Pentland, A. P., Jimi, E., & Ghosh, S. (2013). A role for NF-κB activity in skin hyperplasia and the development of keratoacanthomata in mice. *PLoS ONE, 8*(8), e71887.

31. Relvas, M., Calvão, J., Coutinho, I., & Cardoso, J. C. (2021). Case for diagnosis. A pruritic eruption of keratotic papules over the face and neck. *Anais Brasileiros de Dermatologia, 96*(1), 100–102.

32. Robertson, S. J., Bashir, S. J., Pichert, G., Robson, A., & Whittaker, S. (2010). Severe exacerbation of multiple self-healing squamous epithelioma (Ferguson–Smith disease) with radiotherapy, which was successfully treated with acitretin. *Clinical and Experimental Dermatology, 35*(1), e100–e102.

33. Rotola, A., Musmeci, D., Gentili, V., Reale, D., Borghi, A., Rizzo, R., & Corazza, M. (2019). Generalized eruptive keratoacanthoma of the Grzybowski type: Some considerations on treatment and pathogenesis. *International Journal of Dermatology, 58*(4), e242–e245.

34. Sami, N., & Bussian, A. (2015). Acitretin induces remission in generalized eruptive keratoacanthoma of Grzybowski. *International Journal of Dermatology, 54*(1), e67–e69.

35. Scalvenzi, M., Patrì, A., Costa, C., Megna, M., Napolitano, M., Fabbrocini, G., & Balato, N. (2019). Intralesional methotrexate for the treatment of keratoacanthoma: The Neapolitan experience. *Dermatology and Therapy, 9*(2), 369–372.

36. Simpkin, S., Lamont, D., & Yung, A. (2013). A puzzling case: SCC or not? *Australasian Journal of Dermatology, 54*(4), e74–e77.

37. Stoebner, P. E., Fabre, C., Delfour, C., Joujoux, J. M., Roger, P., Dandurand, M., & Meunier, L. (2009). Solitary subungual keratoacanthoma arising in an MSH2 germline mutation carrier: Confirmation of a relationship by immunohistochemical analysis. *Dermatology, 219*(2), 174–178.

38. Tisack, A., Fotouhi, A., Fidai, C., Friedman, B. J., Ozog, D., & Veenstra, J. (2021). A clinical and biological review of keratoacanthoma. *British Journal of Dermatology, 185*(3), 487–498.

39. Tohya, T., Ogura, T., Nishi, K., Nishi, H., & Kuriwaki, K. (2008). Muir-Torre syndrome associated with endometrial carcinoma. *International Journal of Clinical Oncology, 13*(6), 559–561.

40. Watanabe, I. C., Magalhães, R. F., de Moraes, A. M., Stelini, R. F., Cintra, G. F., Metze, K., & Cintra, M. L. (2015). Keratoacanthoma and keratoacanthoma-like squamous cell carcinoma. *Medicine, 94*(26), e934.

41. Zargaran, M., & Baghaei, F. (2014). A clinical, histopathological and immunohistochemical approach to the bewildering diagnosis of keratoacanthoma. *Journal of Dentistry, 15*(2), 91–97.

42. Zhu, P., & Wang, Y. (2021). Multiple keratoacanthomas in a patient with myelodysplastic syndrome. *The Lancet Haematology, 8*(2), e94.

43. Zito, G., Saotome, I., Liu, Z., Ferro, E. G., Sun, T. Y., Nguyen, D. X., Bilguvar, K., Ko, C. J., & Greco, V. (2014). Spontaneous tumor regression in keratoacanthomas is driven by Wnt/retinoic acid signaling cross-talk. *Nature Communications, 5*, 3543.

44. Zito, P. M., & Mazzoni, T. (2023). Acitretin. In *StatPearls*. StatPearls Publishing.

Chapter

2

CHRONIC RESPIRATORY DISEASES

Contents

Introduction

At the global level, chronic respiratory diseases (CRDs), which can be either communicable or non-communicable, are among the leading causes of death, morbidity, economic and societal burden, and disability-adjusted life years (DALYs). In addition to the airways, parenchyma, and pulmonary vasculature, CRDs have an impact on several other components of the respiratory system. In spite of the fact that non-communicable respiratory diseases like asthma, chronic obstructive pulmonary disease (COPD), interstitial lung disease (ILD), cystic fibrosis (CF), and lung cancer (LC) constitute a significant burden on the healthcare system, the therapies that are currently available are only concerned with alleviating the symptoms of these diseases rather than providing optimal treatment and/or prevention. In addition, tuberculosis (TB), which is considered to be one of the most significant communicable respiratory diseases, is linked to the issue of the growing development of antibiotic resistance in the bacterial pathogen *Mycobacterium tuberculosis* (An et al., 2017). This chapter will provide a summary of the underlying molecular and cellular mechanisms that lead to the characteristic pathophysiology of chronic rheumatic disease (CRD) in light of these potential challenges. Moreover, it will discuss the shortcomings of the therapeutic approaches that are currently in use and investigate alternative methods of drug delivery that have the potential to be more efficient in the treatment of chronic renal disease (CRD).

Orientation and Directional Terms

Term	Definition	Illustration
Lungs	The lungs are a pair of spongy, air-filled organs located on either side of the chest. They are responsible for oxygenating blood and expelling carbon dioxide from the body.	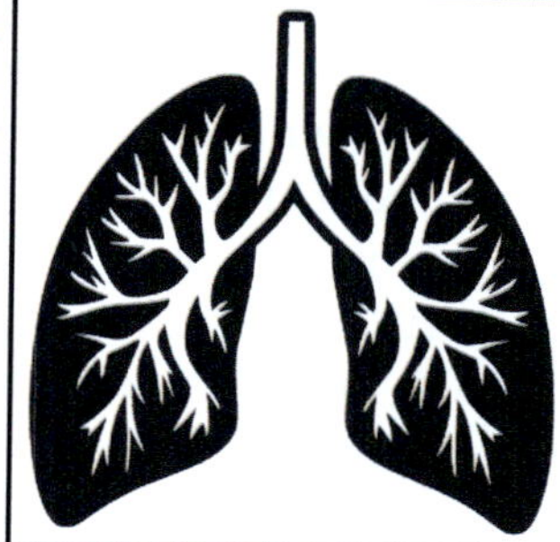
Asthma	A chronic respiratory condition characterized by inflammation and narrowing of the airways, causing difficulty breathing, wheezing, coughing, and shortness of breath.	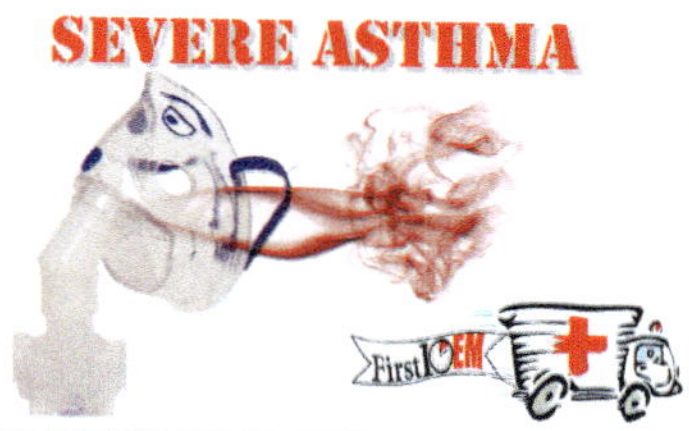
Cystic Fibrosis	A genetic disorder that affects the lungs and digestive system, leading to the production of thick, sticky mucus that clogs airways and causes frequent lung infections.	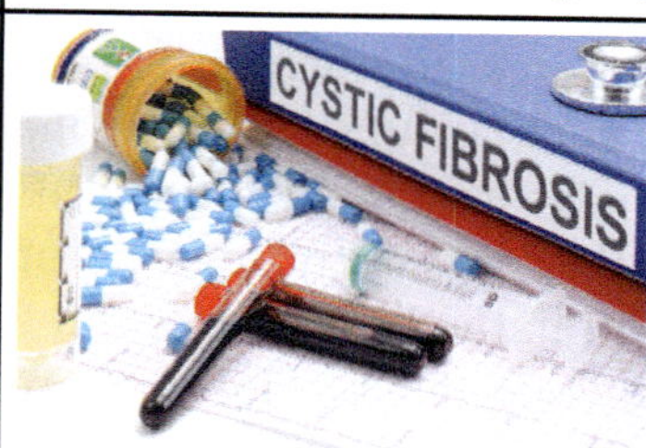
Tuberculosis	A contagious bacterial infection caused by *Mycobacterium tuberculosis*, primarily affecting the lungs but can also impact other parts of the body, leading to serious complications.	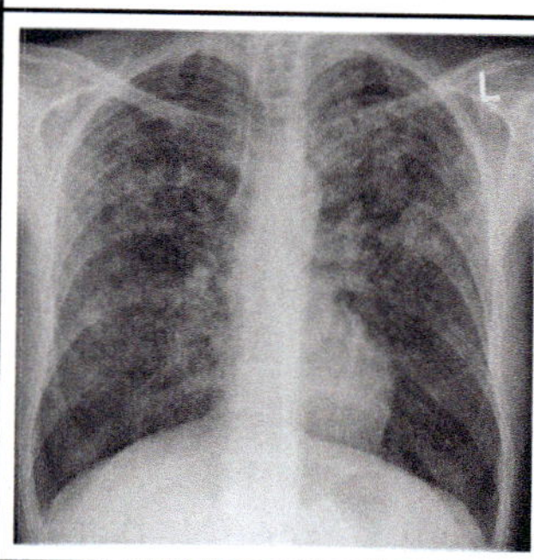
Lung Cancer	A type of cancer that begins in the lungs, often caused by smoking, exposure to carcinogens, or genetic factors, leading to abnormal cell growth and impaired lung function.	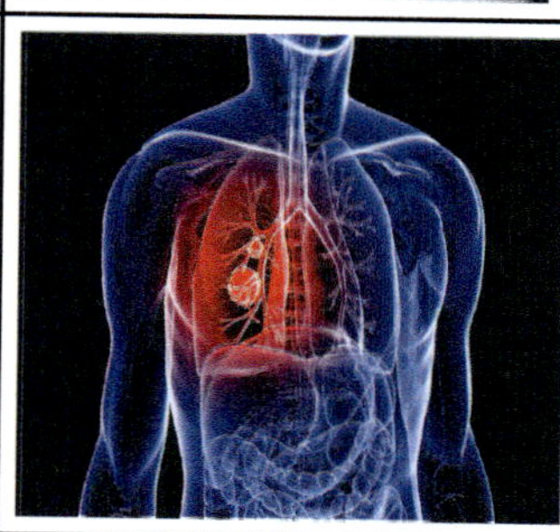

2.1. An Overview

Around the world, the prevalence of chronic respiratory diseases (CRD), which can affect both adults and children, is steadily growing. Although it is not known what causes mortality and morbidity from respiratory diseases, recent statistics published by the World Health Organization (WHO) and other organizations estimate that 400 million people around the world suffer from mild to moderate diseases such as asthma and COPD alone. Not only that, but each year, lower respiratory tract infections brought on by *Haemophilus influenzae* are responsible for the deaths of between 250,000 and 500,000 people. *M. tuberculosis* was the cause of a lower respiratory tract infection that affected 10.4 million people around the world in 2015, and as a result of this infection, 14% of patients passed away. Other non-infectious diseases, such as lung cancer from tobacco use or the inhalation of environmental carcinogens, are responsible for the deaths of 1.6 million people annually, with the number of deaths alarmingly on the rise. Not only are respiratory diseases directly responsible for 10% of all DALYs in the working population, but they are also directly responsible for 90% of all deaths (Bacci et al., 2017).

It is possible to classify respiratory diseases into two broad categories: communicable diseases, which are infectious (such as tuberculosis and pneumonia), and non-communicable diseases (NCDs), which do not have an infectious etiology (such as asthma and COPD, cystic fibrosis, interstitial pulmonary fibrosis, and lung cancer). These differences are based on the pathology of the disease and the mode of transmission. The causes of these respiratory diseases are diverse, and their diagnostic procedures are also quite distinct from one another. On the other hand, the treatment of non-communicable lung diseases is particularly similar. In other words, the treatment of these diseases typically consists of a bronchodilator, corticosteroids, and antibiotics. Furthermore, research into the pathology of COPD has only begun in the past two decades, and there is a lack of a credible disease diagnosis and prevention/management strategy in regions with a high disease burden. This is a matter of particular concern in countries with low and middle incomes, such as India and China, as well as countries in several regions, including the Asia-Pacific region, Latin America, and Africa.

Even though the burden of CRDs is constantly growing, there are not many treatment options available. One of the primary causes is a lack of understanding of the underlying mechanisms that could lead to the discovery of promising molecular or immunological targets. Additionally, the route of administration of existing drugs is also variable, and further research is required to improve the deposition and efficacy of drugs that are currently commonly prescribed (Bragonzi et al., 2017).

2.2. Lungs: Morphology and Physiology

There are two primary components that make up the human respiratory system, the upper respiratory tract (URT) and the lower respiratory tract (LRT). The nasal passages, the mouth, and the first portion of the trachea make up the URT, and the LRT is made up of the trachea, which gradually divides into the bronchi, bronchioles, and finally, the functional units that are referred to as alveoli. The lung parenchyma is responsible for providing support to the airways, and the pulmonary vasculature is responsible for the process of gas exchange, which includes the inhalation of oxygen (O_2) and the exhalation of carbon dioxide (CO_2) and is the most essential function of the respiratory system. The individual membranes of the alveoli are responsible for the gas exchange that brings O_2 and CO_2 into the pulmonary capillaries. Inspiration is the process of taking in air into the lungs, which is primarily accomplished by expanding the chest volume. The air that is inhaled then travels through the airways that are progressively smaller, which are referred to as "conducting" airways. Expiration is the process of taking out air from the lungs, which is the result of the chest volume contracting. The diaphragm and the intercostal muscles are the two types of muscles that are primarily responsible for facilitating the process of inhalation and exhalation. Approximately 50 to 75 square meters make up the lung's internal surface area. A normal human lung weighs approximately one kilogram, with the blood in the pulmonary vasculature accounting for approximately 45 to 50% of the total weight of the lung. The measurements of the volume, as well as the effect of air inhalation and exhalation, are essential for the diagnosis of restrictive and/or obstructive lung diseases like asthma and COPD (Carnell et al., 2018).

To ensure the optimal functioning of the lungs, it is essential to conduct a series of measurements. Lung mechanics involve the efficient exchange of gas, which necessitates the presence of multiple components. Spirometry is a maximal respiratory test that is used to measure the functionality of the lungs. It is safe, practical, reproducible, and is used in almost all clinical laboratories to determine the ventilatory capacity of the lungs. Simultaneously, they offer a real-time graphical representation of the flow-volume curve. Modern spirometers also have the additional benefit of providing the operator with immediate computer-generated feedback on the quality and repeatability of the test. The tidal volume (TV), the inspiratory reserve volume (IRV), the expiratory reserve volume (ERV), and the residual volume (RV) are the standard lung volumes that you will measure. The inspiratory capacity (IC), the functional residual capacity (FRC), the vital capacity (VC), and the total lung capacity (TLC) are the other standard lung capacities that are routinely measured. There is a summary of these lung capacities and volumes displayed in Figure 2.1.

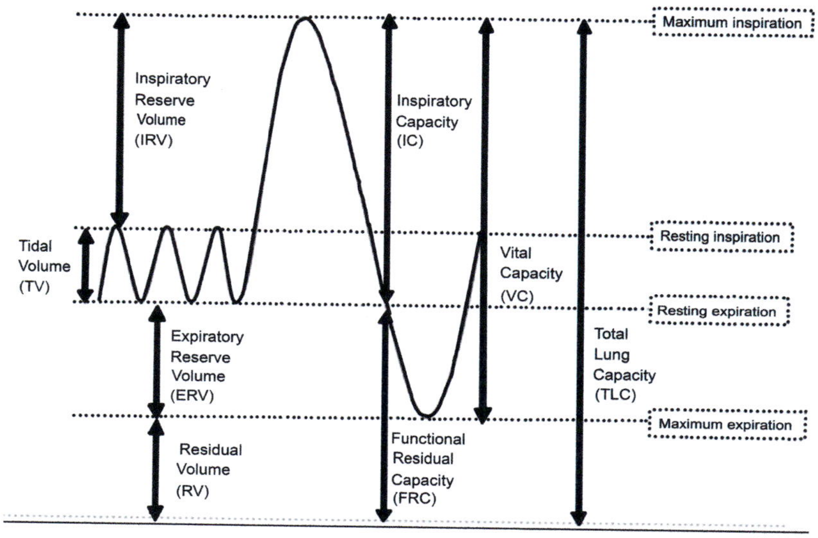

Figure 2.1. *The spirometer trace provides the standard lung volumes and capacities measurement. Specifically, the solid black and gray arrows represent the capacities and volumes of the lungs, respectively.*

Source: Image by Mohamed Faisal Lutfi; reproduced with permission from Lutfi ,M. F., (2017). The physiological basis and clinical significance of lung volume measurements. Multidiscip. Respir. Med., 12(1), 3. doi: 10.1186/s40248-017-0084-5.

Different cell types, each of which performs a highly specialized function, make up a normal human lung. Cell types such as airway epithelial cells, goblet cells, ciliated cells, Clara cells, neuroendocrine cells, basal cells, and type I and type II alveolar cells are among the most significant types of cells. Furthermore, the lung contains immune cells, stem cells, and fat cells in addition to other types of cells (Douglas & Cohen, 2017). There is also a correlation between some respiratory diseases and the presence of one or more specific cell types. An example includes glandular cells in the lungs that are linked to the development of lung adenocarcinomas when risk factors are present. Diseases are more likely to be associated with the functionality of particular cell types, for example, the secretion of surfactant proteins and lipids has been linked to the pathology of respiratory diseases such as neonatal respiratory failure, interstitial lung disease (ILD), alveolar proteinosis, and other uncommon lung diseases (Everaerts et al., 2018). The airway epithelium is not only the first line of defense and a physical barrier that separates the host-environment axis, but it also plays a significant role as a modulator in pulmonary inflammation and immune cell activation, as well as an essential component in the process of pulmonary remodeling and repair. Intimal hyperplasia and smooth muscle hypertrophy/hyperplasia are two additional changes that can occur in the pulmonary vasculature and are most likely the result of chronic hypoxic vasoconstriction of the small pulmonary arteries. In addition, the basal cells of the epithelium that line the airways are becoming increasingly recognized for their significant importance in the remodeling of the airways (Fastres et al., 2017).

The lack of effective treatment and/or management strategies for CRDs continues to be a major cause for concern, particularly for non-communicable diseases such as asthma, COPD, cystic fibrosis, and interstitial pulmonary fibrosis (IPF). This limitation is due to several reasons, including a lack of knowledge regarding the fundamental mechanisms that may be involved in the development and progression of CRDs. The fact that the treatments that are currently available only target the primary symptoms of the disease and do not provide long-term relief, either in terms of prevention or cure, is another indication of inadequate treatments and management strategies. In addition, the drugs that are currently available cannot completely target the biological entities; consequently, more efficient methods of drug delivery are required to alleviate the symptoms of chronic renal disease (CRD). (Faverio et al., 2016)

2.3. Overview of Respiratory Disease

Both the expanding population and the shifting lifestyles of the 21st century have created an environment that is conducive to the spread of a wide range of diseases that are currently posing a threat to the lives of people living in different nationalities. Research has shown that respiratory diseases are the most prevalent among these diseases, and this is true in both middle-income and low-income countries around the world. In spite of the fact that respiratory diseases are extremely common, doctors frequently ignore them or pay them very little attention. The human lung is the only internal organ that is regularly exposed to a wide range of environmental pollutants that are composed of organic, inorganic, and biological agents from a variety of natural and anthropogenic sources. As a result, the human lung is constantly at risk of developing simple to complex lung diseases that can have a negative impact on one's quality of life and ultimately result in death. The following text provides a concise discussion of a few of the respiratory diseases that are currently posing a threat to millions of people all over the world.

2.3.1. Asthma

Asthma is a heterogeneous and complex lung disease that is characterized by variable airflow obstruction, airway (bronchial) hyperresponsiveness, and an increase in airway inflammation as one of the most important symptoms. Asthma affects approximately 10% of the adult population in almost every country, which is equivalent to approximately 300 million people all over the world. Furthermore, it is estimated that asthma is directly responsible for 383,000 deaths across the globe, with greater than 80% of deaths attributed to asthma being reported from countries with low and middle incomes. There is also a significant financial burden associated with asthma, which can amount to up to 3,100 US dollars per person yearly (Florence et al., 2018).

This lung disease is extremely common but has received very little research and can strike people of any age. Indoor pollutants (dust mites and pollution), exposure to allergens found outside (pollen, molds, and pollution), tobacco smoke, occupational exposure to chemical fumes, and air pollution are all factors that can increase the likelihood of developing asthma. In addition to being a complicated illness, asthma can also present itself as an "episodic" disease, which means that it can occur in phases where symptoms appear and then disappear after treatment. The disease can also be "persistent," which is characterized by the presence of clinical symptoms that are typical of asthma. When someone has asthma, the most common symptoms they experience are wheezing, dyspnea (shortness of breath), coughing, and shortness of breath. In addition to exposure to known and unknown allergens, irritants, respiratory infections caused by viruses or bacteria, bacterial sinusitis, physical exertion, thunderstorms, and cold weather, several other factors can aggravate symptoms of asthma.

Recent discoveries in the field of asthma pathophysiology have resulted in the classification of asthma into a variety of phenotypes and/or endotypes. For the treatment of asthma patients to be effective, this is absolutely necessary (GBD, 2015 LRI Collaborators). This has also been recommended by the Lancet Commission, which recently issued a recommendation that suggests the identification of "treatable features" in asthma patients and the targeting of these features in the management of the disease. Asthma can be classified as allergic asthma and non-allergic asthma. Allergic asthma is caused by allergens such as pollen, dust mites, molds, and biological or organic environmental factors, and this classification is mainly based on the triggers that cause the development of the disease. Non-allergic asthma, on the other hand, is linked to several risk factors, including exposure to cold air, infections caused by viruses or bacteria, tobacco smoke, physical activity, and diet. Studies have shown that the majority of asthma attacks are brought on by Th2 responses. These responses involve type 2 T helper cells entering the airways in response to both internal and external triggers. These cells further produce cytokines such as IL-4, IL-5, IL-9, and IL-13 at the highest possible levels. There is a significant role that IL-4 plays in the process of switching IgE cells to B cells, increasing the production of immunoglobulin E. This event then contributes to the production of inflammatory mediators like histamine and cysteinyl leukotrienes. Cytokine IL-5, however, is solely involved in the recruitment of eosinophils, which ultimately results in the development of allergic rhinitis in the upper airways. Both IL-13 and IL-4, in conjunction with inflammatory mediators, are responsible for the contraction of smooth muscle, which in turn causes bronchospasm, an excessive production of mucus, and an increased influx of immune cells. This ultimately leads to a reduction in airway diameter as well as a decrease in airway hyperresponsiveness, which ultimately leads to a reduction in forced expiratory volume in one second (FEV1). It has been discovered that the airway epithelium plays a significant part in the regulation of Th2 responses. This is accomplished through the production of master regulators, such as thymic stromal lymphopoietin (TSLP), interleukin-25 (IL-25), or interleukin-33 (IL33), which regulate the expression of Th2 cytokines and are responsible for the early onset of asthma in children.

In the beginning stages of asthma, wheezing and hyperresponsiveness of the airways to stimuli that are not specific to the condition are the defining characteristics. On the other hand, in later stages (severe forms), airway remodeling and subsequent exacerbations occur as a result of increased inflammation that is promoted by other local (viral or bacterial infections) or systemic factors. In earlier research, observations made in animal models gave the impression that asthma was an allergic, eosinophilic, and Th2-driven inflammatory disease. However, extensive clinical studies conducted on humans have shown that certain types of asthma are associated with fewer or no Th2 responses (Haworth et al., 2017). This demonstrates that there are different phenotypes of asthma. There was a significant increase in the number of neutrophil populations in patients who were suffering from severe asthma, while the number of eosinophil populations either increased or remained the same. In addition, it was discovered that severe asthmatics who are currently or previously being treated with inhaled corticosteroids (ICS) frequently exhibit evidence of neutrophilia, which is an excess of neutrophil populations. This finding raises the question of whether ICS could be the cause of this particular phenotype. When it came to asthmatics who also had neutrophilia, it was discovered that ICS treatment had little to no effect. In order to differentiate between non-allergic asthmatics and allergic asthmatics, clinicians currently rely on the negative result of a skin test. This test involves exposing skin cells to aeroallergens to determine their capability to produce IgE. Additionally, genome-wide association studies of asthma in both adults and children have uncovered a number of significant polymorphisms in IL33, ILRL1, IL18R1, IL2RB, and SMAD3 on chromosome 17q21. These polymorphisms, along with gene expressions of ZPBP2, GSDMB, and ORMDL3, have also been located. It is the responsibility of these genes to ensure that the epithelial barrier continues to function properly and to preserve its integrity (Hewitt & Molyneaux, 2017). There is a lack of understanding regarding the precise genetic markers that are responsible for the development of asthma, whether it be early-onset or adult-onset asthma. Recent research has established a connection between the onset of asthma and the presence of intrinsic factors such as obesity. These studies have also observed that white adipose tissue secretes IL-1, IL-6, and TNF, as well as the generation of oxidative stress from inflammatory macrophages. In addition, the conversion of epithelial tissue to mesenchymal tissue, the thickness of the basement membrane, and the deposition of collagen all contribute to the remodeling of the airways and an increase in airway stress, which in turn exacerbates asthmatic exacerbations that are already present. The results of this study shed light on the diverse nature of asthma and the pressing requirement for the development of novel treatments and approaches to address the issue.

2.3.1.1. Treatments

When it comes to treating asthma patients, clinicians take into consideration more than just one factor. Before beginning treatment, a pulmonary function analysis is carried out in conjunction with a sputum analysis. This analysis considers both pre-existing respiratory conditions and treatments that are currently being administered. While glucocorticoids were the treatment of choice for the majority of asthmatics in the beginning (they suppressed Th2 responses), the use of steroid treatment also had its drawbacks. Dysphonia, candidiasis, osteoporosis, and adrenal suppression are some of the local to systemic side effects associated with prolonged steroid treatment. Conversely, patients with a low Th2 response phenotype or hypersensitivity to neutrophilic asthma may exhibit resistance to such treatments. However, studies have shown that β2-agonists in inhaled corticosteroids (ICS) are effective in managing allergic asthma, such as that triggered by pollen. The treatment of non-allergic patients (viruses/ bacteria) however with systemic corticosteroids (SCS) is a common practice. Additionally, in accordance with EPR-3 regulations, high concentrations of short-acting beta-agonists (SABAs) like albuterol and levalbuterol are administered. Oxygen is the primary treatment for acute asthma; however, in the later stages of the disease, known as chronic asthma, these medications are replaced by epinephrine, magnesium sulfate, non-invasive positive pressure ventilation (NPPV), and hospitalization.

When it comes to the treatment of patients who suffer from severe asthma, azithromycin treatment for an extended period of time has become an increasingly popular option in recent years; however, it continues to be a contentious topic. Gibson and his team demonstrated that the use of azithromycin as an add-on therapy (in conjunction with inhaled corticosteroids) could reduce the number of annual exacerbations experienced by severe asthmatics by 50%, however, the epidemiologic data that was published do not demonstrate that azithromycin is significantly effective in controlling severe asthmatic exacerbations. To draw conclusions and confirm the potential of azithromycin as an effective anti-asthma drug, we require additional human cohorts. Furthermore, an increasing antibiotic resistance to azithromycin was observed in the long term, which is a major limitation of the use of the well-known antibiotic in the treatment of asthma. Conversely, a recent study demonstrated that the use of azithromycin (both antibiotic and macrolide) for an extended period reduced the amount of *H. influenzae* in severe asthmatics.

Over the past decade, the application of monoclonal antibodies in the treatment of diseases has garnered the interest of researchers from all over the world. Biological inhibitors, such as anti-IL-5 (mepolizumab) and anti-IgE monoclonal antibody (omalizumab), which are currently approved for use in humans, have been demonstrated to be effective in controlling exacerbations in severe asthmatics. Omalizumab forms an irreversible complex with immunoglobulin IgE and blocks the production of inflammatory mediators and immune cells (mast cells and basophils), thereby effectively controlling the pathogenesis of the disease. When compared to other groups (placebo and ICS), some researchers demonstrated that the use of omalizumab resulted in a significant reduction in several exacerbations experienced by severe asthmatics. Furthermore, the efficacy and safety of the utilization of omalizumab or other monoclonal antibodies have been officially validated and published. Despite the fact that the utilization of biological inhibitors (mAbs) is efficient and lessens the financial burden of medication, the cost of manufacturing, transportation, and storage of mAbs continues to be a challenge (Lore et al., 2018).

2.3.2. Chronic Obstructive Pulmonary Disease

These lung diseases include emphysema, chronic bronchitis, deterioration of the small airways, and chronic asthma. COPD, which stands for chronic obstructive pulmonary disease, is a collective term that refers to a group of progressive, obstructive-irreversible lung diseases. There were 251 million cases of COPD reported worldwide in the Global Burden of Disease Study, with 90% of those cases occurring in countries with low and middle incomes. During the year 2015 alone, there were an estimated 3.17 million deaths, which accounted for 5% of all deaths. This represents an increase of 11.6% when compared to the year 1990. The Centers for Disease Control and Prevention (CDC) estimated that the economic burden of COPD due to medical costs and lost work time was $32.1 billion by the year 2010, and it is anticipated that this number will increase even further to $49.0 billion by the year 2020 in the United States. This is in addition to the mortality rate. However, the precise number of cases of COPD around the world is still a matter of debate, as the disease was frequently misdiagnosed in the majority of asthma cases in older people. There is also a lack of data from developing or underdeveloped countries in Asia and the Middle East, which could further increase the number of deaths by several million.

Patients who suffer from one form of COPD exhibit a wide range of symptoms, including shortness of breath during everyday activities which is a major indicator that worsens over time. Patients who suffer from severe forms of COPD and asthma experience frequent exacerbations and subsequent visits to the emergency room throughout the year. The partial destruction of the alveoli (emphysema) or the accumulation of excess mucus and inflammatory cells in the bronchioles (chronic bronchitis) is the cause of this condition. This condition is especially prevalent in smokers and ex-smokers who have COPD. This condition reduces the gas exchange capacity of the lungs and obstructs airflow, which ultimately results in decreased oxygen levels in the blood (hypoxemia) and subsequent organ failure. In addition, patients who are suffering from any type of COPD may exhibit common symptoms such as persistent coughing (with or without phlegm), fatigue, wheezing, and chest tightness. In the majority of instances, these symptoms are often mistaken for age-related factors. In certain patients, symptoms do not manifest themselves until the disease has progressed to a more severe stage. Even after decades of tireless research, there is still no treatment that can repair the damaged tissue and improve the function of the lungs. Additionally, COPD is a progressive disease that worsens with age. The treatments that are currently available are designed to provide patients with temporary relief and to slow the progression of the disease and are unfortunately not able to restore the function that has been lost in the areas that have been damaged. According to the data that is currently available, smoking is the most common cause of COPD, where recent studies have shown that long-term exposure to non-cigarette smoke irritants, such as airborne dust particles, geogenic dust, and metal contaminants, is a significant risk factor for its development and exacerbation in non-smokers and smokers, respectively. Regrettably, this is a topic that has received relatively little attention in the scientific community. In addition, studies have demonstrated that hereditary factors and genetic predispositions, such as a lack of alpha-1-antitrypsin (AAT), play a role in the development of chronic obstructive pulmonary disease (COPD). Despite this, the precise mechanisms that are responsible for this condition are still largely unknown. Individuals who are deficient in AAT, on the other hand, are more likely to suffer from respiratory infections.

Genetic factors are responsible for 1% of all COPD cases, with tobacco smoking and air pollutants being the primary causes of the condition. The fact that not all smokers or ex-smokers develop the disease is an interesting fact to consider; in fact, only 20–30% of active smokers or ex-smokers develop the disease over the course of their lifetime. Although the exact mechanisms that are responsible for COPD development are still unknown, the studies found that passive smoking was one of the most significant risk factors (Maiz et al., 2018).

It is primarily the obstruction of airflow and the influx of inflammatory cells, particularly CD8+ T lymphocytes, neutrophils, and macrophages, into the alveoli and peripheral spaces that are responsible for COPD. These occurrences are in response to tobacco smoke or environmental particles or gases. There are, however, a variety of COPD subtypes COPD, each of which triggers a unique immune system response. Chronic bronchitis, which is characterized by excessive mucus production, increased inflammatory cells, overexpression of the MUC5AC gene in response to secreted serine proteases, increased reactive oxygen species (ROS) concentrations from inhaled smoke or activated macrophages, leads to the narrowing of the airspace and subsequent damage to adjacent cells which results in airway remodeling (fibrosis) and thus loss of lung elasticity. Emphysema (centrilobular and panlobular), however, is a direct consequence of cigarette smoke. Smoke inhalation causes inflammation to increase in the territorial bronchioles and alveolar sacs, which ultimately results in the gradual destruction of the alveolar sacs and the smaller airway walls. This ultimately leads to a loss of alveolar structure, function, and back pressure. In patients with COPD, the activation of innate and adaptive immune responses is understudied. Nevertheless, the overexpression of CXC, IL8, and MMP by immune cells, as well as the production of proinflammatory mediators like TNFα, IL1β (Th1 responses), leukotriene B4, and transforming growth factor beta (TGFβ), may result in the development of local fibrosis and an imbalance between ROS and reactive nitrogen species (RNS). These factors have been among the most important contributors to the exacerbation of the disease.

Spirometry that does not involve any invasive procedures and the GOLD staging system, which was developed by the Global Initiative for Chronic Obstructive Lung Disease (GOLD), are frequently utilized by clinicians to diagnose and evaluate the severity of the progression of the disease. To classify a person into one of the following four stages, the GOLD staging system evaluates lung function, which is the ratio between forced expiratory volume and forced vital capacity (FEV1/FVC). This ratio refers to the amount of air that a patient exhales in one second after taking a single deep breath.

- **Stage 1:** If the person has an FEV1/FVC ratio of ≥ 80% of normal, they are classified as having mild COPD.
- **Stage 2:** If the person has an FEV1/FVC ratio between 50% and 80% of normal, they are classified as having moderate COPD.
- **Stage 3:** If the FEV1/FVC ratio is between 30% and 50% of normal, it is severe emphysema.
- **Stage 4:** An FEV1/FVC ratio of 30% of normal or stage 3 with low oxygen levels in the blood is a very severe form of emphysema or COPD.

COPD is a disease that can be prevented but cannot be reversed. There are currently treatments available that aim to alleviate symptoms and slow the progression of the disease; however, they do not aim to completely cure the disease, which is only possible through a lung transplant, an option that is not feasible. In order to relax the muscles of the airways, improve airflow, and reduce inflammation in the lower airways, it is possible to make use of medications such as bronchodilators, corticosteroids, glucocorticosteroids, phosphodiesterase-4 inhibitors, theophylline, and antibiotics. In stages 3 and 4, doctors frequently recommend oxygen therapy to bring blood oxygen levels back to baseline (Maselli et al., 2017). However, this is only a temporary solution, and if the oxygen supply is interrupted, the patient's condition will quickly deteriorate once more. Adopting alterations to one's lifestyle, such as giving up smoking, avoiding exposure to air pollution, and reducing the amount of food consumed, can also slow the progression of the disease.

2.3.3. Interstitial Lung Diseases

There are over 100 different lung diseases that fall under the umbrella of interstitial lung diseases (ILD), which are a large group of lung diseases that cause scarring and fibrosis of the lungs. The manifestations that are characteristic of ILDs are variable and include respiratory symptoms such as coughing and dyspnea, a worsening of lung capacity, abnormalities in chest radiographs, and abnormal fibrosis and inflammation in biopsies. It is possible to categorize ILDs into individual diseases by taking into account a number of these particular clinical, physiologic, radiologic, and histopathologic findings. For instance, the presence of granulomatous inflammation (but not parenchymal fibrosis) is a sign of sarcoidosis. On the other hand, extensive pulmonary fibrosis and distortion of the lung are characteristics that are unique to idiopathic pulmonary fibrosis (IPF). It has become more difficult to accurately estimate the incidence rates of ILDs due to the complexity of making a definitive diagnosis. On the other hand, it seems that IDLs are prevalent all over the world and primarily affect adults. One of the most prevalent ILD is interstitial pulmonary fibrosis (IPF), which is estimated to affect approximately 3 million people worldwide and 130,000 people in the United States. Furthermore, there has been a growing incidence rate reported. Variations in the epidemiology of infectious diseases can occur depending on the disease. For instance, interstitial pulmonary fibrosis (IPF) is most prevalent in individuals who are over the age of 65, whereas sarcoidosis appears to be more prevalent in people of African American and Northern European descent.

There is a wide range of outcomes that can occur as a result of ILD, ranging from partially reversible fibrosis to chronic progressive fibrotic ILD, which includes the possibility of death. A very poor prognosis is associated with interstitial pulmonary fibrosis (IPF), which is the most prevalent form of chronic progressive fibrotic disease, with the median survival time estimated to be only two to five years after diagnosis. Patients with infectious pulmonary fibrosis can alternate between periods of little change and rapid deterioration in lung function, and simultaneously can experience frequent and acute exacerbations, which can be fatal. The progression of interpulmonary fibrosis (IPF) is highly variable both between patients and within individuals, for example in some patients, the disease progresses slowly, while in others, the loss of lung function occurs rapidly. A heterogeneous course and a variable outcome depending on the patient are also characteristics of sarcoidosis, which is another common inflammatory bowel disease (IBD) that is associated with significant morbidity. Sarcoidosis can range from an acute onset with spontaneous regression toward chronic progressive disease. ILDs frequently have comorbidities and/or lack specific symptoms, which can make diagnosis difficult (Miravitlles & Anzueto, 2017). This can result in delays in treatment and compromise the prognosis for the patient. For instance, one study found that the median amount of time it took to diagnose IPF patients was approximately 2.1 years.

Interstitial lung disease (ILD) is characterized by the fact that the cause of the lung injury and the subsequent fibrosis is not known in the majority of cases. Nevertheless, there have been instances in which ILDs have been linked to systemic diseases (for example, an autoimmune disease like rheumatoid arthritis), infections, or exposure to environmental agents that are especially harmful to the lungs (like tobacco smoke or asbestos) among other things. In addition, certain instances of idiopathic lung disease (ILD) have been linked to genetic mutations. The modification of particular genes has been linked to increased fibrosis or has been identified as the cause of ILD, which is also known as Hermansky-Pudlak syndrome. Bronchiolitis obliterans is an extremely uncommon form of inflammatory lung disease (ILD), and it has been demonstrated that patients who have undergone lung transplantation or hematopoietic stem cell transplantation have a higher risk of developing this condition.

There is still a lack of knowledge regarding the mechanisms that are responsible for the development of ILD; however, it appears that these mechanisms are multifactorial and involve both the aging process and damage to the lung epithelium. ILD is characterized by the presence of abnormal inflammation and fibrosis in the lung, which is characterized by an excessive number of inflammatory cells (macrophages, lymphocytes, and so on), as well as abnormal deposition of collagens and other extracellular matrix components in the lung. These are two of the most prominent features of an inflammatory lung disease. Although there is evidence that polymorphonuclear cells infiltrate the lung or that activated macrophages may exhibit profibrotic properties, the contribution of inflammation in idiopathic pulmonary fibrosis (IPF) continues to be a contentious and poorly understood topic. Following chronic injury to the pulmonary alveolar epithelium, the local proliferation of fibroblasts and myofibroblasts, as well as their production of collagen and other extracellular matrix components, appears to be the primary factor that is responsible for the development of fibrosis in the lungs of individuals with interstitial pulmonary fibrosis (IPF). We do not yet have a clear understanding of the mechanisms that are responsible for the accumulation and activation of fibroblasts and myofibroblasts; however, it is possible that multiple pathways with distinct dynamics are involved, which would explain the wide range of clinical manifestations that people experience.

It is common practice to base treatment strategies on the specific diagnosis of ILD as well as the severity of the disease. The avoidance of the precipitating factor is one of the recommended methods for preventing the progression of the disease in patients with ILD for which the cause is known. As was mentioned earlier, however, most cases of ILD are idiopathic, and as a result, they cannot be prevented unless the risk factors that cause them are reduced. These risk factors include cigarette smoking, exposure to environmental and microbial stimuli, and other similar factors. The treatment options for ILD are dependent on the particular disease, and Kim et al. and Richeldi et al. have provided a detailed description of these treatment options. As a means of preserving lung function, reducing the frequency of acute exacerbations, and improving patient survival, they frequently involve the administration of immunosuppressants and/or corticosteroids (like prednisone, cyclophosphamide, or azathioprine, for example). Nevertheless, it does not appear that the administration of these therapies results in long-term improvement for patients who are suffering from the most severe cases of progressive fibrosis. As a result, there is currently no demonstrated treatment for IPF that has the potential to extend the lives of patients. There have been two antifibrotic agents approved for use, nintedanib, and pirfenidone, and it has been demonstrated that they are beneficial in preventing a decline in lung function and slowing the progression of disease in patients who have IPF or other progressive ILDs. It seems that they act on several different signaling pathways, which could be the reason for their effectiveness, however, there is still a lack of comprehension regarding their mode of operation. The intracellular tyrosine kinase receptors that are involved in inflammatory pulmonary disease (IPF) include profibrotic mediators, the platelet-derived growth factor receptor, the fibroblast growth factor receptor, and the vascular endothelial growth factor receptor and can be inhibited by nintedanib. Pirfenidone, on the other hand, appears to possess a wide range of antifibrotic, anti-inflammatory, and antioxidant properties (including a reduction in TGFβ and TNFα). However, these antifibrotic agents have been shown to have some unfavorable effects, including gastrointestinal effects (such as diarrhea), which may lead patients to discontinue treatment if they are not provided with counseling and personalized practical management of these effects. When administered as monotherapy or in combination with corticosteroids or pirfenidone, the antioxidant N-acetylcysteine has shown promising results in improving lung function and slowing the progression of the disease in patients with interstitial pulmonary fibrosis (IPF). Clinical trials, however, have frequently failed to show improvements in patients, despite the fact that there have been some encouraging preliminary results from biological immunomodulatory drugs designed to prevent the progression of interferon-positive pulmonary disease (IPF) (for example, treatment with interferon gamma-1b). There are, however, a great number of treatment options that are still in the clinical trial stage and offer patients hope. For instance, preclinical studies have demonstrated that therapies based on mesenchymal stem cells have shown promising results; however, additional research is required to either confirm or disagree with these findings. Currently, there are no treatments available for patients who are suffering from advanced progressive cases of IDL. The only remaining option for these patients is lung transplantation, which has been demonstrated to increase the likelihood of survival (Polverino et al., 2017). In spite of this, the median survival rate following transplantation continues to be low, with IPF patients having a median survival rate of only six years after transplantation. This highlights the necessity of developing new treatment options.

Generally speaking, ILDs continue to be a significant health problem for which there are frequently no effective treatments. Even though there has been some advancement in the understanding of ILD in recent times, the discovery of a cure for the most aggressive and chronic progressive ILDs is still on the horizon. At this time, medical research on ILDs is a combination of basic research, which includes studies conducted on animals and cell cultures, and clinical research, which includes clinical trials and studies conducted in the real world. The objective of this research is to determine the mechanism and molecular pathways that are involved in the development of abnormal lung inflammation and fibrosis. To improve the quality of life and survival rates of affected patients, the purpose of these studies is twofold: first, to discover new biological markers that will make it easier to diagnose inflammatory lung diseases (ILDs) and to track their progression; second, to develop new therapies for ILDs that are currently incurable.

2.3.4. Cystic Fibrosis

There are mutations in the gene known as the cystic fibrosis transmembrane conductance regulator (CFTR), which are the root cause of the serious genetic disease known as cystic fibrosis (CF).

CFTR is a gene that encodes a protein that assists in the translation of a chloride-containing transmembrane channel. This channel is responsible for regulating anion transport as well as the mucociliary clearance mechanism in the airways. There is a genetic risk factor that is responsible for approximately 70% of cases of CF. The deletion of the amino acid phenylalanine at residue 508 of the predicted 1,480 amino acid CFTR protein is the specific gene that is responsible for causing CF. This deletion typically takes the form of a triple base deletion, which results in the loss of the phenylalanine amino acid. In addition, researchers have discovered over 2,000 mutations that have the potential to influence the function of the CFTR gene in humans. These mutations can be roughly divided into the following categories: Mutations in protein production (class 1) (i.e., nonsense and splicing mutations that impair protein production), mutations in protein processing (class 2) (i.e., mutations that lead to the addition or deletion of amino acids), gating mutations (class 3) (i.e., mutations that cause the CFTR protein to remain closed), conduction mutations (class 4) (malfunction in protein function), and mutations in insufficient protein (class 5). There is a high level of expression of CFTR mRNA transcripts in the epithelial cells of the respiratory tract, including epithelial cells of nasal, tracheal, and bronchial origin. However, the expression of CFTR mRNA in these epithelial cells is quite low, with approximately one to two copies per cell (Polverino et al., 2017).

The condition known as CF affects approximately 70,000 individuals across the globe, primarily children of Northern European descent (approximately 1 in 2,500–3,000 births). There is a high mortality rate associated with the disease, with survival rates ranging from 33 to 50 years in various regions of the world, when considered together. In addition, the consequences of CF on the economy are just starting to be better understood. Patients can expect to pay anywhere from €17,551 per patient yearly in Germany to approximately €48,603 in the United Kingdom for their treatment.

Genetic mutations and bacterial infections that are recurrent and/or persistent are the primary factors that set off the cellular mechanisms that are involved in CF diagnosis and treatment. Despite the fact that mucus is constantly produced by goblet cells and submucosal glands, mucus that is not adequately cleared by the cilia can lead to the formation of mucus plugs. It is important to note that the CFTR mutation causes a protein to be misfolded or to function poorly, which can result in dehydrated mucus and, as a consequence, impaired mucociliary clearance. These mucus plugs can potentially contribute to local tissue hypoxia, particularly on the surface of the epithelial cells. There is also a correlation between local tissue hypoxia and local inflammation and an increased risk of viral infection. On top of that, the most significant risk factors for the progression of CF, particularly in the first few years of life, are bacterial infections of the large airways that are both recurrent and persistent.

There is an inherent need for improved drug delivery mechanisms that can deliver the therapeutic agent to the site of pathology in an efficient manner. The use of common absorption enhancers such as surfactants (bile salts, phospholipids, and fatty acids and derivatives), cationic polymers, enzyme inhibitors, cyclodextrins, and tight junction modulators in conjunction with many different strategies that involve novel routes of drug delivery via the nose and/or lungs could be one way to accomplish this goal. There is also the possibility of conducting research into the effectiveness of nanoparticles functioning as "drug carriers.," such as mucopenetrating polystyrene-based particles (also known as MPP).

2.3.5. Tuberculosis

On a global scale, tuberculosis (TB) is currently the infectious agent that is responsible for the highest number of deaths that can be attributed to a single infectious agent. An estimated 10 million people became ill with the disease in 2018, with a total mortality of 1.5 million people. When it comes to geography, the burden of TB is not distributed evenly. It was found that approximately two-thirds of the cases that were reported by the World Health Organization (WHO) in 2018 were found in the regions of Southeast Asia (44%), Africa (24%), and Africa. On the other hand, the proportion of cases in Europe (3%) and the Americas (3%) was significantly lower. India had the highest number of TB cases in 2018, with 2.69 million cases, followed by China with 866,000 cases and Indonesia with 845,000 cases.

The acid-fast bacterial species *M. tuberculosis* is the primary agent responsible for TB in humans. On the other hand, the animal-adapted species *Mycobacterium bovis* is responsible for a relatively small number of zoonotic cases only (143,000 in 2018). TB from *M. tuberculosis* can be transmitted in aerosols from the lungs of active patients through sneezing, coughing, or spitting, and remain highly infectious. This is despite the fact that it lacks many of the classical virulence factors that are associated with other bacterial pathogens, such as exotoxins. The inhalation of the pathogen into the alveoli of the lower respiratory tract occurs when a susceptible individual is exposed to droplets that contain the bacterium. The resident macrophages, which are typically the first cells of the immune system to come into contact with *M. tuberculosis* in the lungs, are responsible for the internalization of the bacterium (Shiratori et al., 2017).

In an experimental model of TB, the bacterium possesses several virulence genes that, when inactivated, result in a loss of pathogenicity. However, the inactivation of these genes does not hinder the growth of mycobacteria under optimal *in vitro* conditions, also known as conditions in which there is neither stress nor starvation. It is possible to classify the virulence factors of *M. tuberculosis* into the following categories: enzymes involved in lipid metabolism, proteins found in the cell envelope, proteins that inhibit the function of macrophages, protein kinases, proteases, metal transporters, gene regulators, and proteins with an unknown function, such as PE and PE_PGRS particles. Following phagocytosis by alveolar macrophages, *M. tuberculosis* can withstand the activity of reactive oxygen and nitrogen intermediates, as well as prevent phagosome acidification and lysosomal fusion through its ability to resist these processes. In addition to facilitating bacterial replication, tissue dissemination and damage in active tuberculosis cases, and subsequent human-to-human transmission, these functions are essential for the persistence of the pathogen in the host during latent TB. Fibrosis, cavitation, traction bronchiectasis, bronchostenosis, and parenchymal destruction are the various types of structural lung damage that can transpire as a result of pulmonary TB.

The administration of four particular medications for two months—namely, isoniazid, rifampicin, pyrazinamide, and ethambutol—is the standard therapeutic regimen that the WHO recommends for patients with drug-susceptible pulmonary TB. After that, patients should continue taking isoniazid and rifampicin for an additional four months. There was an overall success rate of 85% with this treatment regimen among patients whose TB was detected, reported, and treated in the year 2017. On the other hand, this success rate drops to 56% for cases that are resistant to both isoniazid and rifampicin, also known as multidrug-resistant (MDR) or rifampicin-resistant (RR) cases. MDR/RR-TB accounted for 3.4% of newly diagnosed cases of tuberculosis and 18.0% of cases that had already been treated in 2018. In 2018, there were 484,000 cases of MDR/RR-TB worldwide.

The standard regimen that is recommended by the WHO consists of an intensive eight-month phase with at least four effective second-line TB drugs plus pyrazinamide, followed by a continuation phase with at least three effective second-line TB drugs, extending the treatment duration to a total of 20 months. MDR-TB requires an even longer treatment duration than other types of TB. Moxifloxacin, kanamycin, prothionamide, clofazimine, pyrazinamide, high-dose isoniazid, and ethambutol are the seven medications that are included in the eight- to six-month intensive phase of treatment that is recommended by the WHO. This phase is followed by a five-month continuation phase that includes moxifloxacin, clofazimine, pyrazinamide, and ethambutol (Shiratori et al., 2017).

MDR-TB treatment is not only more expensive than drug-susceptible TB treatment, but it also has a lower success rate and requires a longer treatment duration. The cost per case is estimated to be USD 1,34,000 in the United States and € 57,213 in the 15 countries that make up the European Union (EU). This is in comparison to the cost of USD 17,000 and € 10,282 for drug-susceptible TB, respectively. Methods that can deliver drugs to patients in a more efficient manner, as well as methods that can reduce the cost and/or duration of anti-TB treatment, are therefore required.

The development of drug delivery systems may potentially increase the effectiveness of pre-existing TB medications. In addition to a reduction in adverse effects, these systems allow for improved targeting of tuberculosis drugs, as well as improved release and bioavailability. Regarding the management of TB, new delivery systems have the potential to assist in several ways, including the enhancement of patient adherence to TB treatment, the reduction of the number of untreated TB cases and treatment failures, and the development of new treatment regimens that encompass shorter durations.

The oral administration of isoniazid, rifampicin, ethambutol, and pyrazinamide is the primary method of treatment for drug-resistant TB during the initial phase of treatment. In addition, several drugs that are considered to be second-line treatments for MDR-TB are injectable intramuscularly or intravenously. These drugs include amikacin, kanamycin, and capreomycin. The pulmonary route is currently being investigated as a potential route for the delivery of anti-TB drugs, as the latter are believed to be more effective in reaching the lungs, which are the primary site of TB disease and the primary port of entry for *M. tuberculosis*. In recent times, there has been an investigation into the utilization of a stomach-specific delivery system, which has enabled the administration of multigram doses of TB drugs for a period of several weeks in a porcine model.

The delivery of drugs to treat tuberculosis includes a wide variety of new transportation systems that are being researched. These include the utilization of 1) liposomes, which are typically between 50 and 450 nanometers in size, consisting of phosphatidylcholine and cholesterol, 2) microparticles, which are between 1 and 1,000 micrometers in size, and consist of polylactic acid (PLA) or polylactic-co-glycolic acid (PLGA), and 3) nanoparticles, which are between 1 and 100 nanometers in at least one dimension, and consisting of alginate, PLA, PLGA, or poly-ε-caprolactone (PCL). It has been demonstrated that it is possible to successfully incorporate several anti-TB drugs into liposomes, microparticles, and/or nanoparticles. These drugs include the first-line drugs isoniazid, rifampicin, ethambutol, and pyrazinamide, as well as the second-line drugs levofloxacin, ofloxacin, and capreomycin. One study demonstrated that the use of aerosolized polylactic acid nanoparticles (PLGA nanoparticles) increased the bioavailability of isoniazid, rifampicin, and pyrazinamide. The use of these nanoparticles improved the elimination of *M. tuberculosis* from the lungs of infected guinea pigs more effectively than the use of standard drugs for oral administration.

Although liposomes, microparticles, and nanoparticles are relatively small in size, they have the capability of being taken up by macrophages, which allows them to selectively concentrate TB drugs in the primary host cell of *M. tuberculosis* that is invading the body. The use of these particles also serves to reduce the dose and duration required to achieve eradication of the infection and consequently reduces the toxic side effects that are associated with the current treatment regimens for TB. An additional possibility is the creation of vehicles that are capable of delivering their drug cargo after entering macrophages. Nanoparticles with pH-controlled valves based on cyclodextrin, for instance, have been developed, where they only release isoniazid in an acidic environment, such as the acidified endosomes of human macrophages (Shiratori et al., 2017).

In humans, novel delivery systems that target drugs to the primary site of TB infection and pathology have the potential to significantly advance the control of the disease by reducing the amount of time and dosage that is required for successful chemotherapy. Not only would this bring down the costs of healthcare, but it would also bring down the negative effects that anti-TB drugs have on patients, as well as improve treatment adherence and success rates – the latter is of particular importance. Therefore, it is hoped that additional research and testing of new drug delivery systems will result in the development of improved treatments that are more affordable for both drug-susceptible and drug-resistant TB.

2.4. Lung Cancer

A delayed diagnosis and inadequate treatment are the primary factors that contribute to the mortality rate associated with lung cancer around the world. Around 70% of people who have lung cancer are typically in an advanced stage of the disease, either stage III or stage IV. Among both men and women, it is a malignant disease that is extremely invasive, rapidly metastasizing, and widespread. Lung cancer in the United States has a mortality rate that is higher than the combined mortality rate of the other four leading cancers (prostate, breast, colon, and pancreas), according to statistical comparisons. A history of smoking that is at least 20 years old appears to have a significant association with the occurrence of development and mortality. It is believed that the susceptibility to lung cancer that it causes is highly dependent on competing gene-enzyme interactions at the procarcinogen level, as well as the level of DNA damage that results from these interactions. Therefore, it is generally believed that lung cancer can be prevented by avoiding and quitting smoking altogether. It is necessary to raise public awareness and educate the public to reduce or eliminate cigarette smoking and prevent the inevitable rise in the number of respiratory cancers that will occur in countries where smoking has increased (Smith et al., 2018).

Lung cancer is the leading cause of death worldwide due to cancer, making it the leading cause of death for both men and women. Martin et al. conducted a study in which they found that there were approximately 1.8 million new cases of lung cancer in the year 2012, representing 12.9% of all new cancer diagnoses. Following the research of the Global Burden of Disease Study 2020, the health burden and costs associated with lung cancer were extremely prominent across the globe. According to the findings of one study, there is no correlation between the level of economic progress and the mortality rate from cancer in men. The study revealed, to everyone's surprise, that the level of economic development in a country is connected to the mortality rates of lung cancer in females. By contrast, in developing countries, breast cancer continues to be the leading cause of death because of cancer in females.

The history of smoking cigarettes is significantly associated with both the prevalence of lung cancer and the mortality rate associated with the disease. It is interesting to note that both the prevalence of lung cancer and the mortality rate associated with it have been observed to rise over time. This suggests that there has been an increase in smoking rates, followed by a decrease, which could be a result of the formulation and implementation of comprehensive smoking cessation campaigns. There has been a significant decrease in the mortality rate and the prevalence of lung cancer since the 1990s, according to data collected from the United States of America and the United Kingdom. On the other hand, low- and middle-income countries (LMICs), and in particular the BRICS countries (specifically Brazil, Russia, India, China, and South Africa), have seen a significant increase in the number of people smoking cigarettes, regardless of whether they are male or female. In addition, low- and middle-income countries (LMICs) have a higher mortality rate for lung cancer, even though they have a lower incidence of the disease in comparison to countries with higher incomes. The most likely explanation for this is that access to health facilities is disproportionately difficult, which in turn makes it difficult to diagnose and treat patients in a timely manner. Additional important factors include pollution and/or contamination of the environment, as well as taboos in sociocultural contexts. Consequently, this highlights the importance of preventative measures, such as the WHO Framework Convention on Tobacco Control, which ought to be further strengthened in these countries by implementing taxation policies, smoke-free environments, surveillance, support for quitting smoking, education on the harmful effects of tobacco, and bans on tobacco advertising.

As a result of its origin in various parts of the bronchial tree, as well as the various symptoms and signs that manifest themselves depending on the type of lung cancer and the anatomical location of the disease, lung cancer is characterized by its complex heterogeneity. Small cell lung cancer (SCLC) and non-small cell lung cancer (NSCLC), the early traditional classification of lung cancer, account for 15% and 85% of all lung cancers, respectively. Adenocarcinomas, squamous cell carcinomas, and large cell carcinomas are the three primary subtypes of NSCLCs, and there are specific histopathologic features and reliable immunohistochemical markers that have been added to this specific stratification of lung cancer. These features and markers make it possible to differentiate between invasive adenocarcinomas and preinvasive lesions. In addition, the introduction of molecular characterization of lung cancer and the ever-expanding arsenal of treatments that are currently available have both contributed to a significant shift in the classification of lung cancer in the modern era. Based on the available data, it appears that lung cancer is a collection of diseases that are both histologically and molecularly distinct from one another, even within the same histologic subtype.

Statistically speaking, squamous cell carcinomas are the most significant of all the subtypes of lung cancer. This is due to their higher prevalence (25–30%), their site of origin (main bronchi) located in the lung, and their aggressive metastases (carina bifurcation of the trachea in the bronchi). In comparison, peripherally located adenocarcinomas are responsible for 40% of all lung carcinomas, and they manifest themselves in a localized manner through symptoms such as lobar atelectasis and pneumonitis. Bronchioloalveolar carcinomas (BAC) were also reclassified based on their origin in the alveoli and their local spread to interalveolar compartments. This was done through the process of reclassification. Consequently, this led to the classification of lung carcinomas into two distinct categories: adenocarcinoma in situ (AIS) and minimally invasive adenocarcinoma (MIA). SCLC, as previously noted, accounts for 10–15% of all lung carcinomas. These tumors, which originate from neuroendocrine cells (APUD cells) in the bronchus, also known as Feyrter cells, are considered to be extremely aggressive tumors due to their rapid ability to spread to nearby lymphatic vessels and associated regional lymph nodes (Smith et al., 2018).

More than 70% of patients diagnosed with non-small cell lung cancer are in advanced stages or have metastatic disease. The options and treatment cycle for NSCLC are determined by the location and stage of the tumor, taking into account the patient's involvement and the current state of their performance. Some conventional and current treatments for NSCLC are described below, depending on the stage, metastasis, and recurrence.

1. **Stage I and II – NSCLC:** Surgery is the most common primary treatment for resectable stage I and II disease. Postoperative adjuvant platinum-based chemotherapy is also suggested and shown to be beneficial for stage II NSCLC patients.
2. **Stage III – NSCLC:** Due to the complex heterogeneity of stage III, treatment options are divided into resectable and non-resectable diseases, which are highly dependent on the involvement of regional lymph nodes. The spectrum ranges from resectable tumors with microscopic metastases in regional lymph nodes to non-resectable stage III disease with distant nodal involvement. Traditionally, the treatment of resectable stage IIIA disease consists of surgery followed by chemotherapy alone. In contrast, treatment of non-resectable stage IIIA disease consists of chemotherapy alone or chemoradiation (combined chemotherapy and post-chemoradiation therapy). Traditional treatment of stage IIIB NSCLC consists of either a sequential combination of chemotherapy or external beam radiotherapy.
3. **Stage IV – NSCLC:** Due to the complexity of the disease, 40% of newly diagnosed NSCLC patients have stage IV disease. For this reason, treatment options are usually based on combination therapy in the form of combination chemotherapy, and targeted therapy, as well as external beam radiotherapy with internal endoscopic radiotherapy if necessary.
4. **Recurrent NSCLC:** The recurrence or relapse of NSCLC following the completion of initial treatment (which may include chemotherapy, radiotherapy, or surgery). The chemotherapy treatment plan for patients with stage IV non-small cell lung cancer (NSCLC) generally follows

the same approach for all patients with stage IV NSCLC. The treatment regimen is typically determined based on factors such as the patient's overall health, the specific characteristics of the tumor, and any molecular or genetic mutations present in the cancer cells. On the other hand, patients who experience recurrence after chemotherapy have several treatment options available to them. These include: (1) external palliative radiotherapy, which works to alleviate pain and other symptoms related to the tumor; (2) cytotoxic chemotherapy; (3) EGFR inhibitors (TKIs) in patients who have or do not have EGFR mutations; and (4) an EML4-ALK inhibitor (crizotinib) in patients who have EML-ALK translocations.

Additionally, it has been demonstrated that chemotherapeutic treatment of NSCLC is beneficial for patient survival, in addition to surgical resection. Chemotherapies are currently being used for the treatment of NSCLC patients, and many more classes of chemotherapies are currently being tested. Some important treatment strategies are presented below.

2.4.1. Angiogenesis Inhibitors

Angiogenic signaling pathways are always considered to be a critical target in the treatment of NSCLC since the tumor forms new blood vessels in the desmoplastic stroma for its growth and progression. It is always considered to be of the utmost importance to target a variety of proangiogenic factors, such as vascular endothelial growth factor (VEGF), fibroblast growth factor (FGF), and platelet-derived growth factor (PDGF), to prevent the angiogenesis that is necessary for the growth of tumors. Currently, the monoclonal anti-VEGF antibody known as bevacizumab has been approved for the first-line treatment of advanced NSCLC when combined with platinum-based chemotherapy procedures. In addition, there is evidence from studies that suggest that bevacizumab may also be useful in the treatment of patients who have adenocarcinoma. However, it has been observed that eventually, every single patient will demonstrate resistance to treatment with anti-VEGF agents. Sorafenib, a multiple tyrosine kinase inhibitor (TKI) that targets VEGFR-2/3, PDGFR-β, c-Kit, Raf, and Flt-3, has therefore been developed due to this limitation. It has demonstrated promising responses in several phase I and phase II trials, particularly in patients with NSCLC who have a K-Ras mutation (Smith et al., 2018).

2.4.2. Insulin-Like Growth Factor Inhibitors

Two receptors make up the insulin-like growth factor system, also known as the IGF system. These receptors are the receptor for insulin-like growth factor 1 receptor (IGF-IR) and the insulin-like growth factor 1 receptor (IGF-IIR), along with the intracellular ligands that correspond to each receptor. Numerous types of cancer, including lung cancer, exhibit an overexpression of these ligands. In a phase II trial, Figitumumab, which is an anti-IGF-1R monoclonal antibody, demonstrated a remarkable response in patients with NSCLC who had not been treated before, and who had locally advanced or metastatic disease, in comparison to chemotherapy alone. In addition, cixutumab and dalotuzumab, which are both monoclonal antibodies specific to IGF ligands, are currently undergoing clinical trials.

2.4.3. Histone Deacetylase Inhibitors

In the nucleus of the cell, there is a family of proteins known as histones. These proteins are associated with DNA and help to compact it into chromatin. Histone deacetylases, also known as HDACs, are enzymes that control the expression and activity of a large number of proteins that play a role in the development of cancer as well as the progression of cancer. It has been reported that the acetylation of different intracellular proteins that are involved in cell growth and proliferation can be altered by several HDAC inhibitors that have been developed. These inhibitors target a variety of intracellular proteins that are involved in these processes. Tumor suppressor protein (p53), HSP90, STAT3, subunits of NFκ-B, and α-tubulin are some of the cellular target proteins that involve these individuals. In the treatment of cutaneous T-cell lymphoma, the Food and Drug Administration (FDA) has already given its approval to two HDAC inhibitors: suberoylanilide hydroxamic acid and romidepsin. An assortment of HDAC inhibitors, such as entinostat, pivanex, CI-994, panobinostat, and romidepsin, are currently undergoing clinical trials to treat NSCLC.

2.4.4. Proapopototic Agents

The majority of cancer cells can circumvent the typical apoptotic mechanism by upregulating antiapoptotic factors, downregulating proapoptotic mechanisms, or performing both of these strategies simultaneously. Conatumumab (anti-DR1) and YM155 (antisurvivin), both of which are apoptotic promoters, are currently at the stage of clinical trials for the treatment of NSCLC. When compared to chemotherapy on its own, it has been observed that the combination of these proapoptotic agents and chemotherapy has produced remarkable results.

It is still necessary to conduct additional research to identify early detection and treatment methods for these cancers, which could significantly improve the long-term survival rate of patients. This is the case even though ongoing research and progress are being made in the development of numerous new targeted agents. As a result of the unique physiological environment, improved absorption, and treatment organ, drug delivery through the lungs is becoming an increasingly important method. The delivery of cancer drugs in the lung has been the subject of research and development efforts for the past decade. Pfizer's Exubera, an inhalation powder, received a breakthrough approval, which assisted in the testing of a similar strategy for a wide variety of other potential drugs. Several microscopic (e.g., micrometer- and nanometer-sized) drug delivery systems such as liposomes, polymer conjugates, polymeric micelles, microparticles, and nanoparticles (NPs) are currently being intensively researched to target a wide range of potential anti-cancer therapeutic molecules to the part of the lung that exhibits cancer pathology (Smith et al., 2018).

2.5. Challenges of Current Therapeutic Strategies

Although a great deal of research has been done on the pathology and epidemiology of a variety of infectious and non-infectious respiratory diseases, the development of more effective treatments is still in the trial stage. In both high-income and low-income countries around the world, asthma and COPD are the non-infectious diseases that affect the largest populations. Pathology and progression of disease are highly variable from one population to another and are largely attributable to various aspects of an individual's lifestyle. Bronchodilators, which are commonly used, such as albuterol and ipratropium, as well as recently developed long-acting β2-agonists (LABAs) and long-acting muscarinic antagonists (LAMAs), have proven to be effective in treating patients who exhibit mild to moderate symptoms of chronic respiratory disease. However, it has not been demonstrated that these medications are fully effective in treating patients who suffer from chronic asthma and COPD. In addition, the effectiveness of the therapeutics that are currently available has been diminished as a result of personal lifestyle habits such as smoking or prolonged exposure to dust from the workplace. In addition, the severe forms of the disease are characterized by irreversible damage to the lung tissue, which leads to scarring and cannot be treated with therapeutics that are generally available on the market.

In contrast, respiratory diseases brought on by infectious agents are a significant problem. The majority of these diseases are seasonal and continue to manifest themselves either inside or outside of the human body. New powerful mutants with increased drug resistance have emerged as a result of natural selection, mutations, and the excessive use of antibiotics. These mutations have caused a variety of pandemics all over the world. In addition, recent research has demonstrated that a variety of infectious agents can be passed from one species to another (from animals to humans and vice versa), which has the potential to have a more widespread impact on the population of the entire world. The recent outbreak of COVID-19 is a good example of how a specific member of the coronavirus family can pose a serious threat to the health of people all over the world due to the absence of natural immunity to the newborn mutants (Wenzler et al., 2016).

A Closer Look

Cystic Fibrosis

Cystic Fibrosis (CF) is a life-threatening genetic disorder caused by mutations in the cystic fibrosis transmembrane conductance regulator (CFTR) gene, which encodes for a protein responsible for regulating chloride and bicarbonate ion transport across epithelial membranes. The result is thick, sticky mucus accumulation in various organs, particularly the lungs and digestive system. According to the Cystic Fibrosis Foundation, approximately 30,000 individuals in the United States are affected by CF, with many experiencing significant respiratory and gastrointestinal complications due to the disease's progressive nature.

Recent research has focused on the development of targeted therapies aimed at improving CFTR function. A landmark study by Heijerman et al. (2019) published in the *New England Journal of Medicine* demonstrated the effectiveness of a combination therapy involving ivacaftor and lumacaftor, which significantly improved lung function and reduced pulmonary exacerbations in patients with specific CFTR mutations. This therapy, which addresses the underlying cause of CF rather than just managing symptoms, represents a paradigm shift in CF treatment, with the potential to enhance the quality of life for patients.

In addition to pharmacological advancements, there is growing interest in the role of personalized medicine in CF management. A study by Borowitz et al. (2020) highlighted the importance of genotype-driven treatment strategies, suggesting that tailoring therapies based on individual CFTR mutations can lead to better health outcomes. The research underscores the necessity for clinicians to consider genetic testing as part of routine care for CF patients, allowing for optimized treatment plans that align with the patient's specific genetic profile.

Moreover, the psychosocial impact of CF on patients and their families has garnered attention in recent studies. A systematic review by Quittner et al. (2018) in the journal *Pediatric Pulmonology* examined the emotional and social challenges faced by CF patients, revealing that mental health issues, such as anxiety and depression, are prevalent in this population. Addressing these psychosocial factors is crucial for holistic patient care, emphasizing the need for integrated treatment approaches that encompass both medical and psychological support, ultimately enhancing the overall well-being of individuals living with cystic fibrosis.

Summary

- CRDs encompass a group of long-term conditions affecting the lungs and airways, leading to breathing difficulties and impaired lung function. The most common CRDs include COPD, asthma, interstitial lung diseases, and occupational lung diseases.
- COPD is characterized by persistent airflow limitation due to chronic bronchitis and/or emphysema, often caused by smoking or exposure to pollutants. Asthma is a chronic condition characterized by airway inflammation, bronchoconstriction, and increased mucus production, leading to recurrent episodes of wheezing, breathlessness, chest tightness, and coughing.
- Interstitial lung diseases involve scarring and inflammation of the lung tissue, impairing its ability to expand and contract properly, leading to difficulty breathing. Occupational lung diseases result from exposure to harmful substances in the workplace, such as asbestos, silica, and coal dust, causing lung damage over time.
- CRDs can significantly impact quality of life, leading to symptoms like coughing, wheezing, shortness of breath, and fatigue. These conditions are often diagnosed through a combination of medical history, physical examination, lung function tests, and imaging studies like chest X-rays or CT scans.
- Management of CRDs focuses on symptom control, preventing disease progression, and improving quality of life. This typically involves lifestyle modifications (e.g., smoking cessation, avoiding exposure to pollutants), medications (e.g., bronchodilators, corticosteroids), pulmonary rehabilitation, and in severe cases, oxygen therapy or surgery.

References

1. An, J., Park, S., Ko, I., Jin, J., Hwang, L., Ji, E., Kim, S., Kim, C., Park, S., Hwang, J., et al. (2017). Polydeoxyribonucleotide ameliorates lipopolysaccharide-induced lung injury by inhibiting apoptotic cell death in rats. *International Journal of Molecular Sciences, 18*(9), 1847.
2. Bacci, G., Mengoni, A., Fiscarelli, E., Segata, N., Taccetti, G., Dolce, D., Paganin, P., Morelli, P., Tuccio, V., De Alessandri, A., et al. (2017). A different microbiome gene repertoire in the airways of cystic fibrosis patients with severe lung disease. *International Journal of Molecular Sciences, 18*(8), 1654.
3. Bragonzi, A., Paroni, M., Pirone, L., Coladarci, I., Ascenzioni, F., & Bevivino, A. (2017). Environmental Burkholderia cenocepacia strain enhances fitness by serial passages during long-term chronic airways infection in mice. *International Journal of Molecular Sciences, 18*(12), 2417.
4. Carnell, S., Perry, J., Borthwick, L., Vollmer, D., Biboy, J., Facchini, M., Bragonzi, A., Silipo, A., Vergunst, A., & Vollmer, W., et al. (2018). Targeting the bacterial cytoskeleton of the Burkholderia cepacia complex for antimicrobial development: A cautionary tale. *International Journal of Molecular Sciences, 19*(6), 1604.
5. Douglas, J., & Cohen, N. (2017). Taste receptors mediate sinonasal immunity and respiratory disease. *International Journal of Molecular Sciences, 18*(2), 437.

6. Everaerts, S., Lagrou, K., Vermeersch, K., Dupont, L., Vanaudenaerde, B., & Janssens, W. (2018). Aspergillus fumigatus detection and risk factors in patients with COPD–bronchiectasis overlap. *International Journal of Molecular Sciences, 19*(2), 523.

7. Fastrès, A., Felice, F., Roels, E., Moermans, C., Corhay, J., Bureau, F., Louis, R., Clercx, C., & Guiot, J. (2017). The lung microbiome in idiopathic pulmonary fibrosis: A promising approach for targeted therapies. *International Journal of Molecular Sciences, 18*(12), 2735.

8. Faverio, P., Stainer, A., Bonaiti, G., Zucchetti, S., Simonetta, E., Lapadula, G., Marruchella, A., Gori, A., Blasi, F., Codecasa, L., et al. (2016). Characterizing non-tuberculous mycobacteria infection in bronchiectasis. *International Journal of Molecular Sciences, 17*(11), 1913.

9. Florence, J., Krupa, A., Booshehri, L., Gajewski, A., & Kurdowska, A. (2018). Disrupting the Btk pathway suppresses COPD-like lung alterations in atherosclerosis-prone ApoE–/– mice following regular exposure to cigarette smoke. *International Journal of Molecular Sciences, 19*(2), 343.

10. GBD 2015 LRI Collaborators. (2017). Estimates of the global, regional, and national morbidity, mortality, and aetiologies of lower respiratory tract infections in 195 countries: A systematic analysis for the Global Burden of Disease Study 2015. *Lancet Infectious Diseases, 17*(11), 1133–1161.

11. Haworth, C. S., Banks, J., Capstick, T., Fisher, A., Gorsuch, T., Laurenson, I. F., Leitch, A., Loebinger, M. R., Milburn, H., Nightingale, M., et al. (2017). British Thoracic Society guideline for the management of nontuberculous mycobacterial pulmonary disease (NTMPD). *BMJ Open Respiratory Research, 4*(1), e000242.

12. Hewitt, R. J., & Molyneaux, P. L. (2017). The respiratory microbiome in idiopathic pulmonary fibrosis. *Annals of Translational Medicine, 5*(12), 250.

13. Lorè, N., Veraldi, N., Riva, C., Sipione, B., Spagnuolo, L., De Fino, I., Melessike, M., Calzi, E., Bragonzi, A., Naggi, A., et al. (2018). Synthesized heparan sulfate competitors attenuate Pseudomonas aeruginosa lung infection. *International Journal of Molecular Sciences, 19*(1), 207.

14. Máiz, L., Nieto, R., Cantón, R., Gómez, G., de la Pedrosa, E., & Martinez-García, M. (2018). Fungi in bronchiectasis: A concise review. *International Journal of Molecular Sciences, 19*(1), 142.

15. Maselli, D., Keyt, H., & Restrepo, M. (2017). Inhaled antibiotic therapy in chronic respiratory diseases. *International Journal of Molecular Sciences, 18*(5), 1062.

16. Miravitlles, M., & Anzueto, A. (2017). Chronic respiratory infection in patients with chronic obstructive pulmonary disease: What is the role of antibiotics? *International Journal of Molecular Sciences, 18*(7), 1344.

17. Polverino, E., Goeminne, P. C., McDonnell, M. J., Aliberti, S., Marshall, S. E., Loebinger, M. R., Murris, M., Cantón, R., Torres, A., Dimakou, K., et al. (2017). European Respiratory Society guidelines for the management of adult bronchiectasis. *European Respiratory Journal, 50*(3), 1700629.

18. Shiratori, B., Zaho, J., Okumura, M., Chagan-Yasutan, H., Yanai, H., Mizuno, K., Yoshiyama, T., Idei, T., Ashino, Y., Nakajima, C., et al. (2017). Immunological roles of elevated plasma levels of matricellular proteins in Japanese patients with pulmonary tuberculosis. *International Journal of Molecular Sciences, 18*(1), 19.

19. Smith, S., Rowbotham, N. J., & Regan, K. H. (2018). Inhaled anti-pseudomonal antibiotics for long-term therapy in cystic fibrosis. *Cochrane Database of Systematic Reviews, 2018*(3), CD001021.

20. Wenzler, E., Fraidenburg, D. R., Scardina, T., & Danziger, L. H. (2016). Inhaled antibiotics for Gram-negative respiratory infections. *Clinical Microbiology Reviews, 29*(3), 581–632.

Chapter 3

PNEUMONIA

Contents

Introduction

Pneumonia, despite being a common and often treatable respiratory infection, can manifest in rare forms that pose significant challenges in diagnosis and management. While community-acquired pneumonia affects millions globally each year, rare pneumonias are characterized by their infrequency, diverse etiologies, and often severe outcomes (Albrich et al., 2023).

According to the World Health Organization (WHO), pneumonia is the leading infectious cause of death worldwide, responsible for approximately 2.5 million deaths annually, with the majority occurring in children under five years old and the elderly. Despite advances in healthcare, pneumonia remains a significant global health concern.

Rare forms of pneumonia include those caused by uncommon pathogens such as fungi, parasites, or opportunistic bacteria, which may occur in immunocompromised individuals or those with underlying conditions. Additionally, certain types of pneumonia, such as eosinophilic pneumonia or lipoid pneumonia, are considered rare due to their specific causes and clinical presentations.

The diagnosis of rare cases of pneumonia can be challenging, as they may present with atypical symptoms or radiological findings that differ from typical bacterial pneumonia. The treatment of those rare types of pneumonia often involves specialized care and targeted therapies based on the specific pathogen or underlying cause (Alyacoubi et al., 2018).

Despite their rarity, these forms of pneumonia highlight the importance of considering uncommon etiologies in the differential diagnosis of respiratory infections, especially in patients who do not respond to standard treatments. Continued research and awareness are essential to improve the recognition and management of rare pneumonia cases and reduce their impact on global health.

Orientation and Directional Terms

Term	Definition	Illustration
Pneumonia	Inflammation of the lung tissue, usually caused by an infection (bacterial, viral, or fungal), leading to fluid accumulation in the alveoli.	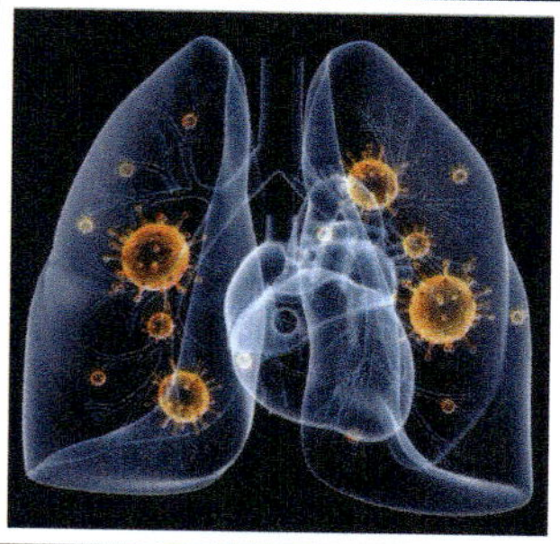
Empyema	Accumulation of pus in the pleural cavity (the space between the lungs and chest wall), usually due to infection.	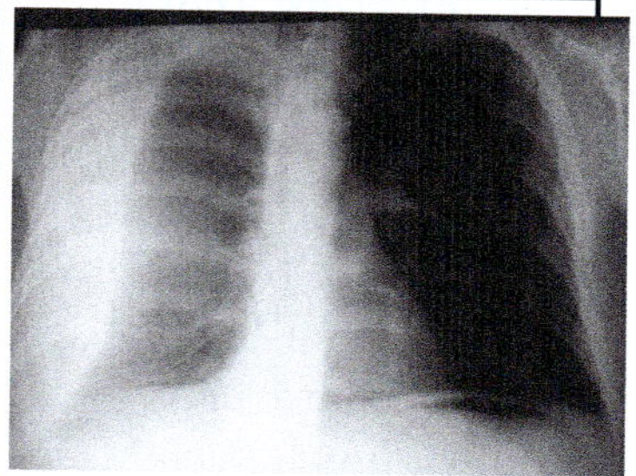
Lung Abscess	A localized area of pus formation within the lung tissue, often resulting from infection and tissue necrosis.	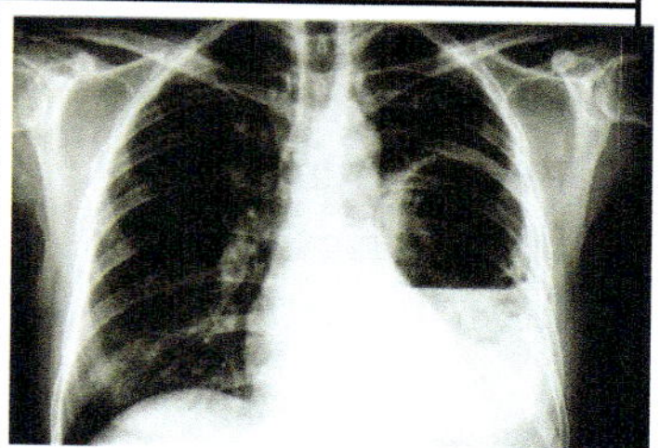
Necrotizing Pneumonia	A severe form of pneumonia where lung tissue becomes necrotic, leading to the formation of cavities in the lung.	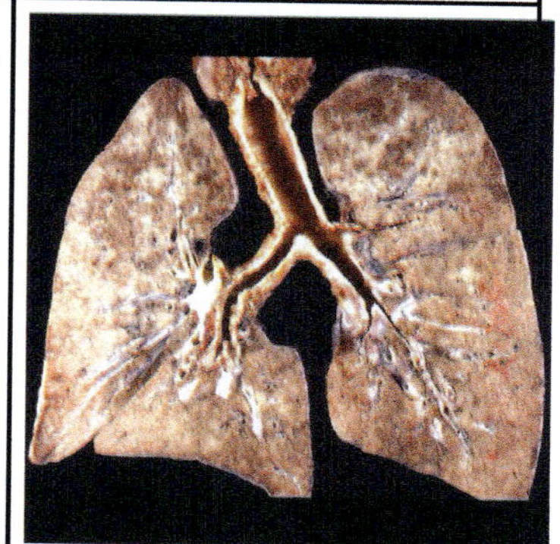
Antibiotic	A substance that inhibits the growth of or kills bacteria, used to treat bacterial infections.	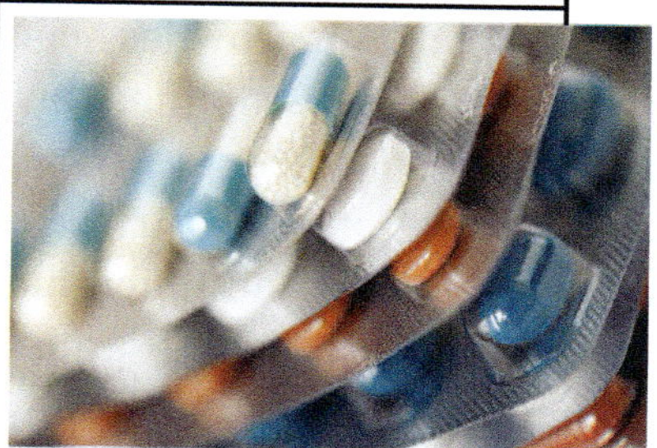

3.1. Pneumonia: Epidemiology and Risk Factors

Pneumonia causes significant morbidity in children worldwide and is one of the main causes of death in children in developing countries. The incidence of pneumonia is highest in children under 5 years of age, and in recent years the incidence of complicated and severe pneumonia appears to be increasing.

The etiologic factors vary according to age, source of infection (community-acquired or hospital-acquired pneumonia), and underlying host defects (for example, immunodeficiency). In preschool children, viruses are the most common etiologic factors, although in many cases more than one pathogen can be identified. Several new pathogens are emerging in community-acquired pneumonia in children: virulent strains of *Streptococcus pneumoniae* not included in currently available vaccines, Panton-Velentine leucocidin-producing *Staphylococcus aureus*, human bocaviruses, and metapneumoviruses are the most important.

In most mild cases of community-acquired pneumonia, the diagnosis is based on clinical assessment alone, as laboratory tests and X-rays do not reveal the etiology. Children with severe pneumonia, hospital-acquired pneumonia, and immunocompromised children require invasive diagnostics (Asti et al., 2019).

Treatment of mild and moderate cases consists of supportive care and antibiotic treatment. The recommended first-line therapy in previously healthy children, regardless of age, is amoxicillin, as it provides adequate protection against the most common invasive bacterial pathogen, *S. pneumoniae*. In hospital-acquired pneumonia, initial empiric treatment should be based on local antimicrobial susceptibility patterns and adjusted appropriately once microbiology test results are available.

Although properly diagnosed and treated pneumonia resolves without permanent changes, in some cases its course may be complicated by pleural effusion and empyema, pneumoatocele, lung abscess, or necrotizing pneumonia due to the virulence of the pathogen and/or the susceptibility of the host. A recognized complication of severe pneumonia is hyponatremia and SIADH (syndrome of inappropriate antidiuretic hormone secretion).

The burden of pneumonia can be reduced by preventive measures ranging from the simplest methods of infection control such as hand washing, limiting exposure to infectious cases, limiting exposure to tobacco smoke, and vaccination to passive immunization in selected cases (Bateman et al., 2016).

3.1.1. Definition

Pneumonia is defined as an inflammation of the lung tissue caused by an infectious agent. The usual clinical operational definition of the WHO is based solely on clinical symptoms (cough or dyspnea and tachypnea). In developing countries, the term "lower respiratory tract infection" (LRTI) is often used instead of pneumonia due to poor access to radiographs and the difficulty of radiologic confirmation of the diagnosis (Bjarnason et al., 2018).

Depending on the site of infection, pneumonia can be divided into:

i. Community-acquired pneumonia (CAP);
ii. Hospital-acquired pneumonia (HAP).

Recently, a third type has been distinguished in adult patients – Health Care Associated Pneumonia (HCAP).

The importance of this classification is based on its clinical utility, as in most cases the pathogens responsible for CAP and HAP are different, justifying a different approach and empirical treatment (Figure 3.1).

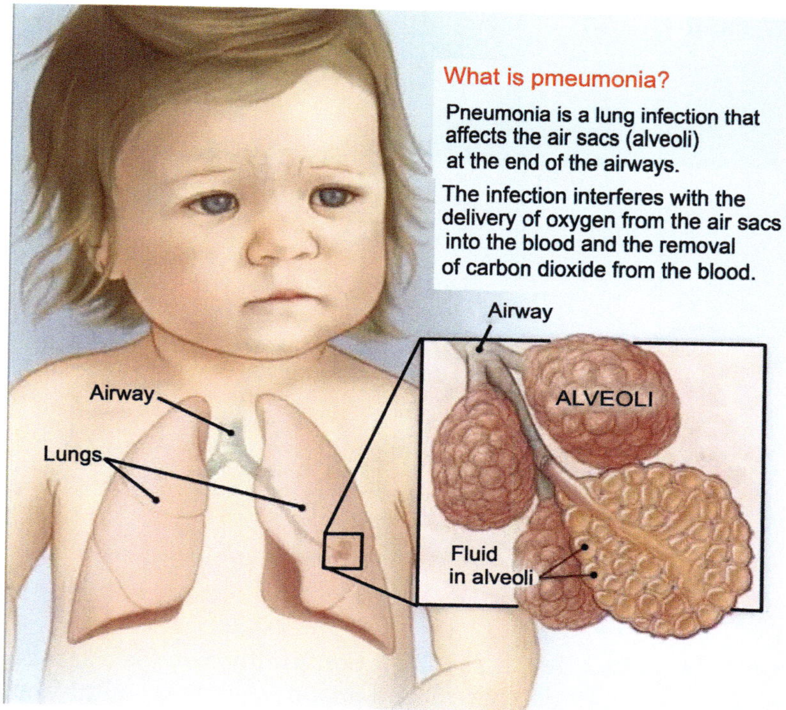

Figure 3.1. *This image demonstrates the disease process within the distal bronchi and alveoli.*

Source: https://onthewards.org/community-acquired-pneumonia-in-children/.

3.1.2. Community-Acquired Pneumonia

CAP can be defined as pneumonia in previously healthy children caused by an infectious agent contracted outside the hospital. The usual clinical practice is to confirm the diagnosis by radiologic findings of consolidations (Bodi et al., 2005).

3.1.3. Epidemiology

Globally, the incidence of pneumonia in children under 5 years of age in developing countries is 0.28 episodes per child per year (150 million/year), compared with 0.05 episodes per child per year in industrialized countries (Breuer et al., 2018). Pneumonia is responsible for 18% of deaths (2 million/year) in young children worldwide, with most cases occurring in impoverished countries with limited access to healthcare. In more affluent societies, pneumonia is rarely fatal but causes significant morbidity. The incidence of radiologically confirmed pneumonia in previously healthy children in Europe is 144-147/100,000 children/year and decreases with age, being highest in children under 5 years of age (328-338/100,000/year and 421/100,000/year in 0–2-year-olds). Rates of hospitalization due to pneumonia in this age group were 122/100,000/year in children ≤ 16 years and 287/100,000/year in children ≤ 5 years. UK studies show that the rate of CAP presenting to the GP in children < 5 years is 191/100,000/year, which is probably due to more seriously ill children presenting directly to the hospital. In a German study, the incidence of hospitalized pneumonia was 300/100,000/year in children aged 0–16 years and 658/100,000/year in children aged 0–5 years. Underlying diseases were present in 23% of these cases and it is possible that many children with bronchiolitis were classified as pneumonia (Brown, 2012) (Figure 3.2).

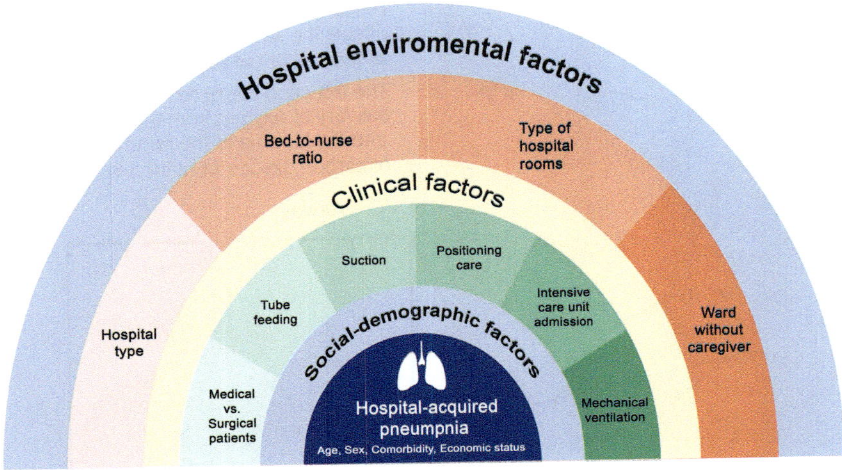

Figure 3.2. *Epidemiology of pneumonia.*

Source: Kim, B. G., Kang, M., Lim, J., et al., (2022). Comprehensive risk assessment for hospital-acquired pneumonia: Sociodemographic, clinical, and hospital environmental factors associated with the incidence of hospital-acquired pneumonia. BMC Pulm. Med., 22, 21. https://doi.org/10.1186/s12890-021-01816-9.

Since the introduction of the conjugate pneumococcal vaccine (PCV7) into national vaccination programs in the US and Europe, the incidence of pneumococcal pneumonia has decreased (by 65% in the US), and hospitalizations with CAP have decreased in children < 1 year of age but seem to be increasing for children > 5 years old. At the same time, the incidence of severe pneumonia requiring hospitalization and complicated pneumonia appears to be increasing. Between 1997 and 2006, the rate of local complications of CAP increased by 77.8% (5.4 or 9.6 cases per 100,000 inhabitants), while Empyema accounted for more than 97% of all local complications (Brown, 2004).

3.1.4. Etiology

The organisms causing pneumonia are diverse and include bacteria, viruses, fungi, and protozoa, with most cases preceded by acute viral bronchitis. Viruses promote infections with pathogenic microorganisms that colonize the nasopharynx, which include *S. pneumoniae*, *Haemophilus influenzae*, and *Moraxella catarrhalis*. Previous colonization with *Streptococcus mitis* and the anaerobic cocci *Peptostreptococcus anaerobius* may have a protective effect against pathogenic strains.

The etiologic factor of pneumonia can be determined in a maximum of 65–86% of patients by combining several diagnostic methods such as culture, serology, and PCR. In daily clinical practice, these methods are rarely used, and treatment remains empirical based on national and international guidelines (Bundesamt für Gesundheit, 2019).

Viruses are responsible for 30–67% of cases of CAP and are most common in children under 2 years of age. Respiratory syncytial virus (RSV), which is isolated in 13–29% of cases, and rhinoviruses (3–45%), either in combination with bacteria or alone, are most commonly identified. Other viruses responsible for pneumonia are adenoviruses (1–13%), influenza (4–22%) and parainfluenza viruses (3–10%), rhinoviruses (3–45%), human metapneumoviruses (5–12%) and human bocaviruses (5–15%). Enteroviruses, varicella viruses, herpes viruses, and cytomegaloviruses are less common. In older children, bacterial infections are more common: *S. pneumoniae* is the frontrunner (30–44% of CAP), followed by *Mycoplasma pneumoniae* (22–36%) and *Chlamydophila pneumoniae* (5–27%). *S. pneumoniae* remains the leading cause of severe pneumonia requiring hospitalization, even in countries with lower rates of invasive pneumococcal disease (Capelastegui et al., 2004). Since the introduction of PCV7, the most common pneumococcal isolates are 1 (primarily responsible for empyema), 19A, 3, 6A, and 7F (all included in the 13-valent vaccine). In contrast to previous reports, *M. pneumoniae* appears to be equally common in school and preschool children. Less common bacterial causes of CAP in children include *Haemophilus influenzae* type B (5–9%), *Staphylococcus aureus*, *M. catarrhalis* (1.5–4%), *Bordatella pertussis*, *Streptococcus pyogenes* (1–7%), *Chlamydia trachomatis* and a pathogen identified in the 1990s – *Simkania negevensis*. Unlike in adults, *Legionella pneumophila* is a rare cause of CAP in children (Costantini et al., 2016).

In the malaria–endemic regions of tropical Africa, multidrug-resistant, non-typhoidal *Salmonella* are a challenging etiologic factor of pneumonia, and in regions where tuberculosis is endemic, they are increasingly recognized as a cause of acute pneumonia.

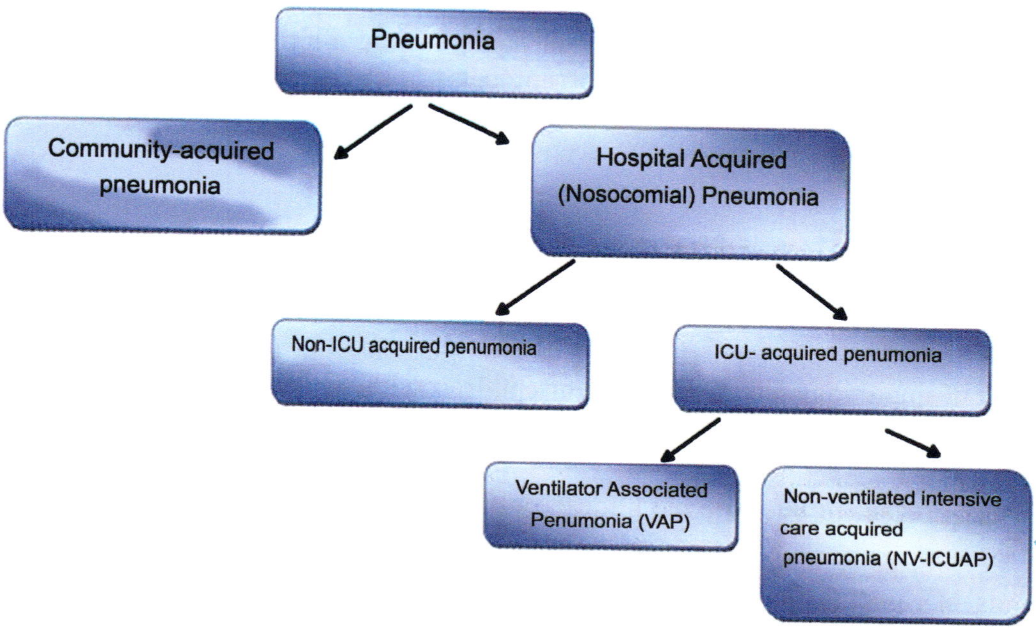

Figure 3.3. *Etiology of pneumonia*

Source: https://pub.mdpi-res.com/ijms/ijms-17-02120/article_deploy/html/images/ijms-17-02120-ag-550.jpg?1569147619.

Around 8–40% of cases are mixed viral-bacterial or bacterial-bacterial infections. A primary viral infection predisposes to bacterial pneumonia: influenza epidemics in industrialized countries coincide with epidemics of *S. pneumoniae* and *S. aureus*, and measles or RSV infections contribute to increased pneumonia mortality in developing countries (Couturier et al., 2014) (Figure 3.3).

3.1.5. Risk Factors for CAP

In addition to immunization status, epidemiological data, and contact with other children, especially preschoolers, there are several known risk factors for CAP that need to be considered. Underlying comorbidities such as diabetes mellitus, asplenia or splenic dysfunction, chronic heart disease, nephrotic syndrome, and severe liver disease are risk factors for invasive pneumococcal disease including pneumonia. Other risk factors for CAP are asthma, history of wheezing episodes, otitis media treated by tympanocentesis in the first 2 years of life (risk factor for children <5), tobacco smoke exposure, malnutrition, immunologic deficiencies (primary or secondary), mucociliary dysfunction (cystic fibrosis, ciliary dyskinesia), congenital malformations of the respiratory tract, swallowing disorders, microaspiration, gastroesophageal reflux, neuromuscular disorders, and treatment with gastric acid inhibitors (a risk factor in adults, while its role in children was confirmed in a study). Environmental factors such as indoor air pollution from cooking and heating with biomass fuels (such as wood or dung), living in confined spaces, and parental smoking also increase a child's susceptibility to pneumonia (Dean et al., 2001). Tobacco smoke exposure has been found to increase the risk of hospitalization for pneumonia in children < 5 years, and the conditions that favor severe pneumonia include being < 5 years and prematurity (24–28 GA). Viral infections, especially influenza, and previous exposure to antibiotics further predispose to pneumococcal and staphylococcal pneumonia. Antibiotics alter the bacterial microflora in the airways and destroy commensal bacteria such as alpha-hemolytic streptococci, while viruses release neuraminidase and other enzymes that promote adherence and the expression of pneumococcal receptors on host cells such as the platelet-activating factor receptor or CD14 (Dixon, 2008).

3.2. Clinical Manifestations

Typical clinical symptoms of pneumonia are:

- Cough (30% of children presenting to the outpatient clinic with cough have radiographic signs of pneumonia after exclusion of children with wheezing, and cough was found in 76% of children with CAP). It should be noted that sputum is rare in preschool children as they tend to swallow it,
- Fever (present in 88–96% of children with radiologically confirmed pneumonia),
- Toxic appearance,
- Signs of respiratory distress: tachypnea (Table 3.1), history of respiratory distress or difficulty breathing – chest indrawing, nasal flaring, grunting, use of accessory respiratory muscles. Tachypnea is a very sensitive marker for pneumonia. Around 50–80% of children with WHO-defined tachypnea have radiologic signs of pneumonia, and the absence of tachypnea is the best single finding to rule out the disease. In children < 5 years, tachypnea had a sensitivity of 74% and a specificity of 67% for radiologically confirmed pneumonia, but its clinical value was lower in the first three days of illness. In infants

< 12 months, a respiratory rate of 70 breaths/min had a sensitivity of 63% and a specificity of 89% for hypoxemia (Dixon, 2011).

Table 3.1. *Tachypnea Defined According to WHO Criteria*

Age	Respiratory Rate/ Minute
0–2 months	“/>60
2–12 months	“/>50
1–4 years	“/>40
≥ 5 years	“/>30

Based on the clinical symptoms, pneumonia can be divided into severe pneumonia, which warrants hospitalization, and non-severe pneumonia (mild and moderate) (El Fahimi et al., 2019). Signs of severe pneumonia vary by age and according to the British Thoracic Society (BTS) include: temperature 38.5°C, respiratory rate > 70 breaths/minute in infants and > 50 breaths/minute in older children, moderate to severe recessions in infants and severe dyspnea in older children, nosebleeds, cyanosis, intermittent apnea, grunting, lack of feeding in infants and signs of dehydration in older children, tachycardia, and capillary refill time ≥2s. Restlessness may also be a sign of hypoxemia. Table 3.2 shows a simplified approach recommended by WHO for developing countries to help local medical staff assess the need for referral to a hospital.

Physical examination:

- Crackles (in 33–90% of children with pneumonia), diminished breath sounds over the affected area, bronchial breath sounds specific for lobar consolidation, absence of breath sounds, and dullness on percussion suggestive of effusion. If the pneumonia is accompanied by pleurisy, a pleural rub may be heard. Crackles and bronchial breath sounds have a sensitivity of 75% and a specificity of 57% in the diagnosis of pneumonia.
- The presence of wheezing, especially in the absence of fever, makes the diagnosis of typical bacterial pneumonia unlikely. However, it is a common sign in viral and mycoplasma pneumonia (up to 30%).
- The combination of several clinical symptoms in a diagnostic algorithm improves the sensitivity and specificity of the diagnosis. The WHO criteria for defining pneumonia (cough or difficulty breathing and tachypnea) examined in a Brazilian study of 390 children have a sensitivity of 94% for children <2 and 62% for children ≥2, with a specificity of 20% and 16%, respectively. The addition of fever improved the specificity to 44% and 50%. In an Australian study of febrile children <5 years presenting to a tertiary emergency department, clinical indicators of pneumonia confirmed radiologically and microbiologically included agitated appearance, fever ≥ 39°C, respiratory distress, chronic illness, prolonged capillary refill time, tachypnea, crackles on auscultation, and lack of pneumococcal vaccination.

It is important to point out that no clinical or radiologic sign, alone or in combination, is sensitive and specific enough to differentiate between viral, atypical, or typical bacterial etiology of pneumonia (Erdede et al., 2010).

Table 3.2. *Severity of Pneumonia – WHO Classification*

Pneumonia/Non-Severe Pneumonia	Cough problems with breathing Tachypnea *No signs of severe pneumonia present
Severe Pneumonia	Signs of pneumonia and ≥1 • Lower chest wall indrawing; • Nasal flaming; • Expiratory grunting. *No signs of very severe pneumonia
Very Severe Pneumonia	Signs of severe pneumonia and ≥1 • Inability to feed; • Cyanosis; • Severe respiratory distress; • Impaired consciousness or convulsions.

3.3. Additional Tests

1. Chest radiography;
2. Pulse oximetry should be performed in all children with pneumonia, as its results facilitate the assessment of severity and thus the need for hospitalization. Pulse oximetry should be performed on all children who are admitted to the hospital;
3. Laboratory tests;
4. Determination of the etiology – microbiological tests.

The determination of the specific pathogen in children with CAP is difficult. Young children do not expectorate sputum, and nasopharyngeal swabs are not reliable as the bacteria present in the upper respiratory tract are not necessarily the same as those that cause pneumonia. Invasive diagnostic tools are effective but are unlikely to be acceptable in otherwise healthy children, most of whom improve with empirical treatment. BTS standards, Pediatric Infectious Diseases Society guidelines, and American Academy of Pediatrics policy statements do not recommend microbiologic testing of children with community-treated pneumonia (Ewig et al., 2009). Microbiologic diagnosis should be attempted in patients admitted to the hospital, especially those in the intensive care unit and those with complications of CAP (Figures 3.4 and 3.5).

- Blood cultures are positive in <10% of patients with pneumonia and <2% of outpatients. They should nevertheless be performed as, if positive, they provide information on the etiology of CAP and antibiotic resistance. In children with complicated pneumonia, the prevalence of bacteremia varies between 7.8% and 26.5% in pneumonia with parapneumonic effusion.

- Nasopharyngeal aspirates or nasal wash samples can help identify respiratory viruses, including respiratory syncytial viruses, parainfluenza viruses, influenza viruses, and adenoviruses by immunofluorescence techniques. The results of these tests are particularly useful for cohorting infected children during outbreaks and for epidemic purposes.
- Sputum is difficult to obtain from young children. A reliable sputum sample, unlike saliva, only contains <10 epithelial cells per low-powered field. Sputum induced by inhalation with 5% hypertonic saline has a much higher bacterial yield and seems to be a valuable tool in microbiological diagnosis in children with CAP.
- Children who require mechanical ventilation should have tracheal aspirates taken for Gram stain and culture at the time of endotracheal tube placement.
- Aspirated pleural fluid should be sent for microscopy, culture, and antigen detection. Cultures are positive in 9%–18% of cases (sensitivity 23%, specificity 100%). Pneumococcal antigen detection in pleural fluid has a sensitivity of 90% and a specificity of 95%. Pleural fluid should be checked for Mycobacteria.
- Pneumococcal antigens detection in urine is not specific, as it is often positive in young children with nasopharyngeal colonization.
- Serological testing: a fourfold rise in antibody titers in complement fixation test is a golden diagnostics standard, but unfortunately it is not useful for treatment guidance. In many laboratories enzyme-linked immunosorbent assays (ELISA) have replaced complement fixation tests as they are less time consuming. Positive anti-Mycoplasma IgM antibody titer 9–11 days from the onset of illness is also suggestive of recent infection. Cross-reactions with adenovirus and *L. pneumophila* have been described. Cold agglutinins measurement value is limited – in school children, the positive predictive value for Mycoplasma of a rapid cold agglutinin test was 70%. In *C. pneumoniae* infection IgM rise is observed after 3 weeks and IgG rise after 6–8 weeks.
- *L. pneumophila* urinary antigen detection remains the golden standard for the diagnosis of legionellosis. The test remains positive for weeks after an acute infection. Urinary antigen is positive only in the case of infection with serogroup 1. Antigens are excreted in urine at the beginning of the second week of illness. Quick diagnostic tests are commercially available with a sensitivity of 80% and specificity of 99–100%. Infection with serogroup 1 can be excluded when the results of 3 consecutive urine samples are negative (Ewig et al., 2016).
- Real-time reverse transcriptase polymerase chain reaction (RT-PCR) can be used for investigating the etiology of pneumonia. The advantage of this method is the availability of results on the same day. It does not, however, provide information on bacterial sensitivity nor is it readily available outside research settings. Pneumolysin-based PCR has been increasingly used to detect *S. pneumoniae* in blood and pleural fluid with a sensitivity of 100% and specificity of 95%. Measuring bacterial load with RT-PCR may help predict the outcome of CAP as adult patients with a bacterial load > 1,000 copies/ml carry a higher risk of sepsis, respiratory insufficiency, and death (Ewig et al., 2021).

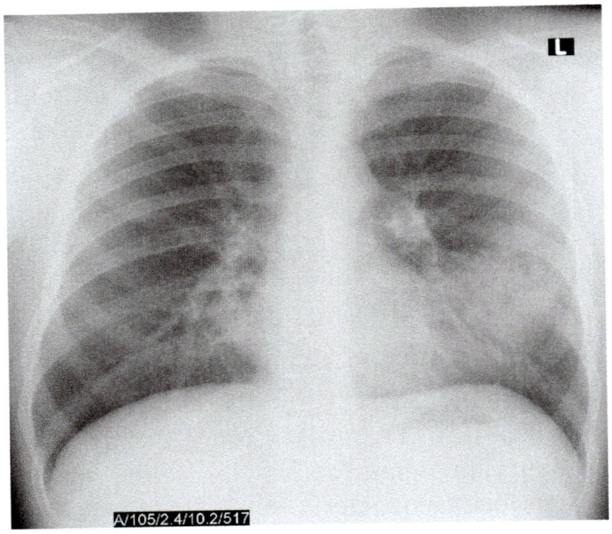

Figure 3.4. *Chest X-ray showing alveolar consolidations in the left lower lobe and in the right lower lobe.*

Source: NCBI.

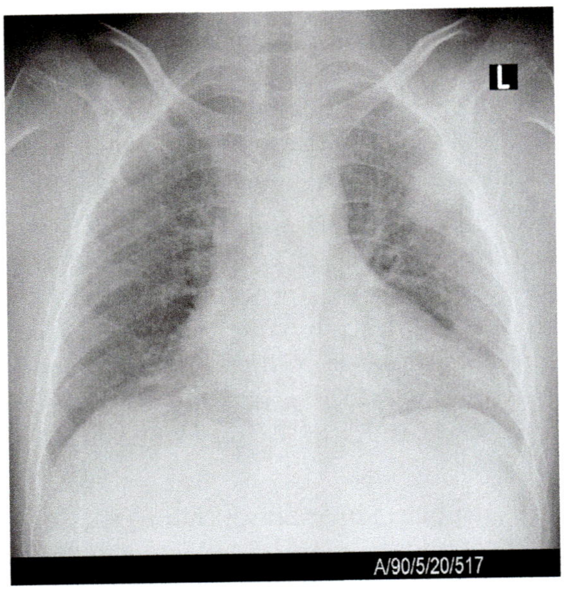

Figure 3.5. *Round focus of consolidation in the left upper lobe – pneumonia.*

Source: NCBI.

3.4. Management

Most children with CAP can be safely treated as outpatients. Indications for hospitalization are:

- Clinical signs of severe pneumonia (see above);

- Signs of sepsis or septic shock;
- Young age – < 6 months of life;
- Hypoxemia – oxygen saturation < 92% (according to BTS) or <90% (according to AAP and PIDS), PaO_2<60 mmHg and $PaCO_2$ >50 mmHg, central cyanosis;
- Underlying diseases for example congenital heart defect, cystic fibrosis, bronchopulmonary dysplasia;
- Diffuse radiological changes: multilobar pneumonia, pleural effusion;
- Outpatient treatment failure;
- CAP caused by pathogens with increased virulence, for example MRSA (PIDS);
- Inability of parents to treat the disease at home.

Children who do not improve despite treatment and who are in respiratory arrest or shock should be admitted to the intensive care unit. The criteria for admission to the intensive care unit are:

- Need for invasive mechanical ventilation or non-invasive positive pressure ventilation;
- Fluid refractory shock;
- Hypoxemia requiring a FiO_2 concentration greater than the inspired concentration or flow possible in the general care area; pulse oximetry measurements ≤92% with an inspired oxygen of ≥0.5 (according to BTS) or ≥0.6 (according to PIDS);
- Altered mental status due to hypercarbemia, hypoxemia, or as a result of pneumonia;
- Recurrent apnea, grunting, or slow irregular breathing;
- Increasing respiratory rate and heart rate with clinical signs of severe respiratory distress, including with or without fatigue.

3.4.1. General Management

All children treated for pneumonia should be re-examined within 48 hours if there is no clinical improvement or worsening, and the fever persists. It is important that parents of children being treated at home are given clear written instructions on managing fever, avoiding dehydration, recognizing signs of deterioration, and continuing access to healthcare professionals (Freund et al., 2017).

Hospitalized hypoxemic children should receive oxygen to maintain oxygen saturation above 92%. Dehydrated children should receive an adequate amount of oral fluids and, if unable to drink, they should be given intravenous fluids. Their electrolytes and creatinine serum levels should be measured daily. To date, there are no studies showing a beneficial effect of chest physiotherapy in children with pneumonia, so chest physiotherapy should not be provided.

Clinical symptoms and laboratory values of inflammatory markers should improve within 48–72 hours of starting appropriate treatment. If there is no improvement, further investigations for possible complications, resistant microorganisms, or alternative diagnoses are required (Grudzinska et al., 2019).

3.4.2. Antibiotic Treatment

Experts disagree on whether all children with CAP should receive antibiotics, however, according to the BTS guidelines from 2011, all children diagnosed with pneumonia should be treated with antibiotics. This contrasts with previous guidelines, which stated that antibiotics could be omitted if a viral etiology was suspected, provided the child was re-examined within 24–48 hours. The reason for this change, despite the obvious concerns about increasing antibiotic resistance in bacteria and potential adverse effects in children who are unnecessarily treated with antibiotics, is that it is impossible to reliably distinguish between viral and bacterial infection based on clinical, laboratory, and radiologic markers, either alone or in combination. In particular, children <2 years of age who have already been vaccinated against conjugate pneumococcus and have mild symptoms of lower respiratory tract infection are unlikely to have pneumonia. Antibiotics can be withheld in these children, provided the child is re-examined if symptoms persist or worsen. In contrast, the PIDS guidelines state that preschool children with CAP do not need to be routinely treated with antibiotics, as pneumonia in this age group is predominantly viral in origin (Huang et al., 2018).

The antibiotic of choice for outpatient treatment of CAP is amoxicillin 90 mg/kg/day, given in two doses over 5–10 days. The results of two randomized trials of short-term (3 days) oral antibiotics in infants in developing countries are difficult to interpret because many of these children had bronchiolitis with wheezing or upper respiratory tract infection and did not require antibiotics at all (Hyams et al., 2020). Amoxicillin is effective against most pathogens responsible for CAP in children and is well-tolerated, and affordable. Alternatives include treatment with coamoxiclav, cefaclor, and macrolides. For penicillin-resistant *S. pneumoniae* with a minimum inhibitory concentration (MIC) of up to 4.0 μg/ml, the preferred treatment is ceftriaxone, and for a MIC greater than 4.0 μg/ml, vancomycin, linezolid, or clindamycin can be used, although resistance to clindamycin appears to be increasing at 15–40% in certain geographic regions. It should be noted that the interpretation of *in vitro* susceptibility testing for penicillin depends on the route of administration. Penicillin administered intravenously can reach tissue concentrations that are effective against organisms with a MIC ≤2.0 μg/ml. It may also be effective against strains with an MIC of 4 μg/ml, but is unlikely to be effective against strains with an MIC ≥ 8 μg/ml. For orally administered penicillin, the corresponding values are <0.06 μg/mL, 0.12–1.0 μg/mL and ≥2.0 μg/mL for resistant strains. Clinical laboratory standards vary by region. The above levels were issued jointly by the Infectious Diseases Society of America (IDSA) and the American Thoracic Society (ATS). The BTS recommends limits for intravenous penicillin of <0.1 mg/L; 0.1–1.0 mg/L and >1.0–4.0 mg/L and the European Respiratory Society (ERS) recommends MIC breakpoints of <0.5 mg/L; 0.5–2.0 mg/L and >2.0 mg/L respectively. PIDS recommends levofloxacin as the preferred choice for oral therapy for children of 6 months of age and older. Macrolide antibiotics may be used for suspected *M. pneumoniae* or *C. pneumonia* if the child's condition does not improve after 24 to 48 hours or in very severe cases. They are not recommended as first-line antibiotics as up to 40% of *S. pneumoniae* strains currently isolated in the US are resistant to macrolides (Jain et al., 2015).

As with the indications for antibiotics in CAP, there is no consensus on how they should be administered. According to the BTS guidelines, antibiotics should be given orally if the child is eating well and not vomiting. Children with moderate pneumonia who are admitted for respiratory distress can be treated with oral antibiotics and discharged once their fever and respiratory distress have subsided. Intravenous administration of antibiotics is reserved for children with severe, complicated pneumonia or sepsis, for whom intravenous administration of amoxicillin, coamoxiclav, cefuroxime, cefotaxime, or ceftriaxone is recommended. However, according to the PIDS guidelines, all hospitalized children should be treated with intravenous antibiotics to obtain reliable blood and tissue concentrations. In hospitalized children with suspected *S. aureus* infection, beta-lactam therapy should be supplemented with vancomycin or clindamycin. Cephalosporins are recommended for children with penicillin allergy, and macrolides, vancomycin, or clindamycin are recommended for type I allergic reactions. Linezolid can be administered to children who cannot tolerate vancomycin or clindamycin. The antibiotic should be changed depending on the results of the culture and sensitivity tests if these tests are positive. As soon as the child's condition improves, a switch to oral antibiotics should be considered (Kamat et al., 2020).

3.5. Complications

3.5.1. Empyema and Parapneumonic Effusion

A parapneumonic effusion is defined as an accumulation of pleural fluid associated with underlying pneumonia, and empyema is defined as the accumulation of purulent fluid in the pleural cavity (Kim et al., 2022). The incidence of parapneumonic effusion is increasing (by 70–100% between the 1990s and the beginning of this century) and affects 0.6% of all children with CAP, 2–10% of pneumonia hospitalizations and 1/3 of pneumococcal pneumonia hospitalizations. The predominant etiologic factors are *S. pneumonia* (serotype 1,3,14,19A), responsible for 10–66% of empyema cases, *S. aureus* including methicillin-resistant *S. aureus* (MRSA) (4–30%), and *S. pyogenes*. Less common are *Haemophilus influenzae*, *Mycobacterium* spp., *Pseudomonas aeruginosa*, anaerobes, *M. pneumonia* and fungi. The accumulation of fluid is usually unilateral. Empyema classically has three stages:

- Exudative – the pleural space contains free-flowing fluid with a small number of white blood cells, a so-called parapneumonic effusion resulting from increased vascular permeability and migration of neutrophils, lymphocytes, and eosinophils during the inflammatory process.
- Fibrinopurulent effusion occurs 5–10 days after the onset of the disease and consists of the deposition of fibrin in the pleural space, leading to septation and the formation of debris. In response to bacterial invasion through the damaged epithelium, the white cell count increases (empyema) and, if left untreated, the disease progresses to organizing.
- Organizing involves the infiltration of fibroblasts and the development of a thick elastic membrane in the pleural cavity (the "shell"). These membranes can impair lung function and prevent the lung from re-expanding. Empyema at this stage may heal spontaneously or chronic empyema may develop.

Some authors distinguish a "pleuritis sicca stage," which precedes the exudative stage but does not necessarily lead to it.

Empyema should be suspected in any child with pneumonia who has a history of persistent fever, tachypnea, pain on palpation of the abdomen, pleuritic chest pain, splinting of the affected side, and persistently high serum C-reactive protein levels. Physical examination may reveal asymmetry of breath sounds, decreased unilateral expansion of the chest wall, and dullness on percussion. In some children with pneumonia, empyema may develop during intravenous antibiotic treatment. One of the identified risk factors for bacterial empyema is previous varicella.

Chest X-rays show a homogeneous opacity of the entire lung (large effusion) (Figure 3.6). Smaller effusions show an ascending rim of fluid along the lateral chest wall (meniscus sign). The obliteration of the chest angle is the first sign of a pleural effusion. It is not possible to distinguish an effusion from empyema based on the X-ray image. One method of choice for the radiologic evaluation of patients with parapneumonic effusion and empyema is ultrasonography. It helps in estimating the amount of fluid, its echogenicity, the detection of localization and fibrin clots, and is used to guide invasive procedures. Chest CT should not be performed routinely, but it can be useful for diagnosing underlying pathology, such as a tumor in the mediastinum or a lung abscess (Koch et al., 2020) (Figure 3.7).

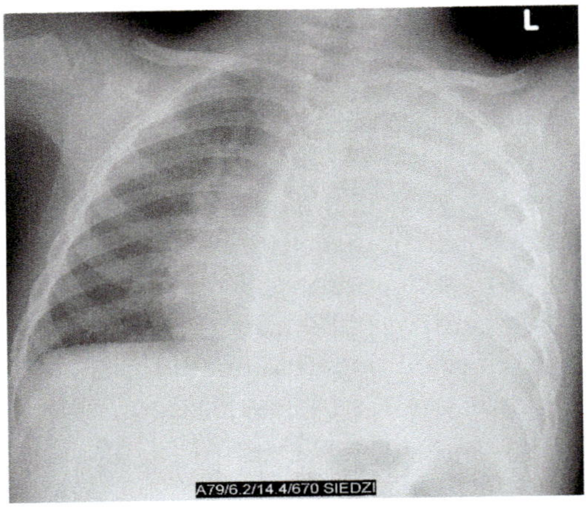

Figure 3.6. *Clouding of the left hemithorax with mediastinal shift to the opposite side. Alveolar consolidation in the central area of the right lobe. Lobar pneumonia with pleural effusion caused by Streptococcus pneumonia.*

Source: NCBI.

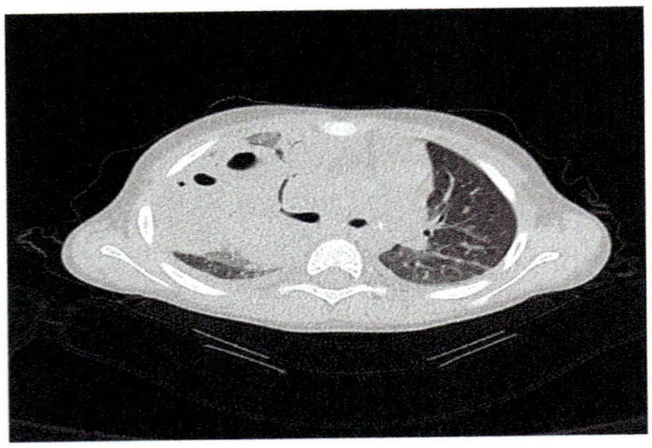

Figure 3.7. *Multiple abscesses in the right upper lobe. Diffuse alveolar consolidations with thickening of the intra-alveolar spaces in the middle and lower right lobe. Fluid in the right pleural space. Staphylococcus aureus pneumonia with lung abscesses and pleural effusion.*

Source: NCBI.

Pleural fluid obtained during thoracentesis or video-assisted thoracoscopic surgery (VATS) should be sent for culture, Gram stain, cytology, and molecular techniques, if available. Bacteriologic studies should always be performed, even if positive in a quarter of cases, as they may provide useful information for antibiotic therapy. Staining for acid-fast bacilli, culture, and PCR should also be performed. In most cases of bacterial empyema, polymorphonuclear leukocytes are the predominant cells. In malignant disease, the fluid may be blood-stained, with a predominance of lymphocytes, although malignant cells may not be present. In tuberculosis, lymphocytes also predominate in the pleural fluid, although the effusion may be neutrophilic in 10% of cases. Mild criteria that are useful for guiding therapy in adult patients have not been properly validated in children and their routine use is not recommended (Levin et al., 2001).

All children with empyema or pleural effusion should be hospitalized. However, there is no consensus on what the optimal treatment for empyema is: antibiotics alone for small to moderate effusions, chest tube insertion with or without fibrinolytics, or VATS for moderate to severe cases (Liapikou & Torres, 2013). The differences in treatment result in part from personal experience and the availability of different treatment modalities, including experienced interventional radiologists and pediatric thoracic surgeons. In general, the two most important factors required for chest drainage are the size of the effusion and the degree of impairment of the child's breathing. There is consensus that due to the invasive nature of the procedure and the need for general anesthesia in younger children, a drain should be inserted instead of repeated needle thoracentesis. According to the PIDS, pleural effusions can be divided into the following categories depending on their size:

- **Small:** < 10 mm on lateral decubitus radiograph or opacifies < ¼ hemithorax.
- **Moderate:** >10 mm rim of fluid and opacifies < ½ hemithorax.
- **Large:** Opacifies > ½ hemithorax.

Conservative treatment with antibiotics is recommended for small effusions. The choice of antibiotic depends on the results of the blood or pleural fluid cultures and, if these are not available, on the treatment guidelines. Many patients do better with conservative treatment alone (Lim et al., 2009). In an American study, over 50% of patients with moderate to severe effusions recovered with antibiotic treatment alone. The treatment of moderate effusions depends on the degree to which the child's breathing is impaired: If the clinical condition is good, treatment with antibiotics is appropriate, and if the child shows signs of respiratory distress, the treatment is the same as for large effusions: the fluid should be removed either by thoracentesis (for non-localized fluid), by chest drainage with fibrinolytics or VATS (both for localized fluid). Once the chest tube is inserted, no more than 10 ml/kg of fluid should be removed in young children, and 1.5 liters of fluid in older children and adolescents to avoid the recurrence of pulmonary edema. Once this volume has been reached, the drain should be clamped for one hour (Lim et al., 2001). There is no clear evidence of a benefit in the clinical outcome of children treated with fibrinolytics compared to VATS. The recommended doses for fibrinolytic agents are:

- Urokinase (not available in the US) 10,000 U every 12 hours for 3 days in children < 1 year and 40,000 U every 12 hours for 3 days in children > 1 year.
- Streptokinase 12,000–25,000 IU/kg/dose daily for 3–5 days.
- Tissue plasminogen activator 0.1 mg/kg; maximum 3 mg three times daily for 3 to 4 days or 4 mg every 24 hours.

There is a risk of hypersensitivity reactions with streptokinase and urokinase. In children who do not improve despite antibiotics, drainage, and fibrinolytics, a VATS examination should be performed to loosen fibrinous adhesions and remove dense, localized fluid. It seems advisable to obtain a surgical opinion if the patient's condition does not improve after 7 days of treatment. Another indication for surgery is a bronchopleural fistula with pyopneumothorax. Formal thoracotomy with decortication should be considered as an alternative to VATS, especially in the case of organized empyema in a child with non-resolving signs of systemic infection with fever. According to the BTS guidelines, clinical signs and symptoms, rather than an abnormal radiologic appearance in an asymptomatic child, are the indication for referral for surgery. Risk factors for failure of tube thoracostomy include symptom duration of more than 7 days before surgery, complex multilocular empyema, pneumatocele, pulmonary necrosis, and underlying disease. A chest tube can be removed if the fluid output is < 1 ml/kg/day, calculated over the previous 12 hours, or 50–60 ml/day and there is no air leak.

A more aggressive approach is to perform a VATS in the first 48 hours of treatment. This offers the chance of a bacteriologic diagnosis, and a shorter hospital stay, although not all studies support the latter observation (Lüthi-Corridori et al., 2023).

The optimal duration of antibiotic treatment for parapneumonic effusion and empyema depends on the clinical response. The recommended route of administration is intravenous administration until the chest tube is removed. Thereafter, it may be switched to oral administration for 1 to 4 weeks or longer if the child has not fully recovered. However, there are no randomized clinical trials to support this approach. Long-term outcomes in children are favorable. Radiographic signs of pleural disease resolve completely in up to 80% of children within 3 months and in all children within 18 months. Pulmonary function test results and exercise tolerance are normal in most patients 12 months after discharge. Conditions that predispose to severe pneumonia with pleural effusion and empyema include immunodeficiencies and cystic fibrosis and should be ruled out during follow-up (Majumdar et al., 2011).

3.5.2. Lung Abscess

A lung abscess is a thick-walled cavity containing necrotic tissue with a diameter of 2 cm or more and is caused by an infection. It can either be primary, which occurs in healthy children without lung abnormalities, or secondary, occurring in children with an underlying condition that predisposes to lung disease. The most important mechanism for the formation of a lung abscess is aspiration, especially in children with neuromuscular disorders. Other risk factors include immunodeficiencies, underlying lung diseases such as congenital malformations, cystic fibrosis, swallowing disorders (for example achalasia), and poor dental care. Abscesses can also be caused by hematogenous spread in septicemia or right-sided bacterial endocarditis, by expansion of foci in the abdominal cavity or the retropharynx, or by obstruction of the airways by foreign bodies (McCabe et al., 2009).

The main causative agents are usually streptococci, anaerobic bacteria, *S. aureus,* and *Klebsiella pneumoniae*, but there are rare reports of other causative agents, including *M. pneumoniae*. Mixed infections are often common. The most frequent sites for the formation of lung abscesses in the supine position are the right upper lobe, the left lower lobe, and the apical segments of both lower lobes. If the patient aspirates in the supine position, the posterior segments of the upper lobes are usually affected (Metlay et al., 2019).

Clinical symptoms include cough, purulent sputum, fever, dyspnea, chest pain, tachypnea, weight loss, hemoptysis, malaise, and lethargy. The physical signs do not differ from those of uncomplicated pneumonia, excluding diminished breath sounds and a muffled sound when tapping may be heard. Symptoms may persist for several weeks.

The diagnosis is usually made by chest X-ray, which shows an inflammatory infiltrate of the lung parenchyma with a cavity containing an air-liquid level. Initially, it may be a solid lesion surrounded by an alveolar infiltrate, and at times, a bulging fissure may be present, representing an increase in the volume of the affected lobe. A CT scan is usually performed to rule out other complications such as empyema, pneumatocoele, and underlying congenital anomalies such as sequestration, bronchogenic cyst, or adenomatoid malformation. Features that distinguish an abscess from other entities include well-demarcated walls, density greater than water, and contrast enhancement in adjacent tissue (Molinos et al., 2015) (Figure 3.8).

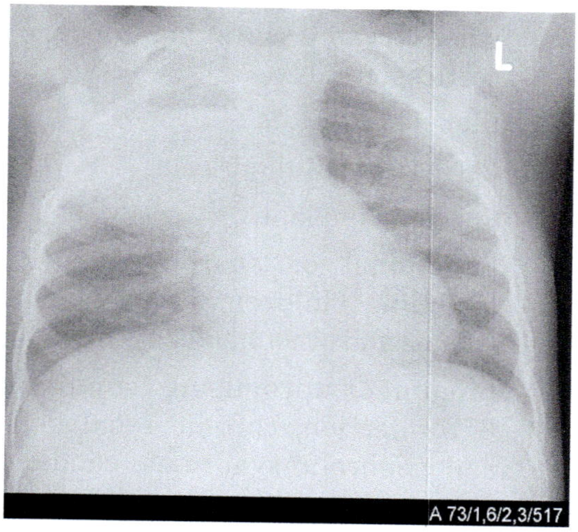

Figure 3.8. *Infiltrate with air-fluid level in the upper field of the right lobe. Lung abscess.*

Source: NCBI.

The mainstay of treatment is conservative antibiotic therapy with a spectrum that includes *S. pneumoniae*, *S. aureus,* and gram-negative bacilli as well as anaerobes in the case of a secondary abscess. In immunocompromised patients, the antibiotics should also cover fungal pathogens. The antibiotic of choice is penicillin with clindamycin or metronidazole. Other experts recommend third-generation cephalosporins as well as flucloxacillin, ticarcillin, ampicillin/clavulanic acid, and piperacillin/tazobactam. The possibility of MRSA infection should be considered, especially if the abscess is complicating pneumonia or has arisen through hematogenous spread from other organs. Generally, 2–3 weeks of intravenous therapy followed by oral treatment for 4 to 8 weeks is recommended. In experienced centers for interventional radiology, CT-guided aspiration of the lung abscess and placement of a pigtail catheter are performed for diagnostic and therapeutic reasons. Surgical intervention is indicated for abscesses that do not improve despite medical treatment (Mortensen et al., 2002).

The overall outcome is favorable, mortality is much lower than in adults: <5% and usually occurs in children with secondary lung abscesses or underlying medical problems. Complications include empyema or pyopneumothorax if the abscess invades the pleural cavity, bronchopleural fistula if the connection between the abscess cavity and the pleural space persists, and localized bronchiectasis (Musher et al., 2013).

3.5.3. Necrotizing Pneumonia

Necrotizing pneumonia (NP), defined as multiple cavitary lesions in consolidated areas, is a rare but increasingly common complication in children. It is characterized by liquefaction and cavitation of the lung tissue. The most common pathogen involved is *S. pneumoniae*, particularly serotypes 3 and 14. Other pathogens involved include group A *Streptococcus*, *S. aureus,* and *M. pneumoniae*. Most patients have no previous medical history. Necrotizing pneumonia should be suspected in patients with complicated pneumonia who do not improve despite optimal medical treatment. The diagnosis can be made by computed tomography. Radiographic criteria for necrotizing pneumonia include loss of the normal architecture of the lung parenchyma and the presence of areas of liquefaction that are replaced by multiple small cavities within 1 to 2 days. Necrotizing pneumonia often occurs together with pleural effusion (Nyamande & Lalloo, 2007).

Treatment consists of prolonged treatment with intravenous antibiotics that are effective against CAP pathogens including resistant strains of *S. pneumoniae*. Interventional procedures are contraindicated in children with NP as they may increase the risk of complications such as bronchopleural fistula formation (O'Kelly et al., 2020). Despite the prolonged hospital stay and associated morbidity, long-term outcomes are favorable in most children. The mortality rate is 5.5–7%.

3.6. Prevention

Various measures can be taken to prevent pneumonia, ranging from general recommendations such as improving diet, housing, and heating systems, reducing exposure to tobacco smoke, and promoting breastfeeding in the first six months of life, to more specific infection control measures such as hand washing, avoiding people with signs of respiratory infection and vaccination. Immunization against the following microorganisms is recommended to prevent pneumonia:

- Influenza virus;
- *S. pneumoniae* (conjugate and non-conjugate vaccine);
- *H. influenzae* (conjugate vaccine);
- Measles virus;
- Varicella virus;
- *Bordatella pertussiss*;
- *Mycobacterium tuberculosis*.

High-risk infants: premature infants (<35 weeks GA), with hemodynamically significant congenital heart disease, bronchopulmonary dysplasia, congenital airway abnormalities, and neuromuscular disease should receive immunoprophylaxis with RSV-specific monoclonal antibodies (palivizumab) during the RSV season (Ogawa et al., 2020).

The AAP recommends routine use of the 13-valent pneumococcal conjugate vaccine (PCV13) for healthy children of 2 to 59 months of age and children of 60 to 71 months of age with an underlying condition that increases the risk of invasive pneumococcal disease (IPD). Underlying conditions that require pneumococcal vaccination include:

- Chronic heart disease, especially cyanotic congenital heart disease, and heart failure.
- Chronic lung disease, including asthma when treated with high-dose oral corticosteroids.
- Diabetes mellitus.
- Cerebrospinal fluid leaks.
- Cochlear implant.
- Functional or anatomic asplenia, including children with sickle cell anemia and other hemoglobinopathies.
- Immunocompromising conditions: HIV infection, chronic renal failure and nephrotic syndrome, conditions associated with treatment with immunosuppressive drugs or radiation therapy (including malignant neoplasms, leukemias, lymphomas, Hodgkin's disease, solid organ transplantation) and congenital immunodeficiencies (including B (humoral) or T lymphocyte deficiencies; Complement deficiencies, in particular C1, C2, C3, and C4 and phagocytosis disorders with the exception of chronic granulomatous diseases).

Healthy children of <5 years of age and children of <6 years of age with underlying diseases who are fully vaccinated with PCV7 should receive an additional single dose of

PCV13. Children between 6 and 18 years of age with diseases favoring IPD (see above) should receive a single dose of PCV13, regardless of whether they have previously received PCV7 or PPSV23 (2 doses of PPSV23 recommended). PCV13, which contains the 6 pneumococcal serotypes (1,3,5,6A,7F,19A) responsible for 63% of cases of invasive pneumococcal disease in children <5 years of age in the US, in addition to the 7 serotypes contained in PCV7 (4,6B,9V,14,18C,19F,23F), was approved by the US Food and Drug Administration in 2010 for use in children of 2 to 71 months of age. Due to its extended coverage, it is intended to replace PCV7 (Ott, 2018).

3.7. Specific Bacterial Causes of Pneumonia

3.7.1. S. pneumoniae

S. pneumoniae is the most common pathogen causing CAP in children and the most common cause of pneumonia mortality in children worldwide. It is responsible for at least 1.2 million infant deaths annually, mainly in sub-Saharan Africa and Asia. There are 92 known pneumococcal serotypes, which are distinguished by the polysaccharide capsule. Serotypes have been found to correlate with different pneumonia outcomes, but study results are inconclusive. In pediatric patients, serotypes 7F, 23F and 3 were associated with the highest risk of death during the course of invasive pneumococcal disease. In another study, serotypes 1, 6, 14, and 19 were most common in children with complicated pneumonia, with serotype 1 causing 24.4% of complicated cases versus 3.6% of uncomplicated cases (Pepper et al., 2019).

S. pneumoniae frequently colonizes the epithelium of the nasopharynx in 20 to 40% of healthy children and more than 60% of infants and children in daycare centers. After colonization, a new strain displaces other competing pneumococcal serotypes and persists in a carrier status for months. Bacteria with a so-called "persistent colonization phenotype" and low risk of tissue invasion are responsible for ongoing transmission in human populations and induce acquired B cell-mediated immunity against reinfection. To facilitate their residence in the nasopharynx and evade host defenses, they use various mechanisms such as surface adhesions, IgA1 protease, and inhibitors of antibacterial peptides. Defects in the host's defense mechanisms can disrupt the balance and lead to infection in immunocompromised hosts (Peyrani et al., 2019). Another phenotype – the so-called "invasive pneumococcal phenotype" – can spread efficiently from person to person through coughing and rapidly trigger the disease. The most important virulence factor is the polysaccharide capsule, which prevents mechanical clearance by mucosal secretions, limits autolysis, reduces exposure to antibiotics, and facilitates invasion and spread. Other virulence factors include the pore-forming cytotoxin – pneumolysin, which, among other pathologic effects, can inhibit cilia movement of epithelial cells and impair the respiratory burst of phagocytic cells. The recent acquisition of an invasive serotype is more important than long-term colonization in terms of further infection and is considered one of the clear risk factors for pneumococcal pneumonia.

Some of the host immune mechanisms that are important in the defense against pneumococcal pneumonia are Toll-like receptors (TLR) (Raith et al., 2017). Children with a genetic deficiency of the common TLR adaptation protein Myeloid Differentiation Primary-Response Protein 88 (MyD88) or interleukin-1 receptor-associated kinase 4 (IRAK4), a kinase that acts directly downstream of MyD88, are particularly susceptible to invasive pneumococcal disease. Another genetic factor predisposing to invasive pneumococcal disease is the polymorphism of genes encoding inhibitors of nuclear factor κB and defects in the complement C3 pathway, which is critical for opsonization and consequently clearance of pneumococci (Roson et al., 2000).

Pneumonia usually begins with a viral infection of the upper respiratory tract. The pathogen most commonly associated with dual infections with streptococcal pneumonia is the influenza virus. Concurrent infection with the influenza virus weakens the host immune response and reduces its ability to clear pneumococci. The influenza virus possesses neuraminidase, which facilitates the adhesion of pneumococci to the epithelium of the respiratory tract by exposing certain receptors. Local innate immune defense systems such as mucociliary clearance, the cough reflex, and antimicrobial peptides normally manage to eliminate the pathogen. If this is not successful, pneumonia occurs. The clinical symptoms are characteristic of bacterial pneumonia with high fever, chills, malaise, cough, and dyspnoea. In older children, the cough becomes productive, with purulent, bloody sputum. Pleural involvement is quite common. Untreated pneumococcal pneumonia can lead to respiratory failure, septic shock, and subsequently death (Said et al., 2013).

The usual radiological picture of pneumococcal pneumonia is lobar pneumonia, often accompanied by a small pleural effusion. The changes may be limited to a single segment, affect several segments or lobes, or occur as bronchopneumonia.

Since the general introduction of the conjugated 7-valent pneumococcal vaccine in 2000, the incidence of pneumococcal pneumonia in children under 5 years of age has decreased. However, there is concern that the serotypes contained in the vaccine may be replaced by previously rare, potentially more virulent serotypes such as serotype 1 or 19A. Fortunately, these serotypes have been included in the newer 13-valent conjugate vaccine (Schuetz et al., 2018).

Increasing antibiotic resistance is a problem – up to 10% of pneumococcal isolates cultured in Europe in 2008 are not susceptible to penicillin, although the impact of *in* vitro resistance on the clinical outcome of patients is not as clear. Fortunately, no increase in mortality or complication rates was observed in children infected with resistant strains.

3.7.2. S. aureus

The incidence of *S. aureus* pneumonia has increased considerably over the last 20 years. An increasing number (up to 76% in Texas) of community-associated *S. aureus* is community-associated MRSA (CA-MRSA) and has become the leading cause of complicated CAP in children in some regions. CA-MRSA was first described in the 1990s as a cause of infection in previously healthy children and adolescents who had not previously been hospitalized or had no experience with chronic healthcare facilities. Nasal colonization of healthy children with MRSA is also increasing significantly – in another study from the USA, 36.4% of healthy children were colonized with *S. aureus* and 9.2% with MRSA. CA-MRSA has a different genotype from hospital-acquired strains. Notably, 22% of MRSA strains had a gene locus for PVL, and in a UK study, 11% of all *S. aureus* isolates from pneumonia patients carried the gene. Although the effect of nasal colonization on pneumonia risk is not clear, as no prior colonization was documented in 1/3 of patients with staphylococcal infection, these data show a wide prevalence of MRSA in the population (Silveira et al., 2012).

Primary *S. aureus* pneumonia occurs by direct invasion of the lungs via the tracheobronchial tree and secondary pneumonia by hematogenous spread. *S. aureus* CAP typically occurs in very young infants: 30% of cases occur in children under 3 months of age and 70% in children under 1 year of age, more frequently in boys. CA-MRSA CAP often occurs in previously healthy children and adolescents, and in many cases is either preceded by influenza or influenza-like illness or skin and soft tissue infection. Severe respiratory symptoms and hypotension develop rapidly. The USA300 clone is associated with venous thrombosis and subsequent septic pulmonary embolism (Sinclair et al., 2013).

S. aureus possesses a variety of virulence factors, including surface proteins (for example, protein A) that promote adherence and thus colonization of host tissue, invasion factors (leukocidin, kinases, and hyaluronidase) that promote bacterial dissemination in tissue, and membrane-damaging toxins (for example, the aforementioned leukocidin). There are several reports of pneumonia in previously healthy children and adolescents caused by Panton–Valentine leukocidin-producing *S. aureus*. The pore-forming toxin, which is encoded by the luk-S-PV and luk-F-PV genes, lyses neutrophil granulocytes and causes an exaggerated, albeit ineffective, inflammatory response. Patients present with rapidly progressive necrotizing pneumonia, manifested by fever, leukopenia, and haemoptysis, and are preceded by a viral infection, usually influenza. Leukopenia is characteristic of PVL and is probably due to the destruction of white blood cells by leukocidin. Radiographically, multiple, usually unilateral, nodular infiltrates are observed, which may progress to cavitary lesions and pneumatocele. The radiographic progression of the infiltrates can be very rapid and should suggest *S. aureus* pneumonia. Another characteristic radiologic sign – pneumatoceles – occurs in more than half of the cases, and both their size and number may change hourly. Staphylococcal pneumonia is often complicated by empyema, lung abscess formation, pneumothorax, and acute respiratory distress syndrome (ARDS) (Strauß et al., 2014).

Given the severe and potentially fatal nature of the infection, prompt initiation of appropriate antibiotic therapy is critical. For hospitalized patients with pneumonia caused by methicillin-susceptible *S. aureus*, PIDS recommends intravenous therapy with β-lactamase-stable penicillin (oxacillin, cloxacillin, flucloxacillin or nafcillin) or a first-generation cephalosporin (cefazolin). For more severe infections, some experts recommend combination therapy with an aminoglycoside or rifampin, although there is no data from controlled clinical trials to support these recommendations. The first-line treatment for hospitalized children with suspected CA-MRSA is vancomycin. However, there are concerns about the appropriate concentration of the drug in the epithelial fluid of the lung – in adults it has been shown to reach 18% of the serum concentration. Alternatives include linezolid and clindamycin, which have the added advantage of blocking the production of PVL toxin and staphylococcal exotoxins, making them the drugs of choice in the treatment of PVL-CA infections. Clindamycin should be used with caution considering local sensitivity data and should not be used in infections with high inoculum, such as empyema, as in this case there is a high risk of the bacteria constitutively producing methylase. Linezolid reaches higher concentrations in the epithelial lining of the lung (Triantafyllidis et al., 2012).

3.7.3. Mycoplasma pneumoniae

Mycoplasmas are the smallest self-replicating organisms that can live outside the host cells. They have a sterol-containing cell membrane, instead of a cell wall and do not stain well with Gram stains. Antibiotics that typically target the bacterial cell wall, such as β-lactams, are ineffective against these organisms. *M. pneumoniae* pneumonia is usually a mild disease, and transmission is by person-to-person contact with an incubation period usually between 1 and 2 weeks. Epidemics occur in cycles of about 4 to 7 years, and recurrent infections are common (Troeger et al., 2018).

Infections with *M. pneumonia* are common, and therefore antibodies are present in 1/3 of all infants aged 7 to 12 months and in over 90% of adolescents. Very few infections occur in infants in the first 6 months of life, which is probably due to the presence of maternal antibodies. Recent studies show that contrary to earlier reports, *M. pneumoniae* CAP is also quite common in children under 4 years of age, and that these microorganisms are responsible for ¼ of the infections in this age group.

The microorganisms are acquired via the respiratory tract and attach to a receptor of the respiratory epithelium via adhesions. Lung damage in *M. pneumoniae* pneumonia is associated with cell-mediated host immunity and is also accompanied by ciliostasis (van der Eerden et al., 2005).

Patients present with symptoms of upper respiratory tract infection, fever, malaise, and headache. The onset of symptoms is insidious. Cough, which is initially unproductive, occurs 3 to 5 days after the onset of the disease. Accompanying symptoms include hoarseness, chills, chest pain, vomiting, nausea, diarrhea, and myalgia. Runny nose is a rare finding, and pleural effusion occurs in 5–20% of patients. On auscultation, crackles, wheezing, and bronchial breathing may be heard. *Mycoplasma pneumonia* may also present extrapulmonarily, for example, with non-exudative pharyngitis, cervical lymphadenopathy, otitis media, conjunctivitis, arthritis, and rash. The disease usually resolves within 3 to 4 weeks but can be more severe in children with sickle cell anemia and Down syndrome. Mycoplasma can lead to exacerbations in asthma patients.

Radiologic findings vary from reticular and interstitial patterns to lobar consolidations. A hilar adenopathy is present in 1/3 of patients, and the poor correlation between clinical symptoms and physical, and radiological findings is characteristic (Viasus et al., 2019).

In rare cases, pneumonia acquired from *M. pneumoniae* can be severe and lead to massive lobar consolidation, pleural effusion, lung abscess, or pneumatocele formation. Occasionally, fever and radiographic changes progress despite standard macrolide therapy. There is one report of successful treatment of refractory pneumonia with methylprednisolone in children. Rare complications – obliterative bronchiolitis and diffuse interstitial fibrosis – have been described. Abnormal findings such as mosaic perfusion, bronchiectasis, bronchial wall thickening, decreased vascularity, and air trapping are observed in one-third of children between 1–2 years after *M. pneumoniae* infection. Extrapulmonary complications further cause signs in a variety of organs and systems, and include:

- **Nervous system:** Meningoencephalitis, transverse myelitis, cranial neuropathy, myeloradiculopathy, a poliomyelitis-like syndrome, psychosis, Guillain-Barré syndrome,
- **Skin:** Erythematous maculopapular or vesicular exanthema, erythema multiforme, Stevens–Johnson syndrome,
- **Heart:** Pericarditis, myocarditis, congestive heart failure, heart block,
- **Gastrointestinal Tract:** Nausea, vomiting, diarrhea, liver dysfunction, jaundice,
- **Hematology:** Hemolytic anemia, thrombocytopenia, disseminated intravascular coagulation,

- **Musculoskeletal Disorders:** Myalgias, arthralgias,
- **Genitourinary:** Glomerulonephritis, interstitial tubulonephritis.

3.8. Hospital Acquired Pneumonia

Hospital-acquired pneumonia (HAP) is defined as pneumonia occurring 48 hours or more when a patient previously had no signs of illness at the time of hospital admission. It can be further subdivided into early-onset pneumonia (48–96 hours after admission), which is usually caused by CAP pathogens, and late-onset pneumonia (>96 hours after admission), which is caused by multidrug-resistant nosocomial pathogens.

Ventilator-associated pneumonia (VAP), a form of HAP that occurs in mechanically ventilated patients, is defined as pneumonia that occurs more than 48 hours after intubation.

A third, and more recently described form, is care-associated pneumonia (HCAP) and occurs in patients who fulfill one of the following conditions:

- Hospitalization for 2 or more days within 90 days prior to infection;
- Stay in a nursing home or long-term care facility;
- Antibiotic therapy or chemotherapy or wound care within 30 days prior to infection;
- Visit to a hemodialysis center.

The definition of HCAP has not been validated in children, although HCAP is a significant problem in this population due to the growing number of pediatric patients with chronic conditions (for example, cerebral palsy, congenital malformation syndromes, chronic lung, heart, and kidney disease) who have frequent contact with healthcare workers.

HAP occurs in 16–29% of pediatric patients and accounts for 10–15% of all nosocomial infections in children and up to 67% of nosocomial infections in children admitted to pediatric intensive care units. VAP occurs in about 3 to 32% of ventilated pediatric intensive care patients. It is the most common nosocomial infection in Europe and the second most common nosocomial infection in children treated in intensive care units in the USA. The mortality rate for HAP is significantly higher than for CAP and is between 10 and 70%, depending on the etiologic factors and concomitant diseases. HAP and especially VAP increase the length of hospital stay and hospital costs (Viasus et al., 2017).

The most common etiologic factors of pediatric HAP are respiratory viruses, including respiratory syncytial virus, adenovirus, influenza, and parainfluenza viruses. Bacteria responsible for late-onset HAP include Gram-negative bacilli: *P. aeruginosa*, *Escherichia coli*, *Klebsiella pneumonia*, *Acinetobacter* spp., and *Serratia* spp. as well as Gram-positive organisms, particularly *S. aureus* and coagulase-negative staphylococci. *P. aeruginosa* is the most common bacterial pathogen in pediatric intensive care units, associated with a mortality rate of up to 80%. Most bacteria responsible for nosocomial infections are multidrug-resistant, including MRSA and ESBL-producing Gram-negative bacilli (extended spectrum β-lactamase). Immunocompromised children are particularly at risk of fungal infections, especially with *Aspergillus*, *Candida*, and *Pneumocystis jiroveci*. In 38% of cases, the etiology of VAP in children is polymicrobial.

Risk factors for hospital-acquired pneumonia include intubation and mechanical ventilation (increases the risk by 6 to 21 times), neuromuscular blockade, length of hospital stays, immunosuppression, recent treatment with antibiotics and H2 blockers, as well as overcrowding and understaffing of hospital wards. Genetic syndrome, female gender, reintubation, transport from the ICU, surgery prior to ICU admission, enteral feeding, and use of anesthetics were found to be independent risk factors for VAP in children.

Nosocomial pneumonia should be suspected in any child who presents with new respiratory symptoms, hypoxemia, increased oxygen or ventilatory requirements, and increased amount or altered nature of respiratory secretions during hospitalization. Most definitions include clinical and radiologic signs, with some adding bacteriologic and laboratory data. According to the Centers for Disease Control's (CDC) National Healthcare Safety Network, HAP can be diagnosed in patients with new radiographic changes (infiltrate, consolidation, cavitation, pneumatocele in infants in the first year of life) and at least three clinical criteria (clinically defined pneumonia) or two clinical and one laboratory criteria. In children with underlying lung or heart disease, the radiologic changes must be confirmed by at least two serial radiographs. The clinical criteria that must be met include:

- Fever > 38°C with no other cause or,
- Leucopenia (<4,000/mm^3) or leucocytosis (≥12,000/mm^3) and at least one (or two for clinically defined pneumonia) of the following:
- New onset of purulent sputum,
- Increase in respiratory secretions,
- Change in the character of sputum or respiratory secretions,
- New onset or worsening of respiratory symptoms: cough, tachypnea, dyspnea,
- Auscultary findings: rales, bronchial sounds,
- Increased oxygen requirements, $PaO_2/FiO_2 \leq 240$.

In children of up to 12 years of age, clinical criteria are slightly different, and at least three (two in infants ≤1 year of age) must be fulfilled. These include:

- Fever > 38°C or hypothermia < 36.5°C (or temperature instability for infants ≤1 year of age) with no other cause or,
- Leucopenia (<4,000/mm^3) or leukocytosis (≥15,000/mm^3) and ≥10% immature forms (infants ≤1 year of age),
- New onset of purulent sputum,
- Increase in respiratory secretions,
- Change in the character of sputum or respiratory secretions,
- New onset or worsening of respiratory symptoms: apnea, cough, tachypnea, dyspnea,
- Nasal flaring with chest wall retractions or grunting, wheezing – infants ≤1 year of age
- Auscultary findings: rales, bronchial sounds,
- Bradycardia (<100 beats/minute) or tachycardia (>170 beats per minute) – infants ≤1 year of age
- Increased ventilation requirements, hypoxemia (Sat <94%) – this condition is

obligatory for infants ≤1 year of age.

Laboratory criteria include positive cultures of blood (not associated with other infections), pleural fluid or lower airway specimens (bronchoalveolar lavage – BAL or protected brushings), intracellular bacteria in ≥5% of cells from BAL on direct microscopic examination, histopathologic evidence of abscess formation, focal consolidations, intense polymorphonuclear cell accumulations in the small airways, lung parenchymal invasion by hyphae or pseudohyphae. The diagnostic value of BAL in children with VAP is 50–72% and the specificity is 80–88%, the quantification of intracellular organisms in the BAL samples is 30–55% and 89–95%, respectively. Laboratory criteria for HAP caused by atypical bacteria (*Mycoplasma* spp., *Chlamydophila* spp., *Legionella* spp.) or viruses include positive culture from respiratory secretions, positive detection of antigen or antibody in respiratory secretions, a 4-fold increase in IgG in paired sera, positive PCR, detection of *L. pneumophila* serogroup 1 antigens in urine (Waterer et al., 1999).

Bacteriological diagnosis is often difficult, as hospitalized patients are frequently colonized with pathogenic flora. Therefore, a quantitative criterion for bacterial yield (≥104 cfu/mL or ≥104 cfu/g tissue in the case of lung parenchyma samples) has been introduced to facilitate the etiologic diagnosis of pneumonia. The applicability of invasive diagnostic techniques (lung biopsy) remains controversial due to the risk of complications in unstable or severely ill patients and the lack of data confirming their impact on clinical outcomes or mortality.

Patients with HAP are usually debilitated individuals with multiple underlying conditions. HAP is a serious disease with a high mortality rate. Therefore, the diagnosis should be made as soon as possible, using a wide range of diagnostic tools and techniques, and empirical treatment should be given immediately, pending cultures and other microbiological investigations. The spectrum of antibiotics should be broad enough to cover both Gram-negative and Gram-positive bacteria, taking into account previous antibiotic exposures, local flora, antimicrobial susceptibility patterns, and infectious disease specialist guidelines. Risk factors for the acquisition of antibiotic-resistant Gram-negative bacteria in pediatric intensive care unit (PICU) patients include younger age, severe general condition (assessed by PRISM score {pediatric mortality risk}), intravenous antibiotic administration in the past 12 months, past PICU admission, and contact with chronic care facilities. Inappropriate antibiotic treatment is associated with increased mortality in patients with HAP. Children with early-onset HAP can be treated like children with CAP unless they have specific risk factors for HCAP, VAP, or colonization with multidrug-resistant bacteria. PICU patients should receive protection against *P. aeruginosa* (aminoglycoside with an appropriate β-lactam: piperacillin, ceftazidime, or cefepime), and in-hospital units where the incidence of methicillin-resistant staphylococci or ESBL-producing Gram-negative bacilli exceeds 5%, vancomycin and carbapenems or ureidopenicillin-drug therapy should be used. Ureidopenicillin derivatives combined with β-lactamase inhibitors should be included in the empirical treatment regimen. In children with immunodeficiencies, antifungals should be administered. Once the causative organism and its susceptibility are known, therapy should be tailored to the narrowest spectrum agent available. Antibiotics should be administered intravenously and, if possible, switched to oral administration as soon as the patient's condition improves (World Health Organization, 2016).

Infection control measures that should be carefully implemented to reduce the number of HAP include:

- Appropriate hand hygiene, use of gloves,
- Personal protective equipment – face masks, especially during periods of increased incidence of respiratory viruses,
- Cohorting of patients infected or colonized with resistant microorganisms,
- Care practices: semi-recumbent position for ventilated patients, oral care,
- Use of non-invasive ventilation instead of mechanical ventilation in appropriate patients,
- Care of medical equipment: ventilator circuits, suctioning devices, pulmonary function testing equipment,
- Avoidance of overcrowding and understaffing,
- Avoidance of H2 antagonists,
- Judicious use of antibiotics,
- Immunization practices (as described above for CAP).

A Closer Look

Empyema

Empyema is a serious complication of pneumonia characterized by the accumulation of pus in the pleural cavity. It typically arises after a bacterial infection, with Streptococcus pneumoniae and Staphylococcus aureus being the most common causative agents. The condition can lead to significant morbidity and mortality if not diagnosed and treated promptly. A study by López-Campos et al. (2017) highlighted that the incidence of empyema is on the rise, particularly among older adults and individuals with predisposing factors such as chronic lung disease or immunosuppression. The research emphasized the importance of early identification and management of pneumonia to prevent the progression to empyema.

Diagnostic modalities for empyema include chest X-rays, ultrasound, and computed tomography (CT) scans. The utilization of thoracentesis, both for diagnostic and therapeutic purposes, is a key component of management. Wang et al. (2019) conducted a meta-analysis showing that ultrasound-guided thoracentesis is associated with higher diagnostic accuracy and fewer complications compared to blind procedures. Their findings support the need for imaging guidance in the diagnosis of pleural effusions, which aids in distinguishing between simple and complicated effusions that may indicate empyema.

The treatment of empyema can vary based on its stage—exudative, fibrinopurulent, or organizing. Dey et al. (2020) outlined that the management approach often begins with the use of broad-spectrum antibiotics, with the addition of drainage procedures for more advanced cases. In patients with complex empyema, video-assisted thoracoscopic surgery (VATS) has emerged as a preferred intervention, as evidenced by a study showing it reduces hospital stay and improves recovery times compared to traditional open surgery. This study underlines the importance of tailoring treatment plans to individual patient needs and disease severity.

Long-term outcomes for empyema patients can be influenced by timely intervention and appropriate management strategies. A cohort study by Kakkar et al. (2021) revealed that delayed treatment significantly correlates with increased morbidity, including persistent pleural infection and the need for surgical interventions. Furthermore, this research emphasizes the necessity for follow-up care in empyema patients to monitor for potential complications and to ensure complete resolution of infection. Overall, the growing body of evidence underscores the importance of an early and multidisciplinary approach to the management of empyema, improving patient outcomes and reducing healthcare burdens.

Summary

- Pneumonia is a serious infection that inflames the air sacs in one or both lungs. The air sacs may fill with fluid or pus, causing cough with phlegm or pus, fever, chills, and difficulty breathing. In severe cases, it can lead to hospitalization and even death, especially in high-risk groups such as infants, the elderly, and those with weakened immune systems.
- Pneumonia can be caused by bacteria, viruses, or fungi. The most common cause is the bacterium S. pneumoniae, but other bacteria such as M. pneumoniae and viruses such as influenza and respiratory syncytial virus (RSV) can also lead to pneumonia. Fungal pneumonia is less common but can occur in people with weakened immune systems.
- The diagnosis of pneumonia is typically based on symptoms, physical examination, and chest X-ray. Treatment depends on the underlying cause and severity of the illness. Bacterial pneumonia is usually treated with antibiotics, while viral pneumonia may improve with antiviral medication. In some cases, hospitalization and supportive care, such as oxygen therapy and intravenous fluids, may be necessary.
- Prevention of pneumonia includes vaccination against common pathogens, such as the pneumococcal vaccine and the influenza vaccine. Good hygiene practices, such as washing hands frequently and avoiding close contact with sick individuals, can also help prevent the spread of pneumonia-causing pathogens.

References

1. Albrich, W., Kahlert, C., Blanco, N. B., Hauser, C., Pedrazini, B., Ott, S., & Swiss Society for Infectious Diseases. (2023). Pneumonie/Ambulant-Erworbene Pneumonie CAP. *SSI Guidelines*. Available online: https://ssi.guidelines.ch/guideline/3007 (accessed on 9 September 2024).
2. Alyacoubi, S., Abuowda, Y., Albarqouni, L., Böttcher, B., & Elessi, K. (2018). Inpatient management of community-acquired pneumonia at the European Gaza Hospital: A clinical audit. *The Lancet, 391*(Suppl. S2), S40.
3. Asti, L., Bartsch, S. M., Umscheid, C. A., Hamilton, K., Nachamkin, I., & Lee, B. Y. (2019). The potential economic value of sputum culture use in patients with community-acquired pneumonia and healthcare-associated pneumonia. *Clinical Microbiology and Infection, 25*, e1–e1038.
4. Bateman, R. M., Sharpe, M. D., Jagger, J. E., Ellis, C. G., Solé-Violán, J., López-Rodríguez, M., Herrera-Ramos, E., Ruíz-Hernández, J., Borderías, L., Horcajada, J., et al. (2016). 36th International Symposium on Intensive Care and Emergency Medicine: Brussels, Belgium, 15–18 March 2016. *Critical Care, 20*, 94.
5. Bjarnason, A., Westin, J., Lindh, M., Andersson, L. M., Kristinsson, K. G., Löve, A., Baldursson, O., & Gottfredsson, M. (2018). Incidence, etiology, and outcomes of community-acquired pneumonia: A population-based study. *Open Forum Infectious Diseases, 5*, ofy010.
6. Bodí, M., Rodríguez, A., Solé-Violán, J., Gilavert, M. C., Garnacho, J., Blanquer, J., Jimenez, J., de La Torre, M. V., Sirvent, J. M., Almirall, J., et al. (2005). Antibiotic prescription for community-acquired pneumonia in the intensive care unit: Impact of adherence to Infectious Diseases Society of America guidelines on survival. *Clinical Infectious Diseases, 41*, 1709–1716.

7. Breuer, O., Picard, E., Benabu, N., Erlichman, I., Reiter, J., Tsabari, R., Shoseyov, D., Kerem, E., & Cohen-Cymberknoh, M. (2018). Predictors of prolonged hospitalizations in pediatric complicated pneumonia. *Chest, 153*(1), 172–180.

8. Brown, J. S. (2012). Community-acquired pneumonia. *Clinical Medicine, 12*(6), 538–543.

9. Brown, P. D. (2004). Adherence to guidelines for community-acquired pneumonia: Does it decrease cost of care? *Pharmacoeconomics, 22*(6), 413–420.

10. Bundesamt für Gesundheit. (2019). Bericht zur Grippesaison 2018/19. *BAG-Bulletin, 29*, 9–21. Available online: https://www.bag.admin.ch/dam/bag/de/dokumente/mt/infektionskrankheiten/grippe/saisonbericht-grippe-2018-19.pdf.download.pdf/saisonbericht-grippe-2018-19-de.pdf (accessed on 9 September 2024).

11. Capelastegui, A., España, P. P., Quintana, J. M., Gorordo, I., Ortega, M., Idoiaga, I., & Bilbao, A. (2004). Improvement of process-of-care and outcomes after implementing a guideline for the management of community-acquired pneumonia: A controlled before-and-after design study. *Clinical Infectious Diseases, 39*(7), 955–963.

12. Costantini, E., Allara, E., Patrucco, F., Faggiano, F., Hamid, F., & Balbo, P. E. (2016). Adherence to guidelines for hospitalized community-acquired pneumonia over time and its impact on health outcomes and mortality. *Internal and Emergency Medicine, 11*(7), 929–940.

13. Couturier, M. R., Graf, E. H., & Griffin, A. T. (2014). Urine antigen tests for the diagnosis of respiratory infections: Legionellosis, histoplasmosis, pneumococcal pneumonia. *Clinics in Laboratory Medicine, 34*(2), 219–236.

14. Dean, N. C., Silver, M. P., Bateman, K. A., James, B., Hadlock, C. J., & Hale, D. (2001). Decreased mortality after implementation of a treatment guideline for community-acquired pneumonia. *The American Journal of Medicine, 110*(6), 451–457.

15. Dixon, N. (2008). *Getting Clinical Audit Right to Benefit Patients.* Healthcare Quality Quest: Romsey, UK.

16. Dixon, N. (2011). What is clinical audit's purpose: Quality assurance or quality improvement? *FDJ, 2*(2), 79–83.

17. El Fahimi, N., Calleja, M. A., Ratnayake, L., & Ali, I. (2019). Audit of a multidisciplinary approach to improve management of community-acquired pneumonia. *European Journal of Hospital Pharmacy, 26*(4), 223–225.

18. Erdede, M., Denizbasi, A., Onur, O., & Guneysel, O. (2010). Do we really need blood cultures in treating patients with community-acquired pneumonia? *Bratislavské Lekárske Listy, 111*(5), 286–289.

19. Ewig, S., Birkner, N., Strauss, R., Schaefer, E., Pauletzki, J., Bischoff, H., Schraeder, P., Welte, T., & Hoeffken, G. (2009). New perspectives on community-acquired pneumonia in 388,406 patients. Results from a nationwide mandatory performance measurement programme in healthcare quality. *Thorax, 64*(12), 1062–1069.

20. Ewig, S., Höffken, G., Kern, W. V., Rohde, G., Flick, H., Krause, R., Ott, S., Bauer, T., Dalhoff, K., Gatermann, S., et al. (2016). Behandlung von erwachsenen Patienten mit ambulant erworbener Pneumonie und Prävention—Update 2016. *Pneumologie, 70*(3), 151–200.

21. Ewig, S., Kolditz, M., Pletz, M., Altiner, A., Albrich, W., Drömann, D., Flick, H., Gatermann, S., Krüger, S., Nehls, W., et al. (2021). Behandlung von erwachsenen Patienten mit ambulant erworbener Pneumonie—Update 2021. *Pneumologie, 75*(10), 665–729.

22. Freund, Y., Lemachatti, N., Krastinova, E., van Laer, M., Claessens, Y. E., Avondo, A., Occelli, C., Feral-Pierssens, A. L., Truchot, J., Ortega, M., et al. (2017). Prognostic accuracy of Sepsis-3 criteria for in-hospital mortality among patients with suspected infection presenting to the emergency department. *JAMA, 317*(3), 301–308.

23. Grudzinska, F. S., Aldridge, K., Hughes, S., Nightingale, P., Parekh, D., Bangash, M., Dancer, R., Patel, J., Sapey, E., Thickett, D. R., et al. (2019). Early identification of severe community-acquired pneumonia: A retrospective observational study. *BMJ Open Respiratory Research, 6*(1), e000438.

24. Huang, D. T., Yealy, D. M., Filbin, M. R., Brown, A. M., Chang, C. C. H., Doi, Y., Donnino, M. W., Fine, J., Fine, M. J., Fischer, M. A., et al. (2018). Procalcitonin-guided use of antibiotics for lower respiratory tract infection. *The New England Journal of Medicine, 379*(3), 236–249.

25. Hyams, C., Williams, O. M., & Williams, P. (2020). Urinary antigen testing for pneumococcal pneumonia: Is there evidence to make its use uncommon in clinical practice? *ERJ Open Research, 6*(1), 00223–2019.

26. Jain, S., Self, W. H., Wunderink, R. G., Fakhran, S., Balk, R., Bramley, A. M., Reed, C., Grijalva, C. G., Anderson, E. J., Courtney, D. M., et al. (2015). Community-acquired pneumonia requiring hospitalization among U.S. adults. *The New England Journal of Medicine, 373*(5), 415–427.

27. Kamat, I. S., Ramachandran, V., Eswaran, H., Guffey, D., & Musher, D. M. (2020). Procalcitonin to distinguish viral from bacterial pneumonia: A systematic review and meta-analysis. *Clinical Infectious Diseases, 70*(3), 538–542.

28. Kim, P., Deshpande, A., & Rothberg, M. B. (2022). Urinary antigen testing for respiratory infections: Current perspectives on utility and limitations. *Infection and Drug Resistance, 15*, 2219–2228.

29. Koch, C., Edinger, F., Fischer, T., Brenck, F., Hecker, A., Katzer, C., Markmann, M., Sander, M., & Schneck, E. (2020). Comparison of qSOFA score, SOFA score, and SIRS criteria for the prediction of infection and mortality among surgical intermediate and intensive care patients. *World Journal of Emergency Surgery, 15*, 63.

30. Levin, K. P., Hanusa, B. H., Rotondi, A., Singer, D. E., Coley, C. M., Marrie, T. J., Kapoor, W. N., et al. (2001). Arterial blood gas and pulse oximetry in initial management of patients with community-acquired pneumonia. *Journal of General Internal Medicine, 16*(9), 590–598.

31. Liapikou, A., & Torres, A. (2013). Current treatment of community-acquired pneumonia. *Expert Opinion on Pharmacotherapy, 14*(10), 1319–1332.

32. Lim, W. S., Baudouin, S. V., George, R. C., Hill, A. T., Jamieson, C., Le Jeune, I., Macfarlane, J. T., Read, R. C., Roberts, H. J., Levy, M. L., et al. (2009). BTS guidelines for the management of community-acquired pneumonia in adults: Update 2009. *Thorax, 64*(Suppl. 3), iii1–iii55.

33. Lim, W. S., Macfarlane, J. T., Boswell, T. C., Harrison, T. G., Rose, D., Leinonen, M., & Saikku, P. (2001). Study of community-acquired pneumonia aetiology (SCAPA) in adults admitted to hospital: Implications for management guidelines. *Thorax, 56*(4), 296–301.

34. Lüthi-Corridori, G., Boesing, M., Roth, A., Giezendanner, S., Leuppi-Taegtmeyer, A. B., Schuetz, P., & Leuppi, J. D. (2023). Predictors of length of stay, rehospitalization, and mortality in community-acquired pneumonia patients: A retrospective cohort study. *Journal of Clinical Medicine, 12*(14), 5601.

35. Majumdar, S. R., Eurich, D. T., Gamble, J. M., Senthilselvan, A., & Marrie, T. J. (2011). Oxygen saturations less than 92% are associated with major adverse events in outpatients with pneumonia: A population-based cohort study. *Clinical Infectious Diseases, 52*(3), 325–331.

36. McCabe, C., Kirchner, C., Zhang, H., Daley, J., & Fisman, D. N. (2009). Guideline-concordant therapy and reduced mortality and length of stay in adults with community-acquired pneumonia: Playing by the rules. *Archives of Internal Medicine, 169*(16), 1525–1531.

37. Metlay, J. P., Waterer, G. W., Long, A. C., Anzueto, A., Brozek, J., Crothers, K., Cooley, L. A., Dean, N. C., Fine, M. J., Flanders, S. A., et al. (2019). Diagnosis and treatment of adults with community-acquired pneumonia. An official clinical practice guideline of the American Thoracic Society and Infectious Diseases Society of America. *American Journal of Respiratory and Critical Care Medicine, 200*(7), e45–e67.

38. Molinos, L., Zalacain, R., Menéndez, R., Reyes, S., Capelastegui, A., Cillóniz, C., Rajas, O., Borderías, L., Martín-Villasclaras, J. J., Bello, S., et al. (2015). Sensitivity, specificity, and positivity predictors of the pneumococcal urinary antigen test in community-acquired pneumonia. *Annals of the American Thoracic Society, 12*(10), 1482–1489.

39. Mortensen, E. M., Coley, C. M., Singer, D. E., Marrie, T. J., Obrosky, D. S., Kapoor, W. N., & Fine, M. J. (2002). Causes of death for patients with community-acquired pneumonia: Results from the Pneumonia Patient Outcomes Research Team cohort study. *Archives of Internal Medicine, 162*(9), 1059–1064.

40. Musher, D. M., Roig, I. L., Cazares, G., Stager, C. E., Logan, N., & Safar, H. (2013). Can an etiologic agent be identified in adults who are hospitalized for community-acquired pneumonia: Results of a one-year study. *Journal of Infection, 67*(1), 11–18.

41. National Institute for Health and Care Excellence (NICE). (2022). *Pneumonia in Adults: Diagnosis and Management*. London, UK: NICE. ISBN 9781473108646.

42. Nyamande, K., & Lalloo, U. G. (2007). Poor adherence to South African guidelines for the management of community-acquired pneumonia. *South African Medical Journal, 97*(7), 601–603.

43. O'Kelly, B., Rueda-Benito, A., O'Regan, M., & Finan, K. (2020). An audit of community-acquired pneumonia antimicrobial compliance using an intervention bundle in an Irish hospital. *Journal of Global Antimicrobial Resistance, 23*, 38–45.

44. Ogawa, H., Kitsios, G. D., Iwata, M., & Terasawa, T. (2020). Sputum Gram stain for bacterial pathogen diagnosis in community-acquired pneumonia: A systematic review and Bayesian meta-analysis of diagnostic accuracy and yield. *Clinical Infectious Diseases, 71*(2), 499–513.

45. Ott, S. R. (2018). Ambulant erworbene und nosokomiale Pneumonie. *Swiss Medical Forum, 18*(34), 569–574.

46. Pepper, D. J., Sun, J., Rhee, C., Welsh, J., Powers, J. H., Danner, R. L., & Kadri, S. S. (2019). Procalcitonin-guided antibiotic discontinuation and mortality in critically ill adults: A systematic review and meta-analysis. *Chest, 155*(6), 1109–1118.

47. Peyrani, P., Mandell, L., Torres, A., & Tillotson, G. S. (2019). The burden of community-acquired bacterial pneumonia in the era of antibiotic resistance. *Expert Review of Respiratory Medicine, 13*(2), 139–152.

48. Raith, E. P., Udy, A. A., Bailey, M., McGloughlin, S., MacIsaac, C., Bellomo, R., & Pilcher, D. V. (2017). Prognostic accuracy of the SOFA score, SIRS criteria, and qSOFA score for in-hospital mortality among adults with suspected infection admitted to the intensive care unit. *JAMA, 317*(3), 290–300.
49. Rosón, B., Carratalà, J., Verdaguer, R., Dorca, J., Manresa, F., & Gudiol, F. (2000). Prospective study of the usefulness of sputum Gram stain in the initial approach to community-acquired pneumonia requiring hospitalization. *Clinical Infectious Diseases, 31*(4), 869–874.
50. Said, M. A., Johnson, H. L., Nonyane, B. A. S., Deloria-Knoll, M., O'Brien, K. L., Andreo, F., Beovic, B., Blanco, S., Boersma, W. G., Boulware, D. R., et al. (2013). Estimating the burden of pneumococcal pneumonia among adults: A systematic review and meta-analysis of diagnostic techniques. *PLoS ONE, 8*(4), e60273.
51. Schuetz, P., Wirz, Y., Sager, R., Christ-Crain, M., Stolz, D., Tamm, M., Bouadma, L., Luyt, C. E., Wolff, M., Chastre, J., et al. (2018). Effect of procalcitonin-guided antibiotic treatment on mortality in acute respiratory infections: A patient-level meta-analysis. *The Lancet Infectious Diseases, 18*(1), 95–107.
52. Silveira, C. D., Ferreira, C. S., & Corrêa, R. d. A. (2012). Adherence to guidelines and its impact on outcomes in patients hospitalized with community-acquired pneumonia at a university hospital. *Jornal Brasileiro de Pneumologia, 38*(2), 148–157.
53. Sinclair, A., Xie, X., Teltscher, M., & Dendukuri, N. (2013). Systematic review and meta-analysis of a urine-based pneumococcal antigen test for diagnosis of community-acquired pneumonia caused by *Streptococcus pneumoniae*. *Journal of Clinical Microbiology, 51*(7), 2303–2310.
54. Strauß, R., Ewig, S., Richter, K., König, T., Heller, G., & Bauer, T. T. (2014). The prognostic significance of respiratory rate in patients with pneumonia: A retrospective analysis of data from 705,928 hospitalized patients in Germany from 2010 to 2012. *Deutsches Ärzteblatt International, 111*(30), 503–508.
55. Triantafyllidis, C., Kapordelis, V., Papaetis, G. S., Orphanidou, D., Apostolidou, M., Nikolopoulos, I., & Pefanis, A. (2012). Guidelines adherence for patients with community acquired pneumonia in a Greek hospital. *European Review for Medical and Pharmacological Sciences, 16*(1), 1–9.
56. Troeger, C., Blacker, B., Khalil, I. A., Rao, P. C., Cao, J., Zimsen, S. R., Albertson, S. B., Deshpande, A., Farag, T., Abebe, Z., et al. (2018). Estimates of the global, regional, and national morbidity, mortality, and aetiologies of lower respiratory infections in 195 countries, 1990–2016: A systematic analysis for the Global Burden of Disease Study 2016. *The Lancet Infectious Diseases, 18*(11), 1191–1210.
57. Viasus, D., Calatayud, L., McBrown, M. V., Ardanuy, C., & Carratalà, J. (2019). Urinary antigen testing in community-acquired pneumonia in adults: An update. *Expert Review of Anti-Infective Therapy, 17*(2), 107–115.
58. Viasus, D., Vecino-Moreno, M., de La Hoz, J. M., & Carratalà, J. (2017). Antibiotic stewardship in community-acquired pneumonia. *Expert Review of Anti-Infective Therapy, 15*(4), 351–359.
59. Waterer, G. W., Jennings, S. G., & Wunderink, R. G. (1999). The impact of blood cultures on antibiotic therapy in pneumococcal pneumonia. *Chest, 116*(5), 1278–1281.
60. World Health Organization. (2018). *Global Health Estimates 2016: Deaths by Cause, Age, Sex, by Country and by Region, 2000–2016*. Geneva, Switzerland: WHO. Available online: https://www.who.int/data/gho/data/themes/mortality-and-global-health-estimates (accessed on 9 September 2024).

Chapter

INFANT LEUKEMIA

4

Contents

Introduction

Infant leukemias are a rare and distinct subgroup of pediatric acute lymphoblastic leukemia (ALL) and acute myeloid leukemia (AML) that occur in children under one year of age. About 35% of all childhood cancers are acute leukemias, of which 80% are ALL and 15 to 20% are AML. Infant leukemias account for 2 to 5% of pediatric patients with ALL and about 10% of pediatric patients with AML. The specific clinical and biological features of acute leukemia in infants differ markedly from those of older children. These patients usually present with a high white blood cell count at onset, massive organomegaly, early central nervous system (CNS) involvement, and cutaneous leukemia. Infantile leukemias are usually more aggressive and have a poorer prognosis. Congenital leukemia refers to development within the first few months of life. This chapter will focus on analyzing the clinical, cytological, and cytogenetic features of childhood leukemias (Andersson et al., 2015).

Orientation and Directional Terms

Term	Definition	Illustration
Leukemia Cutis	A rare condition where leukemic cells infiltrate the skin, causing lesions or nodules. It typically occurs in patients with certain types of leukemia, such as AML or CLL.	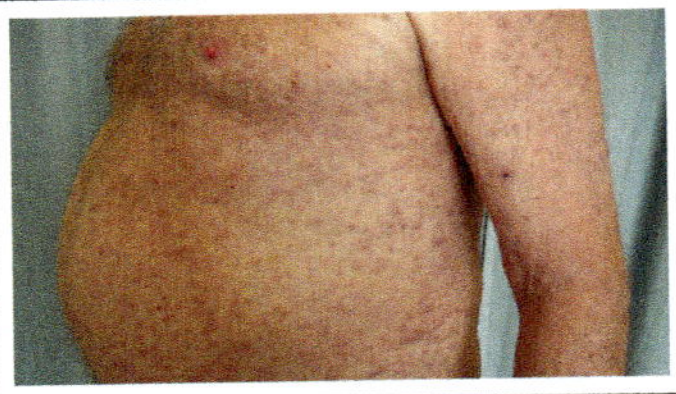
Liver	A vital organ responsible for metabolic processes including detoxification, protein synthesis, and the production of biochemicals necessary for digestion, such as bile.	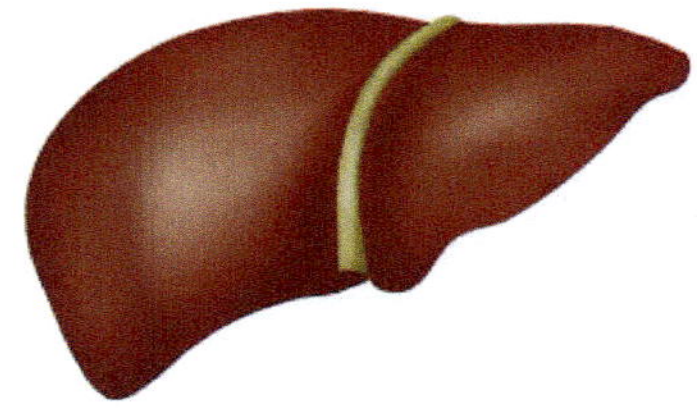
Central Nervous System (CNS)	The part of the nervous system consisting of the brain and spinal cord, responsible for processing sensory information and controlling most bodily functions and activities.	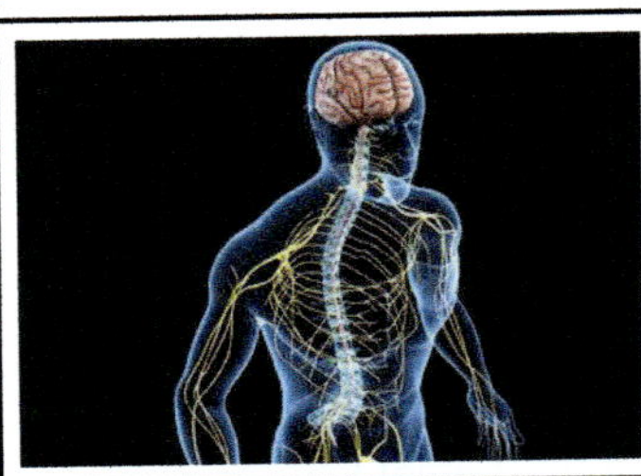
Cytology	The study of cells, especially their structure, function, and chemistry, commonly used in medical diagnostics to examine cells for signs of disease, including cancer.	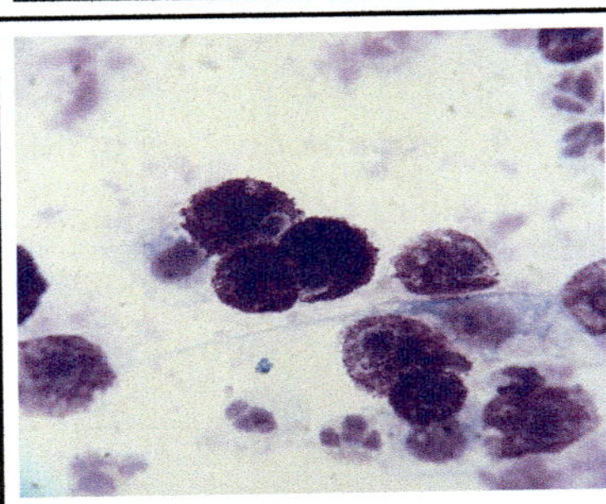
Hairy Cell Leukemia	A rare, chronic type of leukemia characterized by abnormal, "hairy" looking white blood cells that accumulate in the bone marrow, blood, and spleen, affecting immune function.	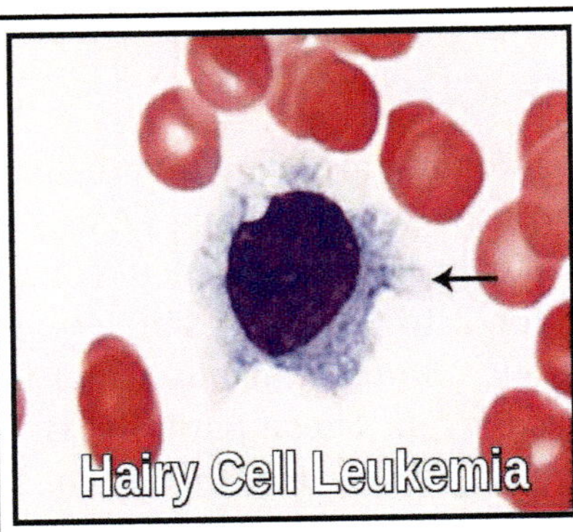

4.1. Incidence

Every year, about 6,500 children and adolescents in the United States are diagnosed with acute leukemia. AML accounts for only about 15–20% of these cases. The incidence of pediatric AML is estimated to be 5 to 7 cases per million people per year, with a peak of 11 cases per million people per year at age 2. Brown reported that the estimated incidence of infant leukemia in the United States is 41 cases per million people. The incidence of ALL in infants is significantly lower than in children aged 1 to 14 years. On the other hand, the incidence of AML in infants is about twice as high as in older children and adolescents. Women have a higher risk of developing infant leukemia than men. Juvenile myelomonocytic leukemia and the associated myeloproliferations associated with congenital syndromes such as Down syndrome and Noonan syndrome are the best known in the literature. AML in infants associated with Down syndrome is an important component of this particular subgroup (Annesley et al., 2019).

4.2. Clinical Characteristics

The typical symptoms of leukemia, such as anemia, bleeding, febrile neutropenia, organomegaly, and bone pain, are frequently observed in acute childhood leukemia. Patients usually present with more aggressive symptoms, including high initial leukocyte counts, massive organomegaly, early CNS involvement, and leukemia cutis. The developmental stage, fetal hematopoiesis, and their different origins may play a role in these different clinical features of childhood leukemias. Few researchers retrospectively analyzed 59 patients with congenital leukemia reported between 2001 and 2016 and found the following clinical features: leukemia cutis, hepatosplenomegaly (47.5%), CNS involvement (blast cells in CSF 25.4%), and spontaneous remission (11.9%). Hyperleukocytosis was found in 62.7% of cases with an average white blood cell count of 68.5 x 109 /L (normal range 4–10 x 109 /L), but anemia was less common at 35.7%. Blast cells were found in the peripheral blood and bone marrow of most patients. The risk of early death is critically high due to severe bleeding and leukostasis in patients with hyperleukocytosis (>100,000/µl). Emergency strategies include exchange transfusions and leukapheresis treatments, and they should be performed as soon as possible (Attarbaschi et al., 2006).

4.2.1. Leukemia Cutis

Leukemia cutis is a distinctive feature of neonatal AML and is frequently observed in infants with AML, whereas it is rare in ALL. Cutaneous infiltrates are present in about two-thirds of patients and may occur without peripheral blood or bone marrow involvement. Leukemia cutis typically presents as multiple papules, nodules, plaques, or subcutaneous myeloid sarcomas (Figure 4.1). These lesions may be blue, red, brown, or purple in color, and the appearance has been described as a blueberry muffin rash. Leukemia cutis is frequently observed in FAB-M4 and FAB-M5 AML. The prognosis in these cases is very poor. In the French ELAM02 cohort, skin involvement was significantly more frequent in young children, namely in 14.5% of children younger than two years compared to 2.6% of older children. One hypothesis is that chemotherapy may not be sufficient to penetrate the skin, leading to a higher incidence of relapse in these patients. On the other hand, spontaneous remissions are specific to this period, which is associated with a significant shift of hematopoiesis from liver to bone marrow, emphasizing the importance of the developmental stage in AML in the absence of known adverse prognostic factors (Boer et al., 2021).

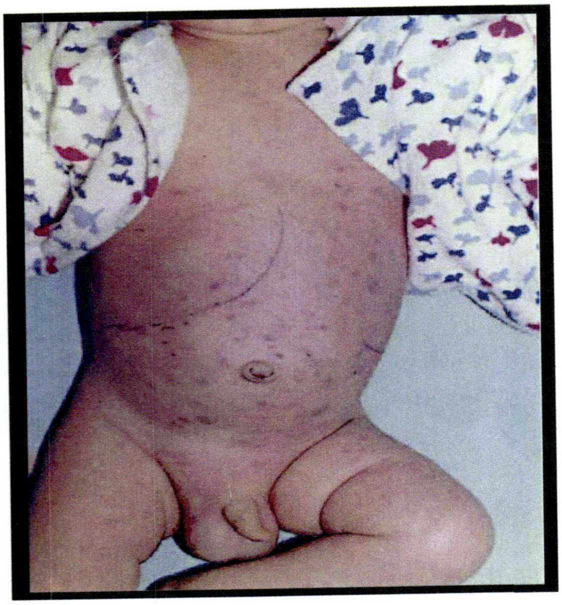

Figure 4.1. *The picture of a 4-month-old boy with infantile leukemia shows hepatosplenomegaly, leukemia cutis and scrotal swelling.*

Source: https://www.ncbi.nlm.nih.gov/books/NBK586204/figure/Ch2-f0001/.

4.2.2. Liver

Liver involvement in congenital leukemia can be prominent and sometimes dominate the clinical presentation. There are only a few documented cases where the liver was reported as the primary site of involvement in congenital leukemia. For instance, a case described a four-week-old infant diagnosed with acute megakaryoblastic leukemia, who presented with ascites due to massive infiltration of the hepatic sinusoids by leukemic cells associated with the cytogenetic abnormality t(1;22)(p13;q13).

Initially, both the bone marrow and peripheral blood smear did not show any blasts. Bone marrow fibrosis developed after the liver infiltration and liver fibrosis. Diagnosing leukemia can be challenging if the bone marrow is not affected. Additionally, patients have been reported with symptoms such as jaundice, ascites, pleural effusions, cardiopulmonary complaints, seizures, and disseminated intravascular coagulation (Bolouri et al., 2018).

4.2.3. Central Nervous System

CNS involvement is more common in childhood leukemia. According to a study by the Children's Oncology Group (COG), 35–45% of patients with CNS involvement are CNS3 (>5 blasts in the CSF or symptoms of the CNS at diagnosis). A bulging fontanel, papilledema, retinal hemorrhages, impaired consciousness, and seizures are observed. Diseases of the CNS are also more common in infants than in AML (35%–45%) and ALL (14%–41%) (Breese et al., 2021).

4.3. Cytology

Childhood leukemias have specific morphologic and immunophenotypic features. The subgroups of acute myeloblastic (FAB-M4), acute monoblastic (FAB-M5), and acute megakaryoblastic (FAB-M7) leukemia of infancy are striking features of AML according to the French–American-British (FAB) classification (Figure 4.2). AML can be diagnosed when ≥20% of blasts with myeloid markers are present in the bone marrow and are associated with the presence of recurrent cytogenetic abnormalities. Acute megakaryoblastic leukemia (AMKL) is very common in infants, but the diagnosis very challenging as the number of megakaryoblasts is quite low and difficult to detect in the peripheral blood (Brown, 2013). Bone marrow aspiration is also difficult due to fibrosis. Megakaryoblasts show cytoplasmic opacities, cell clumping, and binucleation (very rare). Megakaryoblasts are immunophenotypically positive for CD33, CD36, CD41, CD42b, and CD61. In infants with ALL, L1 subtypes are observed more frequently than L2 subtypes, while L3 subtypes do not occur. The latter are CD19-positive, HLA-DR-positive, and CD10-negative and are minimally differentiated early B-cell precursors. On the other hand, childhood leukemia patients may have an indeterminate lineage, either due to a mixed phenotype (acute leukemia with mixed phenotype) or due to a lack of differentiation markers (acute undifferentiated leukemia) (Brown et al., 2019).

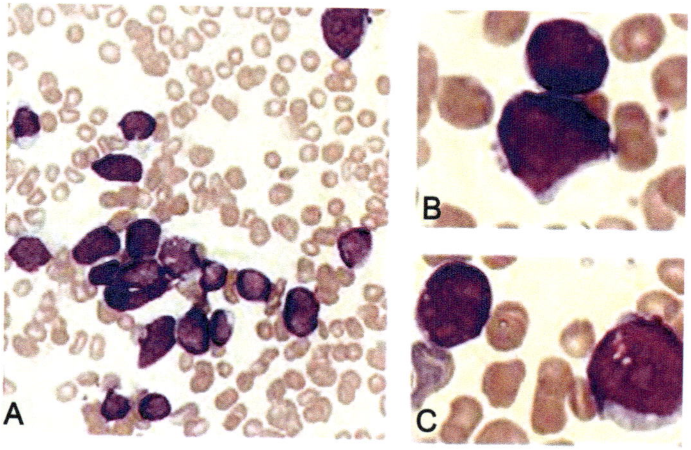

Figure 4.2. *Bone marrow smears. (A) Bone marrow smear of acute monoblastic leukemia. May-Grünwald-Gemsa staining, X100. (B) Bone marrow smear of acute myelomonoblastic leukemia. May-Grünwald-Giemsa staining, X160. And (C) at high magnification, the megakaryoblasts.*

Source: https://www.ncbi.nlm.nih.gov/books/NBK586204/.

4.4. Etiopathogenesis of Infant Leukemias

In the last 10 years, the etiopathology of leukemogenesis has been intensively researched. Genome sequencing data has enabled a better understanding of childhood leukemia. There are many remarkable publications on this topic in the literature. Many childhood leukemias show similar genetic variation to acute lymphoid or myeloid leukemias. It is clear that leukemia in neonates and infants is the result of leukemogenic events that occur in utero, with studies providing findings of indirect evidence for this hypothesis conducted on identical twins with leukemia. Monozygotic twins essentially share a hematopoietic system in utero through vascular anastomoses, and they have a concordance rate of nearly 100% for leukemia, as well as the same genetic lesion identified in both twins. Fraternal twins, who have a completely separate vascular system, do not show this extreme concordance (Brown et al., 2021). Many childhood leukemias have similar genetic alterations that indicate either lymphatic or myeloid differentiation. Cytogenetic analysis provides important information for the diagnosis, prognosis, and follow-up of patients, as well as for determining the most effective treatment protocols with minimal side effects.

4.4.1. KMT2A Rearrangements

Structural abnormalities affecting the long arm of chromosome 11, region 2, band 3 (11q23) are cytogenetic alterations that are repeatedly observed in hematopoietic malignancies, and they are the most common genetic lesion observed in childhood leukemia. A high proportion of childhood leukemia cases are characterized by chromosomal translocations affecting the histone lysine methyltransferase 2A gene (KMT2A gene, formerly known as MLL "Mixed Lineage Leukemia gene") on chromosome 11q23. KMT2A rearrangements (KMT2A-r) result in the fusion of the N-terminus of the KMT2A gene with the C-terminus of a partner gene; approximately 135 different KMT2A partner genes have been identified. KMT2A-r, which was first discovered in patients with ALL and then AML, is the most common cytogenetic abnormality in childhood leukemias (Caslini et al., 2007). The KMT2A gene regulates hematopoietic differentiation and plays an important role in leukemogenesis. The t(4;11)(q21;q23) or t(11;19)(q23;p13) occurs in most cases of ALL, while t(9;11)(q22;p23) is the most frequent translocation in patients with AML. KMT2A-r is observed in approximately 40–60% of infants with AML, and rare translocations have also been identified for this age group, including t(1;22) and t(7;12) (Cheung et al., 2023).

KMT2A fusion proteins are potent oncoproteins that regulate leukemogenesis in infants with few cooperating mutations; fetal and neonatal hematopoietic progenitors may be more sensitive to KMT2A proteins. In childhood ALL, four partner genes were identified in 93% of patients: aFF1 (49%), MLLT1 (22%), MLLT3 (17%) and MLLT10 (5%). In childhood AML, three partner genes were identified in 66% of patients: mLLT3 (22%), MLLT10 (27%), and ELL (17%). Most of these KMT2A rearrangements in AML are morphologically classified as FAB-M4 or FAB-M5. A KMT2A fusion can also be observed in AMKL. KMT2A-r leukemias frequently occur in two distinct clinical presentations: (i) in infants with de novo acute AML or ALL and (ii) in patients with treatment-related AML after exposure to DNA topoisomerase II inhibitors. The growing fetus is more sensitive to the effects of potential DNA damage in the early stages of pregnancy. Transplacental exposures to DNA topoisomerase inhibitors may be related to the etiology of acute leukemias in children with KTM2A-r. Topoisomerase inhibitors include chemotherapeutic agents, benzene metabolites such as benzoquinone, isoflavones, flavonoids, lignans, podophyllin resin, quinolone antibiotics, and some pesticides (Clements et al., 2020).

KMT2A has different prognostic implications for ALL in infants less than 12 months of age depending on the presence or absence of KTM2A-r. Infants with ALL and KMT2A-r do not achieve remission, while the prognosis and survival of ALL infants without KMT2A-r are comparable to ALL in older children. In patients with CMT2A-r ALL, additional independent prognostic factors include age and white blood cell count at diagnosis – younger infants and those with higher white blood cell counts have a poorer prognosis. In childhood AML, KMT2A-r is not a significant risk factor, and are morphologically classified as FAB-M4 or FAB-M5. KMT2A-r is also frequently associated with megakaryoblastic leukemia in infants (Clesham et al., 2020).

Acute megakaryoblastic leukemia is common in infants with AML and is associated with other chromosomal translocations such as t(1;22)(p13; q13) and inv(16)(p13.3, q24.3). The fusion of GLIS2 with CBFA2T3 as a result of inv(16)(p13.3, q24.3) is the most frequently identified chimeric oncogene in AMKL patients to date. Patients with a CBFA2T3-GLIS2 fusion gene are only found in patients aged <3 years, and it is the second most common gene in cases aged less than one year (Diaz-Flores et al., 2019). Core-binding factor rearrangements are uncommon in infants. Infants with Down syndrome have an increased risk of leukemia, particularly acute megakaryoblastic leukemia, which usually resolves spontaneously and is referred to as transient neonatal myelopoiesis or transient abnormal myelopoiesis. The underlying genetic lesion is a mutation in the N-terminal region of the erythroid/megakaryocytic transcription factor GATA-1, which is located on the short arm of chromosome X. A mutation of GATA-1 is pathognomonic for transient leukemia and acute megakaryoblastic leukemia in children with Down syndrome.

Dysregulation of HOX genes is a common feature of AML.hOX genes play a key role in the regulation of hematopoietic development. In leukemia, dysregulated HOX gene expression can occur due to chromosomal translocations affecting upstream regulators such as KMT2A. Translocations of 11q23 occur in approximately 5–10% of adult AML, one to three years after treatment with chemotherapy regimens containing anthracyclines or other topoisomerase II inhibitors.

Transient neonatal myelopoiesis is a rare disease in the neonatal period that is associated with trisomy of chromosome 21. It is characterized by a high number of blast cells in the peripheral blood and bone marrow, and usually disappears within 1 to 3 months without specific therapy. Some reported a transient leukemia with an isolated pericardial effusion in a phenotypically normal newborn. Trisomy 21 was found on blast cells. Congenital leukemia associated with trisomy 21 on blast cells has a good prognosis. Independent unfavorable prognostic features are age < 1 month, leukemia cutis, initial high white blood cell count, poor response to induction chemotherapy, and the presence of KMT2A-r. Due to the destructive nature of childhood leukemia, no curative results could be achieved with standard chemotherapy regimens (Dreyer et al., 2015).

4.4.2. Other Factors

Maternal alcohol consumption during pregnancy, marijuana use, and paternal smoking one month before pregnancy are associated with an increased risk of childhood leukemia. Ross et al. showed that high birth weight is a significant risk factor for the development of childhood leukemia. Insulin-like growth factor 1 is important for blood formation and regulation and has been shown to stimulate the growth of myeloid and lymphoid cells in culture. It has been postulated that high levels of insulin-like growth factor-1 could produce large babies and contribute to the development of leukemia. Emerenciano et al. reported that there is a significant association between the risk of leukemia in infants and maternal hormone intake during pregnancy (Du et al., 2021).

4.5. Hairy Cell Leukemia

Hairy cell leukemia (HCL) is a rare, indolent B-cell neoplasm. It is characterized by the progressive infiltration of mature lymphocytes with typical "hairy" projections in the peripheral blood (PB), bone marrow (BM) and spleen, leading to pancytopenia, splenomegaly and susceptibility to infection. A characteristic molecular feature of the disease, which occurs in ≥95% of cases, is the somatic BRAFV600E mutation. It is important to distinguish between classic HCL and HCL-like diseases, which include unclassifiable splenic B-cell lymphoma/ leukemia, as well as the variant form of HCL (HCL-v) and diffuse splenic red cell lymphoma (SDRPL). Monocytopenia is characteristic of classic HCL.

In HCL-v, the neoplastic lymphoid cells are hybrids with an intermediate morphology between prolymphocytes and hair cells. In SDRPL, the villous lymphoid cells have a polar distribution in the villi and a small or undetectable nucleolus in the PB. HCL-v is characterized by lymphocytosis with relatively large lymphoid cells, prominent nucleoli and cytopenias without monocytopenia. In HCL-v and SDRPL, the neoplastic cells do not express CD25 or CD123, and the BRAFV600E mutation is absent. However, the relationship between HCL-v and SDRPL remains unclear. In this chapter, we focus on the pathogenesis, laboratory and clinical features and treatment of classical HCL (El Chaer et al., 2020).

4.5.1. Epidemiology

Hairy cell leukemia accounts for less than 2% of all leukemias. The incidence is 0.3 cases per 100,000 people with an average male-to-female ratio of 1.5–2:1 and a median age at diagnosis of 58 years. The incidence in the white population is about three times higher than in the black population. The incidence of HCL-v is estimated at 0.2 cases per 100,000. HCL-v mainly affects older patients with an average age of 71 years (Fazio et al., 2021).

4.5.2. Pathogenesis

The pathogenesis of HCL is not fully understood. Exposure to ionizing radiation, pesticides, and agricultural activity have been mentioned as possible causes, and cases of HCL in family members with the same HLA haplotype have been reported. In most patients, HCL arises from a late-activated memory B cell harboring a single somatic point mutation in the DNA sequence of v-Raf murine sarcoma viral oncogene homolog B (BRAF), a kinase-encoding proto-oncogene (BRAFV600E).

The BRAFV600E mutation is detected in up to 80–90% of classic HCL patients. The mutation is a thymine-adenine transversion at a nucleotide in exon 15 of BRAF at position 1799 of the gene coding sequence on chromosome 7q34. The exchange leads to an amino acid change from valine (V) to glutamate (E) at position 600 (V600E) of the protein sequence, which ultimately leads to abnormal activation of BRAF kinase and downstream MEK-ERK signaling. In fact, the BRAFV600E mutation has been found more or less ubiquitously in studies of hundreds of classical HCL patients. The BRAFV600E mutation itself is clonal and heterozygous, although a minority of patients lose the wild-type allele as a result of concomitant 7q deletion. The mutation remains stable throughout the course of the disease, from initial diagnosis to relapses, which can occur many years after initial presentation. The mutation is responsible for continuous BRAF activation, which in turn activates the RAS–RAF–MEK–ERK signaling pathway, whose abnormal activation causes a particular phenotype and promotes HCL cell survival (Ford et al., 1993).

Besides the BRAFV600E mutation, the most common genetic alteration in classical HCL is a loss of the copy number of chromosome 7qchromosome7q. A mutated gene profile of the immunoglobulin heavy chain variable region (IGHV) is detected in 90% of HCL patients. The absence of a BRAF mutation (BRAFWT) is associated with the activation of mutations in the mitogen-activated protein kinase 1 (MAP2K1) gene by non-mutated IGHV and VH4-34 rearrangements; this small subset of classical HCL patients has a poor prognosis and responds poorly to nucleoside purine analogs (PNAs). In addition, a whole-exome sequencing study in patients with classical HCL confirmed the presence of several cancer-associated genes, including EZH2 and ARID1A, as well as novel inactivating mutations of the cell cycle inhibitor CDKN1B. CDKN1B is the second most frequently mutated gene in HCL (Forgione et al., 2020).

4.5.3. Clinical Presentation

In most cases of HCL, patients are asymptomatic, with pancytopenia discovered incidentally during a routine blood count. When they are symptomatic, they typically present with symptoms related to worsening pancytopenia (fatigue, bruising, bleeding gums, epistaxis, menorrhagia), splenomegaly (abdominal fullness, increasing discomfort after eating), and recurrent infections. Rare clinical manifestations include polyarteritis nodosa, cutaneous leukocytoclastic vasculitis, bone involvement, or CNS involvement.

The typical hair cells are usually found in the peripheral blood and BM smear (Figures 4.3 and 4.4). These are medium-sized lymphoid cells with abundant pale blue cytoplasm, small cytoplasmic projections, and a mature-looking nucleus that gives the cell the appearance of a "fried egg." However, it is often difficult to aspirate BM as it is highly fibrotic due to the infiltration of leukemic hair cells (dry tap). A trephine biopsy is indicated to confirm a diagnosis of HCL. The BM biopsy specimen typically shows massive infiltration by cells characterized by a broad rim of pale-stained cytoplasm surrounding and separating the drab, bland hair cell nuclei, as well as well-preserved cytoplasmic margins that enhance the "fried egg" appearance (Figure 4.5). The characteristic pattern of infiltration, which is interstitial, diffuse, or patchy, allows differentiation from other B-cell lymphoid malignancies, in which lymphoid cells with densely packed nuclei usually aggregate or form focal nodules. The nucleus is round, oval, or slightly jagged. The Ki-67 value is very low. Silver staining shows an increase in reticulin fibers. Infiltrating hair cells often disrupt the bone marrow microvasculature, leading to extravasation of red blood cells and the formation of pseudosinus and blood lakes. A more accurate assessment of the extent of infiltration can be made by immunohistochemical staining. HCL cells are typically positive for B cell-associated antigens such as CD20, but also for Annexin-1 and VE1. Cases with hypocellular BM have also been reported, and therefore special caution is required to avoid misdiagnosis with aplastic anemia (George et al., 1973).

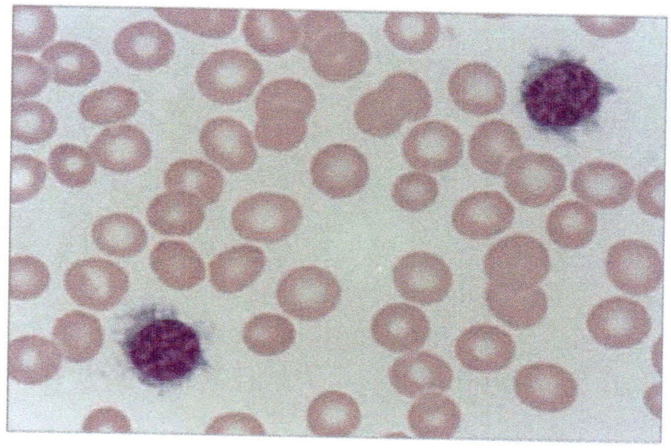

Figure 4.3. *Morphological features of classic HCL cells with small- to medium-sized cells with oval to indented nucleus and circumferential cytoplasmic projections.*

Source: https://www.ncbi.nlm.nih.gov/books/NBK586203/figure/Ch3-f0001/.

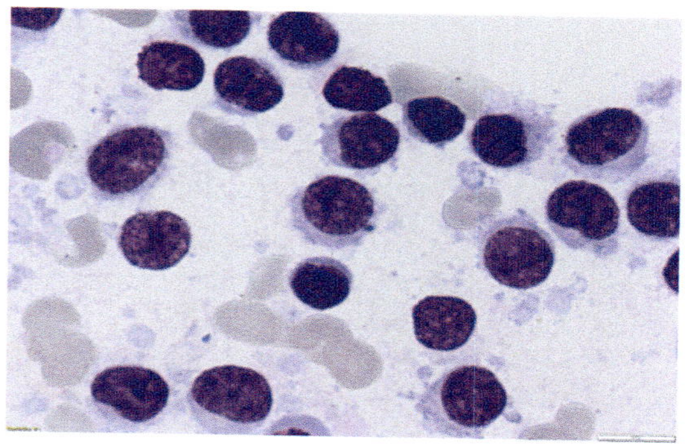

Figure 4.4. *Bone marrow smear in classic HCL.*

Source: https://www.researchgate.net/publication/364588454/figure/fig2/AS:11431281185043144@1693506505063/Bone-marrow-smear-in-classic-HCL.png.

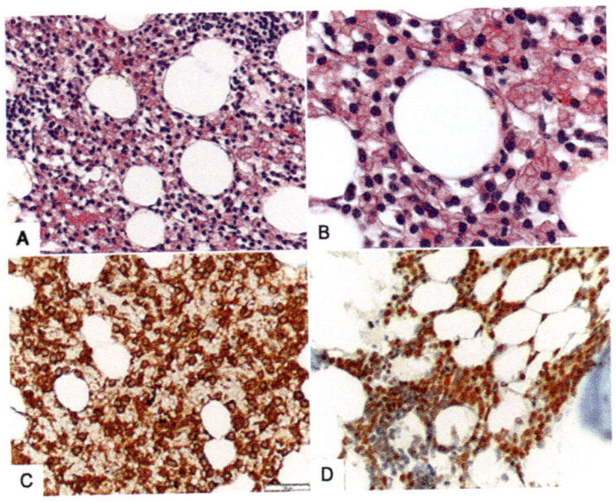

Figure 4.5. The histology of bone marrow involved by hairy cell leukemia with diffuse infiltration by regular, small cells (A, B); strongly expressing CD20 (C); and CD25 (D).

Source: https://www.researchgate.net/publication/364588454/figure/fig3/AS:114312811849895 45@1693506505297/The-histology-of-bone-marrow-involved-by-hairy-cell-leukemia-with-diffuse-infiltration-by.ppm.

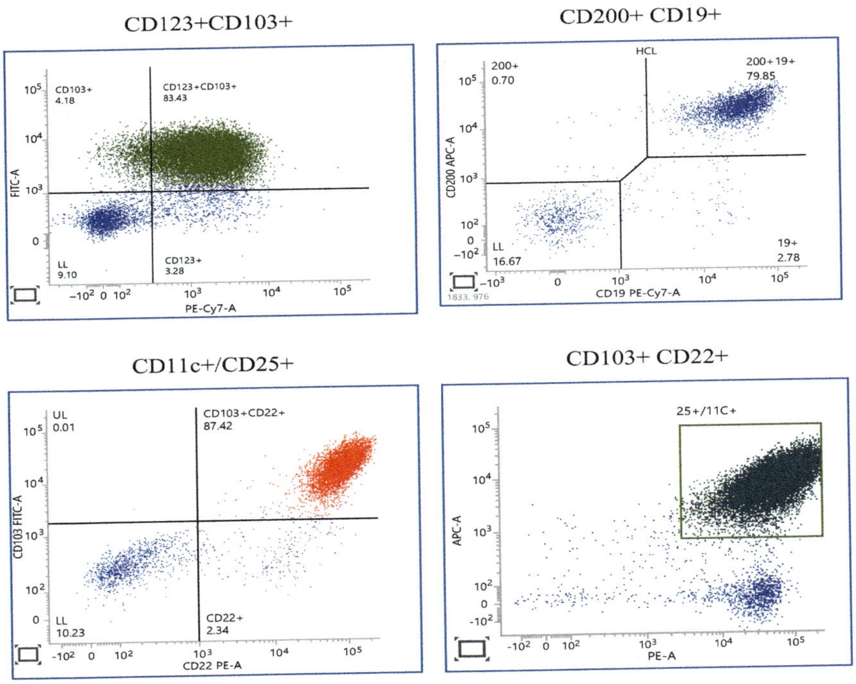

Figure 4.6. Classic HCL-phenotype on flow cytometry: CD11c+, CD103+, CD123+CD22+, CD25+, and CD200+ cells.

Source: https://www.ncbi.nlm.nih.gov/books/NBK586203/figure/Ch3-f0004/.

Immunophenotypic analysis is crucial for the diagnosis. HCL cells show a mature B-cell phenotype, with immunoglobulins on the surface with restricted light chains. They strongly express pan-B cell antigens, including CD19, CD20, and CD22, as well as the hair-specific antigens CD11c, CD25, CD103, and CD123 (light) (Figure 4.6). The staining for CD200 is intense. A large proportion of HCL also expresses annexin A1, which is not expressed in any other type of B-cell neoplasm. HCL-v is usually negative for annexin A1, which can be a helpful distinguishing feature. However, since it is also expressed by myeloid cells and some T cells, staining for annexin A1 must be interpreted in conjunction with staining for a B cell antigen (Gore et al., 2018).

Although 96% of patients with HCL have an enlarged spleen, diagnostic or therapeutic splenectomy is rarely performed nowadays due to the obvious BM involvement. Histologically, the disease is associated with enlargement of the red pulp areas and severe atrophy of the white pulp. The normal splenic architecture of cords and sinusoids is destroyed by the infiltration with hair cells, which leads to the formation of blood lakes and pseudosinus. The HCL infiltrate is histologically similar to that described in the bone marrow. The lymph nodes are rarely enlarged and are therefore rarely examined by pathologists. Infiltration of the nodes is usually limited to retroperitoneal and abdominal nodes. Hairy cells infiltrate the cortex and the medullary cord regions, while the sinuses are typically intact and the follicular structures are spared (Gruber et al., 2022).

4.5.4. Treatment of Classic HCL

The diagnosis of HCL does not necessarily mean that treatment is initiated in all patients. In fact, asymptomatic patients with moderate pancytopenia may remain stable and asymptomatic for years. Such cases should be carefully monitored as outpatients until the blood cell count begins to decline. The frequency of visits must be adapted to the patient's clinical condition. To ensure safe monitoring, the patient should also have a broad knowledge of the symptoms (Guenther et al., 2005).

However, symptomatic patients should receive treatment for HCL. Indications for initiating treatment include symptomatic splenomegaly, constitutive symptoms, recurrent infections, and/or at least one significant cytopenia (absolute neutrophil count <1,000/μL, hemoglobin concentration <11 g/dL or platelet count <100,000/μL). Given the myelosuppressive effect of PNAs, it seems advisable to start treatment before the values fall to a dangerous level (Guest et al., 2022).

4.5.5. First-Line Treatment

The purine nucleoside analogs cladribine (2-chlorodeoxyadenosine, 2-CdA) and pentostatin (deoxycoformycin, DCF) remain the standard first-line treatment for HCL, and their development is still considered one of the greatest achievements in cancer therapy (Table 4.1). Although 2-CdA and DCF have never been directly compared, the two agents show similar long-term efficacy and toxicity results.

However, 2-CdA is more comfortable for patients due to the shorter duration of treatment and is therefore used more frequently than DCF. In a study conducted at the Scripps Clinic in San Diego in 1990, all 12 patients responded to treatment, and 11 achieved complete remissions (CR). Retrospective studies report overall response rates (ORR) of > 95% and a complete remission (CR) rate of > 75%, with median relapse-free survival (RFS) of up to 15 years. Many patients who were first treated with PNA are still alive 30 years later and are in their first CR. A recently published European multicenter meta-analysis confirmed the high efficacy of 2-CdA as a first-line treatment. Data from 384 patients treated between 1969 and 2018 showed an ORR of 94, which was comparable to previous analyzes, and a median OS of 25 years. The median PFS was

13 years, but more importantly, 43% of patients were still free of disease progression after 22 years (Guest et al., 2022).

Table 4.1. *Selected Clinical Trials of First-Line Treatment with PNAs with Prolonged Follow-Up in Classical Hairy Cell Leukemia*

Study	Treatment	No. of pts/ Follow-Up	Response	Response Duration and OS
Saven et al. (1998)	2-CdA 0.087 or 0.1 mg/kg/d ci × 7 days.	349/ median 52 m	ORR 98%, CR 91%, PR 7%	Median PFS for all responders 52 m, for CR 53 m, for PR 37 m.
Goodman et al. (2003)	-C A 0.1 mg/kg/d ci × 7 days.	207/NA	ORR 100%, CR 95%, PR 5% 95%/ Median 98 m.	Median PFS for all responders 98 m, OS 97% at 108 months.
Cheson et al. (1998)	2-CdA 0.1 mg/kg/d ci × 7 days.	861/ median 52 m	CR 50%, PR 37%	Median PFS > 44 m (range 1–63 + m)
Broccoli et al. (2022)	2-CdA sc or iv	384/ median 8.5 yrs	CR 72%, PR 22%	Median PFS 13 years, median OS not reached at 25 years.
Inbar et al. (2018)	2-CDA i.v. (62%) or sc (38%) × 5 days.	203/ median 5.2 yrs	NR.	OS at 10-year 94%, and at 20 yrs 75%
Broccoli et al. (2021)	2-CdA 0.14 mg/kg sc or iv, for 5–7 days or once a week for 5 weeks.	122/ followed between 1986 and 2018	ORR 86%, CR 54%	Median TTNT – 8.2 years, for PR 5.3 years; for CR median NR at 25.8 years, median OS NR; probability of 65.7% alive at 25 years.
Grever et al. (1995)	DCF 2–4 mg/m^2 iv biweekly	154/ median 57 m	OR 79%, PR 76%	Median RFS 82 m
Else et al. (2009)	DCF 4 mg/m^2 iv biweekly	188/ median 14.0 yrs	OR96%, CR82%	Median PFS 10.5 yrs; Median RFS 16 yrs; OS at 15 yrs 78%.

Cladribine is administered according to different regimens and by different routes. Initially, 2-CdA was administered at a dose of 0.1 mg/kg/d over seven days as a continuous intravenous infusion (Hilden et al., 2006). However, the plasma concentration of 2-CdA does not differ between a two-hour and a continuous infusion, so in most cases, the drug is administered as a two-hour intravenous or subcutaneous infusion. In addition, treatment with weekly 2-CdA infusions is as effective as the standard 5-day administration of 2-CdA. Currently, 2-CdA is usually administered at a dose of 0.12–0.14 mg/kg/day as a two-hour intravenous infusion over five to seven days or at a dose of 0.12–0.15 mg/kg/day as a two-hour intravenous infusion once a week over six doses.

Treatment with 2-CdA may be complicated by fever occurring during or shortly after therapy without other infectious symptoms or marked worsening of the general clinical condition; this is usually attributed to the release of cytokines associated with the rapid lysis of circulating hair cells. In addition, neutropenia and infections may occur as symptoms of the natural course of the disease. On the other hand, these symptoms may also occur as a consequence of the administration of PNA and its myelosuppressive and/or immunosuppressive effects (Ibrahimova et al., 2021). A complete diagnostic work-up and the immediate use of broad-spectrum antibiotics in combination with granulocyte colony-stimulating factor are usually indicated. Cladribine is contraindicated in patients with an active infection, and it is recommended to treat infections before starting treatment with PNA if possible. If immediate initiation of treatment is required, DCF at a reduced dose or interferon alpha (IFN-α) must be considered. Recently, BRAF inhibitors have been reported to be effective and safe in patients with newly diagnosed classical hairy cell leukemia and active infection.

If PNAs are contraindicated, the BRAF inhibitors vemurafenib or dabrafenib can be used off-label in patients with neutropenia and infections. They can also be used prior to PNA therapy; in such cases, PNA therapy should be considered after improvement in blood cell counts and recovery from infection to achieve the best possible response in the treatment of HCL.

Another option for the treatment of HCL patients is the use of 2-CdA administered concurrently with eight weekly doses of rituximab, or with rituximab administered at least six months later, depending on minimal residual disease (MRD) status. In patients treated with 2-CdA and rituximab at the same time, the cure rate was 94%, and MRD was undetectable for a median of 6.5 years. However, this treatment is more recommended for patients who have relapsed or are refractory to PNA monotherapy (Isoyama et al., 2002).

Pentostatin is usually administered at a dose of 4 mg/m^2 as an intravenous bolus injection or diluted in a larger volume and administered over 20 to 30 minutes once every two weeks. In the absence of severe toxicity and sustained improvement, treatment should be continued until hematologic CR, with two additional doses after CR. In patients with active infection or other increased risk of mortality or morbidity due to myelosuppression, the pentostatin dose may be reduced to 2 mg/m^2 until clinical improvement occurs, with subsequent administration of standard doses.

Today, there are only limited indications for the use of IFN-α in first-line treatment. The responses induced by IFN-α are partial and short-lived. Most patients eventually relapse, with the median duration of response ranging from 6 to 25 months. IFN-α can be used temporarily to increase neutrophil counts and cure infections before initiating treatment with PNA. Another potential indication for IFN-α treatment is the COVID-19 pandemic to avoid the severe immunosuppression associated with the use of PNA and rituximab. Splenectomy is a life-saving procedure for splenic rupture due to splenomegaly. In patients who are refractory to IFN-α, it can also be performed during pregnancy.

4.5.6. Treatment of Relapsed/Refractory HCL

Despite the remarkable success of PNA, half of the patients suffer at least one relapse of the disease later in life (Issa et al., 2023). Therefore, new therapeutic strategies are still needed to further improve PFS. In case of relapse, the same indications for treatment apply as for first-line therapy, including symptomatic disease or progressive cytopenias. Patients with early relapse are candidates for alternative therapies, preferably with new drugs or in clinical trials. After 24–60 months of remission, re-treatment with PNA in combination with rituximab should be considered. The addition of rituximab to 2-CdA at the standard dose of 375 mg/m^2 weekly for 6–8 doses, either simultaneously or sequentially one month after 2-CdA, may improve the outcome. Finally, patients who have been in CR for more than five years (> 60 months) can be continued on the original therapy (Karol et al., 2019).

Bendamustine (70 mg/m^2 or 90 mg/m^2) in combination with rituximab (375 mg/m^2), administered intravenously on days 1 and 15, for six cycles at four-week intervals, showed efficacy in 12 heavily pretreated HCL patients. The overall response rate was 100%, with seven CRs. MRD was undetectable in six patients with CRs after 30–35 (median 31) months of follow-up.

4.5.7. Moxetumomab Pasudotox

Moxetumomab pasudotox (Moxe) was originally discovered by Ira Pastan and Robert Kreitman at the National Cancer Institute, Center for Cancer Research. Moxe is an anti-CD22 recombinant immunotoxin produced by fusing a toxin fragment, *Pseudomonas* exotoxin A (PE38), with the Fv of the murine anti-CD22 antibody, thereby delivering the toxin directly to the tumor cell. The drug was effective and well tolerated in phase 1 and 3 studies in relapsed/refractory patients with HCL. In the phase 1/2 study, Moxe was used at a dose of 50 μg/kg every other day for three doses in four-week cycles. In the 33 patients analyzed, the OR rate was 88%, with 64% CR. The duration of CR was longer in MRD-negative patients. The median CR duration was 13.5 months in nine MRD-positive CRs and 42.1 months in 11 MRD-negative CRs (Keating et al., 2019).

In a phase 3 study, 80 patients were treated with Moxe at a dose of 40 μg/kg by 30-minute intravenous infusion on days 1, 3, and 5 of a 28-day cycle. Treatment was either continued for up to six cycles or until CR with MRD negativity, disease progression, or unacceptable toxicity. After a median follow-up of 24.6 months, 60 patients (75%) had responded to treatment, 27 of whom had an MRD-negative CR. The rate of durable CR with a hematologic response of more than 180 days was 36% and CR of more than 360 days was 33%. A longer median hematologic remission was observed in MRD-negative patients (62.8 months) than in MRD-positive patients (12.0 months). Poorer results were observed in splenectomized patients. There is a single report of successful re-treatment with Moxe in relapsed patients (Khaw et al., 2016).

The most common adverse events (AEs) were easily manageable nausea, peripheral edema, headache, and pyrexia. Hemolytic uremic syndrome (HUS) and capillary leak syndrome (CLS) are black box warnings for Moxe, which occurred in eight patients (10%) before or on day 8 of treatment and led to discontinuation of the drug. Therefore, careful clinical and laboratory monitoring is required during treatment. Adequate oral and intravenous hydration is recommended to avoid life-threatening complications. All patients should receive intravenous fluids two to four hours before and after Moxe administration. On days 1 to 8 of each 28-day cycle, all patients should be provided with oral fluids, 250 ml per hour, and should not go more than two to three hours without drinking at night. Thrombosis prophylaxis with low-dose aspirin is also considered.

Moxe was approved by the US Food and Drug Administration (FDA – September 2018) and the European Medicines Agency (EMA – February 2021) for the treatment of adult patients with relapsed/refractory HCL who have received at least two prior systemic therapies, including treatment with purine analogs. However, in July 2021, the European Commission withdrew the marketing authorization for Moxe in the European Union. The withdrawal was made at the request of the marketing authorization holder, AstraZeneca, for commercial reasons. Moxe is still commercially available in the USA (Koh et al., 2015).

4.5.8. BRAF Inhibitors

The BRAFV600E mutation, the driving genetic event in HCL, provided the scientific basis for the therapeutic use of BRAF-MEK pathway inhibitors in patients with classical HCL. The BRAF kinase inhibitors vemurafenib and dabrafenib are active drugs in patients with refractory and relapsed HCL; they can be used as monotherapy or in combination with CD20 antibodies or MEK inhibitors (Table 4.2). In a single-arm multicenter phase 2 study conducted in Italy and the US, vemurafenib was administered as a single agent at a dose of 960 mg twice daily for a median of 16–18 weeks. Most of the patients responded to treatment. The overall response rate was 96% after a median of eight weeks in Italian patients and 100% after a median of 12 weeks in the USA. The complete response rate was 34.6% and 41.7%, respectively. However, all CRs were MRD-positive and the median RFS was only nine months after discontinuation of treatment (Kosaka et al., 2004).

Table 4.2. *Larger Clinical Trials with Novel Agents in Hairy Cell Leukemia*

Study	Treatment Regimen	No. of pts/ Characteristics	Response	Response Duration and OS
Kreitman et al. (2018, 2021)	Moxetumomab pasudotox 40 µg/kg i.v. on days 1, 3, and 5 every 28 days for ≤6 cycles.	80/cHCL or HCL-v after ≥2 prior therapies.	ORR – 80%, CR – 41%; CR MRD negative – 85%.	Median PFS 71.7 m for CR lasting ≥ 60 months, CR with HR ≥ 360 days –33%.
Tiacci et al. (2015)	Vemurafenib 960 mg p.o. twice daily for 16 or 18.	50/cHCL, R/R after PNA.	Italian study: ORR – 96%, CR – 35%, U.S. study: OR –100%, CR –42%.	Italian study: RFS 19 m; U.S. study: 1-year PFS 73% and 1-year OS 91%.
Dietrich et al. (2016)	Vemurafenib 240–1920 mg/d p.o. for median 90 days.	21/cHCL, median TFD 8 yrs.	ORR 95%, CR 40%.	Median EFS 17 m, OS at 12 m –88%.
Tiaccci et al. (2021)	Vemurafenib 960 mg p.o. twice daily for 8 weeks + rituximab 375 mg/m^2 i.v. every two weeks.	30/c HCL with a median of 3 previous therapies.	CR – 26/30 (87%), MRD negative CR 17 (65%).	PFS for median follow-up of 37 m 78%, RFS for median follow-up of 37 m 85%.

Tiaccci et al. (2021)	Dabrafenib 150 mg p.o. twice daily for 8–12 weeks.	10/RR cHCL, median 3.5 prior there therapies.	ORR 80%, CR 30%, PR – 50%.	OS 90% at median follow-up 64 m.
Kreitman et al. (2018)	Dabrafenib 150 mg p.o. twice daily) + trametinib 2 mg p.o. once daily.	43/RR cHCL (49% received ≥ 4 prior treatments).	ORR – 32/41 (78%); CR – 20 (49%), PR 12 (29%).	PFS and OS at 1 year – 97.6%.
Rogers et al. (2021)	Ibrutinib: 420 mg – 840 mg p.o. daily-10.	37/ cHCL –28 (76%) HCL-v – 9(24%).	ORR (CR and PR) at 32 weeks 24% and at 48 weeks 54%.	Estimated 3 yrs. – PFS rate – 73% and OS rate – 85%, median OS – 69 months.

Drug-related adverse effects were mostly grade 1–2 and included skin toxicity (rash, photosensitivity), arthralgia, fever, and increased bilirubin levels. All adverse events were reversible and easily managed by dose adjustments and symptomatic treatments, including low-dose steroids and non-steroidal anti-inflammatory drugs. However, approximately 50% of patients required dose adjustment due to adverse events. Originally, the dosing and scheduling of BRAF inhibitors was extrapolated from standard melanoma treatment and remains controversial. Based on retrospective analysis of patients treated with variable dosing regimens outside of clinical trials, we already know that BRAF inhibitors induce hematologic remission in all HCL patients, regardless of the dose used. However, higher doses of BRAF inhibitors (vemurafenib > 480 mg BID, dabrafenib > 150 mg BID) improve the quality of responses and prolong the time to the next treatment (TNT) compared to low-dose BRAF inhibitors. Re-treatment with BRAF inhibitors is only as effective after the second cycle, but the response decreases with each subsequent cycle, with a median TNT of less than four months. In cases where BRAF inhibitors are the only available treatment option, continuous treatment with low-dose BRAF inhibitors should be considered as it may allow stabilization of the disease for more than one year (Kotecha et al., 2014).

A deeper and longer response can be achieved when vemurafenib is combined with rituximab. In a phase 2 study in patients with refractory or relapsed HCL, vemurafenib was administered at a dose of 960 mg BID for eight weeks and rituximab at a dose of 375 mg/m^2 every two weeks for eight weeks. A CR was achieved in 26 out of 30 patients. In addition, 17 of 26 patients with CR were found to have undetectable MRD. MRD negativity correlated with longer survival without relapse (Krivtsov et al., 2019). This excellent response correlated with PFS, which was 78% at a median follow-up of 37 months. In addition, this drug combination appears to be effective in patients previously treated with Moxe. In a Phase 2 study, vemurafenib was also combined with Obinutuzumab in previously untreated HCL patients. Vemurafenib was administered at a dose of 960 mg twice daily for four months, Obinutuzumab at a dose of 1,000 mg intravenously on days 1, 8, and 15 of the second month, and on day 1 of months 3 and 4. MRD-negative CR was achieved in seven patients and PR was observed in two patients at the end of treatment. All patients remained in remission with a median follow-up of 9.7 months (Leahy et al., 2022).

Another BRAF inhibitor, dabrafenib, was investigated in a phase 2 study in relapsed/refractory patients with classical HCL. Dabrafenib was administered at a dose of 150 mg twice daily for eight weeks. If no CR was achieved after this time, patients received a further four weeks of treatment. The ORR was 80% and the CR was 30%. The combination of BRAF inhibitors with MEK inhibitors is another strategy to improve treatment efficacy. In a phase 2 study, dabrafenib was administered continuously at a dose of 150 mg BID with tramentinib 2 mg, once daily. A response was achieved in 78% of patients (Lee et al., 2022). The PFS and OS rates after 12 months were 97.6% each, and the PFS rate after 18 months was 50%. However, side effects led to a dose reduction in 42% of patients and an interruption of treatment in 56 months.

4.5.9. Ibrutinib

The B cell receptor signaling pathway is a critical pathway of B cells, both for their survival and for surface-mediated activation, proliferation, and differentiation. The BCR signaling pathway is also involved in the pathogenesis of HCL. Recently, ibrutinib was evaluated in a Phase 2 study in 37 HCL patients, including 28 with classical HCL and nine with HCL-v. Ibrutinib was administered at a dose of 420–840 mg daily until disease progression or unacceptable toxicity. The response rate was 24% after 32 weeks and 36% after 48 weeks. The OR rate at each time point was 54%, including seven CR, 13 PR, and 10 patients with stable disease. Similar response rates were observed in patients with classic HCL and HCL-v. Estimated 36-month PFS was 73% and OS was 85%, with no differences between HCL and HCL-v. Although the results are not as spectacular as with other new drugs, ibrutinib remains an option for patients for whom other treatments are not an option (Li et al., 2023).

4.6. Hairy Cell Leukemia Variant

Variant hairy cell leukemia (HCL-v) is a rare lymphoproliferative B-cell neoplasm that occurs or is localized mainly in the spleen; it is biologically distinct from classical HCL, is more aggressive, and responds poorly to PNAs. In the fifth edition of the WHO classification of hematolymphoid tumors (2022), HCL-v and prolymphocytic B-cell leukemia are reclassified as splenic B-cell lymphoma/leukemia with prominent nucleoli. The clinical course of HCL-v is more aggressive than that of classic HCL with a median OS of 7–9 years. Morphologically, HCL-v cells show hybrid features between classical HCL cells and prolymphocytes. The nuclei have a prominent nucleolus, similar to prolymphocytes, and the cytoplasm often has a variable number of cytoplasmic projections. Patients are usually symptomatic, with symptoms of anemia and/or bleeding depending on the cytopenia and with abdominal discomfort associated with splenomegaly (Mann et al., 2010). The white blood count is elevated, with lymphocytosis in the PB smear, accompanied by anemia and thrombocytopenia. The absolute monocyte count is normal in contrast to classic HCL. The BM is hypercellular and can be easily aspirated. Peripheral lymphadenopathy is rare, but central lymphadenopathy with enlarged abdominal and retroperitoneal lymph nodes can be detected on CT scans. Hepatomegaly is reported in 20–30% of cases.

A crucial aspect of HCL-v diagnosis is the immunophenotype. Leukemic cells strongly express the pan-B-cell markers CD19, CD20, CD22 and FMC7. The surface immunoglobulins are strongly expressed, although CD5 and CD23 are usually negative. In contrast to classical HCL, CD25 and CD123 are negative, but CD11c is always positive and CD103 is positive in 2/3 of HCL-v cases (Maude et al., 2018).

HCL-v lacks the expression of annexin A1 and the BRAFV600E point mutation that characterizes classical HCL. A subset of patients also exhibit activating mutations in MAP2K1, a gene encoding MEK1, a downstream component of the BRAF-MEK-ERK signaling cascade. While there is no genetic mutation diagnosis for HCL-v, potential therapeutic targets have been identified through genetic profiling (that is MAP2K1, KDM6A, CREBBP, ARID1A, CCND3, U2AF1, KMT2C).

PNAs are less active with HCL-v than with classical HCL. In addition, patient responses are poor and short-lived: only about half of patients achieve PR, and the median duration of response is 15 months. The current treatment of choice for previously untreated HCL-v patients is combined immunochemotherapy with 2-CdA and rituximab. In a phase 2 study, 2-CdA was administered intravenously at a dose of 0.15 mg/kg for five consecutive days, together with eight weekly doses of rituximab at levels of 375 mg/m^2 in 20 patients, eight of whom were previously untreated and 12 of whom had relapsed/refractory disease. The CR rate was 95% and MRD-negative CR in 80% of patients six months after the end of treatment. The 5-year PFS was 63.3% and the 10-year PFS was 44.3%. The duration of response was longer in MRD-negative patients (Meyer et al., 2018).

Ibrutinib is effective in the treatment of HCL-v. Recently published data from Rogers et al. show that ORR increases over time, from 24% at 32 weeks to 36% at 48 weeks, for both HCL-v and classical HCL. Splenectomy remains an option in the treatment of HCL-v as it corrects cytopenias due to hypersplenism and removes a large proportion of the disease. Historical results show that 74% of PRs last 1–10 years (median: four years). Rituximab can be used as consolidation therapy after splenectomy. In addition, spleen irradiation can be considered in older patients with a high surgical risk.

4.7. Flow Cytometry in the Diagnosis of Leukemias

Leukemia is a heterogeneous group of hematological malignant neoplasms characterized by the proliferation of abnormal lymphoid or hematopoietic cells in the bone marrow (BM) and often also affect the peripheral blood (PB), spleen, lymph nodes, and other organs. Leukemia can be classified as acute or chronic leukemia, depending on how quickly it progresses. Acute leukemia progresses rapidly, and the patient's condition deteriorates quickly without treatment. In contrast, chronic leukemia progresses slowly, and patients can suffer from the disease for a long period of time without treatment. Acute leukemia is a malignant disease of the lymphatic or hematopoietic precursor cells (blasts). Depending on the cell origin, acute leukemia can be classified as acute lymphoblastic leukemia, AML, or acute leukemia of unknown origin. These acute leukemias can be divided into numerous subtypes based on further clinical, phenotypic, and genetic information (Meyer et al., 2023). Chronic leukemia is a malignant disease of mature or maturing lymphoid or hematopoietic cells. Most maturing myeloid malignancies present as chronic leukemia. Although there are many types of lymphomas with extensive BM and/or PB involvement, the terminology "leukemia" is used only for a few mature B-cell and T/NK-cell neoplasms, which usually have predominant BM and/or PB involvement. The diagnosis of leukemia is made based on clinical information and laboratory test results.

Flow cytometry (FCM) is a technology that enables rapid multi-parameter analysis of single cells or particles. It simultaneously measures physical characteristics (size and complexity) and multiple surface and intracellular markers of individual cells, enabling rapid and accurate phenotypic characterization of a cell population. Together with histomorphology and other information, multiparametric FCM can enable rapid diagnosis of leukemia and accurate classification of leukemia as a subtype according to the WHO classification. FCM study can also assess clonality of mature B cells by evaluating immunoglobulin light chain (Ig) expression and clonality of mature αβ-T cells by evaluating T cell receptor (TCR) Vβ repertoire or TCR β-chain constant 1 (TRBC1) expression. In addition, FCM can measure DNA content and determine the DNA ploidy of a cell population, which is also helpful for diagnosis and/or prognosis prediction. The fast turnaround time of FCM testing allows for rapid diagnosis or timely selection of appropriate additional tests (Moskop et al., 2022).

Compared to immunohistochemistry (IHC), FCM is not only faster but also able to correlate multiple parameters on a single cell easily and efficiently. In addition, FCM can detect antigen intensity and aberrant antigen expression patterns. The main disadvantage of FCM is the lack of correlation with histomorphology. In addition, FCM requires viable, fresh samples, and reduced viability of certain neoplasms often precludes accurate FCM analysis. This chapter provides an overview of the principles and the important role of FCM in the diagnosis of leukemias.

4.7.1. Principles and Key Elements of Flow Cytometry

Due to the enormous improvement in equipment and reagents over the last decades, FCM has become a very powerful instrument that is used in many areas of research and clinical practice for a variety of purposes.

4.7.1.1. Flow Cytometer

FCMs consist of three main systems: Fluidics, Optics, and Electronics (Figure 4.7(A)). The fluidics system is responsible for transporting the samples to the flow cell, where the cells form a single stream and cross the laser beam. A solution stream (sheath fluid) surrounding the sample is introduced into the device at a higher pressure so that the cells in the sample form an approximately single-row stream due to the phenomenon of hydrodynamic focusing. The cells or particles in the single-row stream travel through the interrogation point where they are illuminated by one or more lasers. Finally, the liquid stream is discharged into a waste container (Figure 4.7(A)).

The optical system consists of light sources (lasers), lenses, filters, and detectors. The lasers illuminate the cells or particles, and dichroic mirrors (DMs) and optical filters (OFs) are used to direct the resulting light signals to the corresponding detectors. DMs allow light of the appropriate wavelengths to pass through while reflecting light of other wavelengths. OFs further limit the wavelengths that reach a detector (Myers et al., 2023). The detectors are usually photomultiplier tubes (PMTs) or photodiode arrays (PDAs), which convert the signals into electrical pulses that are measured by electronics and converted into digital information. The digital information is recorded and interpreted by analysis software. The connected computer system is directly linked to the FCM and controls its functions. Data analysis can be performed either on the computer connected to the FCM or on other computers that have access to the data.

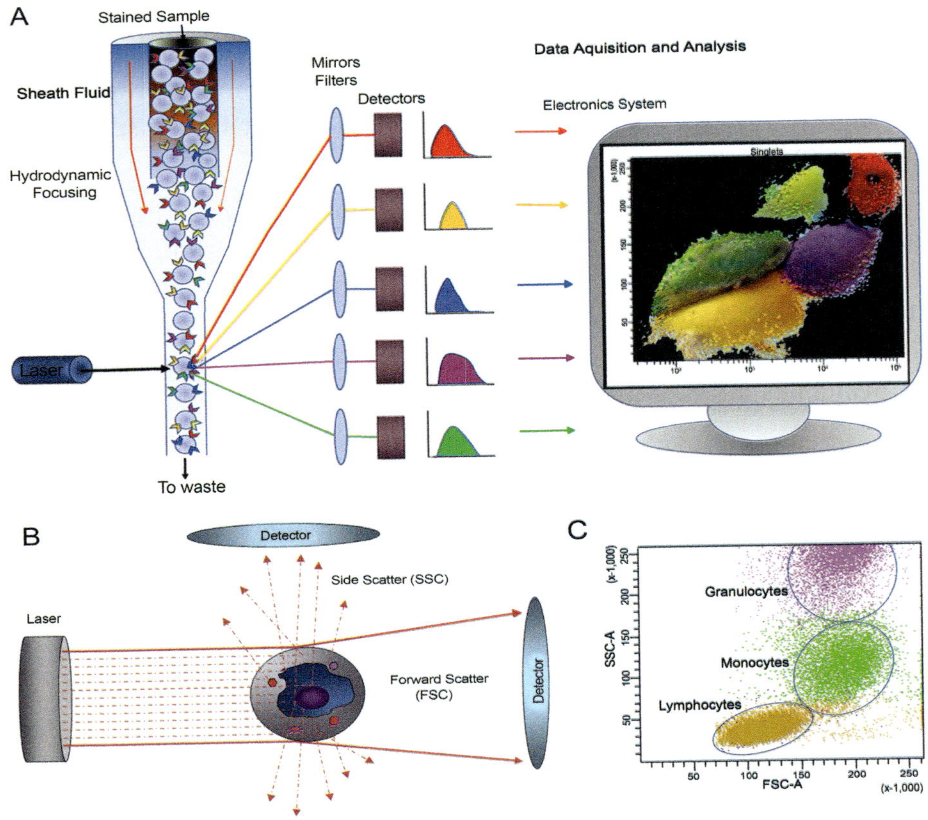

Figure 4.7. *Schematic diagram of how flow cytometry works and light scatter of cells.* ***A,*** *After a liquid sample with stained cells is injected into a flow cytometer, the cells are forced to form a single file stream through hydrodynamic focusing. The cells in a single file stream are illuminated as they travel through a laser beam, and the optical and fluorescence signals of each cell are generated and detected by proper detectors that convert photons to electrical impulses. The electronics system measures the electrical impulses and converts these signals to digital information that is gathered and analyzed by specific software in a computer.* ***B,*** *Illustration of forward light scatter (FSC) and side light scatter (SSC) of a cell.* ***C,*** Differentiation of peripheral blood *leucocytes according to forward and side scatter properties.*

Source: https://www.ncbi.nlm.nih.gov/books/NBK586209/figure/Ch4-f0001/.

4.7.1.2. Specimens and Reagents/Antibody Panels

Samples suitable for FCM analysis include PB, BM, CSF, serous effusions, fine needle aspirates (FNAs) and fresh unfixed tissue (Pieters et al., 2019). PB and BM aspirates must be anticoagulated. Sample preparation for FCM analysis varies depending on the sample type and the antigens to be analyzed. The cell suspension resulting from tissue grinding should be filtered to remove large particles that could clog the cytometer tubes and/or bind antibodies non-specifically. For all samples containing a large amount of PB, the red blood cells should be removed by a lysis procedure using a commercially available reagent or a home-made ammonium chloride solution before the sample is analyzed in an FCM (Pieters et al., 2007).

The most important reagents for FCM studies are fluorochrome-conjugated antibodies against cell surface, cytoplasmic or nuclear antigens. Table 4.3 lists the antigens commonly tested in the investigation of hematologic malignancies. How many antibodies and how many tubes are used for a sample depends on the clinical indication and the type of flow cytometer used. A flow cytometer with a laser can evaluate three to five antigens simultaneously in addition to the light scattering properties. An FCM with several lasers can evaluate more antigens simultaneously. Eight- to ten-color diagnostic antibody panels for hematologic neoplasms are currently widely used in the United States. The combination of antibodies in a tube should be selected according to the antigens on the cells of interest, the fluorochrome properties, and the clinical purpose. In general, the antibody to a weakly expressed antigen should be conjugated to a bright fluorochrome to increase the probability of detecting that antigen. Color matching to minimize overflow between different fluorochromes is very important in multicolor tubes (Pilheden et al., 2022). For diagnostic purposes, antibodies are usually combined as panels to answer specific questions about a cell population. The screening panels should contain sufficient antigens to distinguish a neoplastic cell population from normal/reactive cells with high sensitivity.

Table 4.3. *Surface or Intracellular Antigens Commonly Assessed by Flow Cytometry for Lineage Classification and Immunophenotyping of Hematolymphoid Malignant Neoplasms*

Lineage	**Antigens**
Stem cells	CD34, CD38, CD45
B-cells	CD5, CD10, CD19, CD20, CD22, CD23, CD25, CD34, CD38, CD43, CD45, CD79a, CD103, CD200, FMC2, cIgM, Kappa, Lambda, LEF1, TdT
Plasma cells	CD19, CD20, CD38, CD45, CD56, CD117, CD138, cKappa, cLambda
T-cells/NK cells	CD1a, CD2, CD3, CD4, CD5, CD7, CD8, CD10, CD16, CD25, CD26, CD30, CD34, CD45, CD56, αβ-TCR, γδ-TCR, TdT, TRBC1
Myelomonocytic cells	CD4, CD7, CD10, CD11b, CD11c, CD13, CD14, CD15, CD16, CD33, CD34, CD36, CD38, CD45, CD56, CD64, CD65, CD71, CD117, CD123, cMPO, cLyso, HLA-DR
Erythroblasts	CD34, CD36, CD38, CD45, CD71, CD117, CD235a
Megakaryoblasts	CD33, CD34, CD38, CD41, CD42, CD45, CD61, CD117, HLA-DR

The antigens in bold are lineage-specific markers. cIgM, cytoplasmic IgM; cKappa, cytoplasmic kappa; cLambda, cytoplasmic lambda; cLyso, cytoplasmic lysozyme; cMPO, cytoplasmic peroxidase; TCR, T-cell receptor; TdT, terminal deoxynucleotidyl transferase; TRBC1, TCR β chain constant 1.

4.7.1.3. Light Scatter and Fluorescence Signals

Light scattering and fluorescence are the two types of signals that are generated and collected for a cell as it passes through the laser beam. Light scattering is used to measure the physical properties of a cell. Forward scatter (FSC) refers to the light scattered at narrow angles to the laser beam and is collected by a detector positioned in line with the laser beam on the opposite side of the sample stream (Figure 4.8(B)). The FCS is proportional to the surface area or size of the cell. Lateral scattering (SSC) refers to the light refracted or reflected from cytoplasmic organelles or nuclei of the cells and is detected by a detector positioned at approximately 90º to the laser beam.

The SSC is proportional to the granularity and internal complexity of the cell (Figure 4.8(B)). Together, the FSC and SSC signals allow the separation of cells in a sample containing heterogeneous cell populations, for example, three types of leukocytes (granulocytes, monocytes, and lymphocytes) in PB, which can be easily separated based on the FSC and SSC characters (Figure 4.8(C)). When a cell crosses the laser beam, the fluorescent dye or fluorochrome attached to the cell is excited by light of a specific wavelength (excitation wavelength), further absorbs the energy, is excited, and emits light (fluorescence) at a longer wavelength (emission wavelength). In an FCM, the fluorescence signals from PMTs are detected after they have been filtered by DMs and OFs. The intensity of the fluorescence signal is proportional to the expression level of the antigen to which the corresponding fluorescently labeled antibody binds (Place et al., 2018).

4.7.1.4. Data Acquisition and Analysis

Data acquisition refers to the process of running the stained cells through a flow cytometer and illuminating them with laser light, and the resulting signals are captured by the optical system. The number of cells, also referred to as events, required for evaluation depends on the purpose of the test and the type of sample. For example, when evaluating a PB sample with predominantly leukemic cells, a relatively small number of viable cells (for example 20,000/tube) is sufficient to characterize the leukemia phenotype. In contrast, the detection of MRD usually requires a much larger number of viable cells (for example >500,000/tube) to increase the sensitivity for the detection of a very small population of malignant residual cells (Qasim et al., 2017).

The analysis of FCM data requires specially developed software. Each FCM usually has associated software for data acquisition and analysis. Independent software such as FCS Express and FlowJo with more features is also commercially available. The data can be displayed as histograms, representing a single parameter or dot plots, representing two parameters with each dot denoting a cell or particle. The stronger the signal, the further along the scale the data is displayed.

An antigen is called positive if the corresponding fluorescence signal is above the negative control (background signal). Since most samples contain heterogeneous cell populations, an internal negative control can easily be found and used for most antigens. However, due to the possible differences between non-specific binding and autofluorescence levels, the internal control can be misleading. The addition of non-specific Ig of the same isotype can serve as a better negative control and is used in some FCM tests (Qasim et al., 2017).

Gating refers to the process of isolating cell populations within a heterogeneous cell sample according to their physical and phenotypic characteristics as well as searching for the abnormal cell population. Since normal leukocytes and hematopoietic progenitor cells usually show consistent and reproducible patterns in the SSC vs. CD45 dot plot, SSC vs. CD45 gating is the most commonly used first step to separate different PB or BM cell populations. An abnormal cell population is identified by the difference(s) in its phenotype from normal. These differences include: (i) abnormal increases or decreases in antigens normally expressed on the cells of interest; (ii) homogeneous expression patterns of antigens that normally exhibit variable expression patterns; (iii) asynchronous antigen expression; and (iv) abnormal expression of antigens from other cell types. To recognize these abnormalities, flow cytometrists must be familiar with the normal antigen expression pattern of all cell populations in the sample.

Strict quality assurance (QA) must be performed in an FCM laboratory to ensure the consistency of FCM results, and Quality control (QC) measures must be performed and documented regularly to ensure optimal instrument performance. Any change to reagents, panels, instruments, or protocols must be carefully validated to ensure that the change has no impact on the results. Clinical FCM laboratories should participate in available proficiency testing programs for the tests they perform to ensure that their results are comparable to those of others (Roberts et al., 2018).

4.7.2. Flow Cytometry in the Diagnosis of Acute Leukemias/ Leukemias of Blasts

Acute leukemia is a hematologic malignancy composed of abnormally proliferating lymphoid or hematopoietic precursors (blasts). The definition of acute leukemia is the presence of a significant number of abnormal blasts in the BM according to the WHO classification. For the diagnosis of AML, a value of ≥20% myeloblasts in the total nucleated cells is required. According to the WHO classification, the 20% threshold for AML diagnosis is not required if the blasts carry PML::RARA, RUNX1-RUNX1T1, CBFB-MYH11, DEK::NUP214, RBM15::MRTFA, KMT2A rearrangement, MECOM rearrangement, NUP98 rearrangement or NPM1 mutation. In many treatment protocols, a level of ≥25% lymphoblasts is required to establish a diagnosis of ALL. If the abnormal progenitor cells are predominantly localized in the tissue and form a solid mass lesion without significant BM involvement, the diagnosis should be made as lymphoblastic lymphoma (LBL) or myeloid sarcoma, depending on the type of blast. LBL have the same morphology, immunophenotype, and biology as their ALL counterparts, which is why LBL and the corresponding ALL are combined as one group (ALL/LBL) according to the current WHO classification (Schneider et al., 2023). FCM analysis can be used to efficiently identify abnormal blast populations, assign blasts to a specific lineage, further WHO classification, and sometimes provide prognostic information.

4.7.2.1. *Identification of Blast Population*

Identification of a large blast population, as in the ALL cases in Figure 4.9 and the AML cases in Figure 4.10, is usually straightforward. Blasts usually have low SSC and weak to moderate CD45 expression and thus fall into the so-called blast region (low SSC and weak CD45) on the CD45 vs. SSC dot plot. However, not all cells in the blast region are blasts.

Basophils and plasmacytoid dendritic cells are also found here, and normal B-cell progenitors (hematogones) and early myeloid progenitors are also found here. The leukemic cells of certain acute leukemias may be found outside the blast region, for example, acute promyelocytic leukemia (APL), which typically has intermediate to high SSC (Figure 4.10(B)). Therefore, careful evaluation of the antigen expression profile is always required for the identification or separation of abnormal blast populations, especially in samples with low numbers of blasts (Shi et al., 2024). Blasts often differ from mature cells by expressing immature markers and lacking antigens typically present in mature cells. For example, myeloblasts can be distinguished from mature or maturing myeloid cells by the expression of immature markers such as CD34 and CD117 and the absence of maturation markers such as CD11b, CD15, and CD16. Neoplastic blasts often exhibit an abnormal phenotype that differs from that of normal hematopoietic progenitor cells. Phenotypic abnormalities include an altered expression level or pattern of antigens, aberrant expression of markers from a different cell lineage, and asynchronous or dyssynchronous expression of antigens. For example, leukemic cells of B-cell ALL (B-ALL) usually show increased CD10 levels, decreased CD38 levels, aberrant expression of the myeloid markers CD13 or CD33, and dyssynchronous co-expression of CD34 and CD20 compared to hematogones (normal B-cell precursors in the bone marrow). Knowledge of normal progenitor antigen expression patterns is particularly important for the evaluation of post-treatment samples, which often contain normal regenerative progenitors and very low levels of residual leukemia (Silverman et al., 1997).

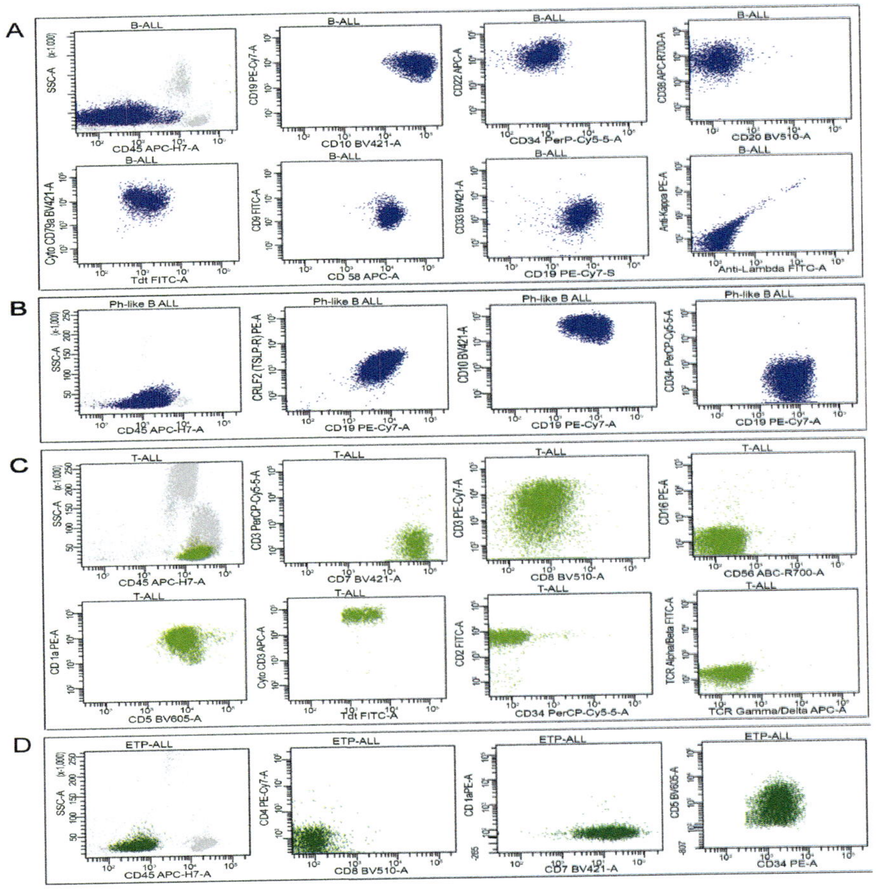

Figure 4.8. *Representative dot plots of acute lymphoblastic leukemia (ALL).*

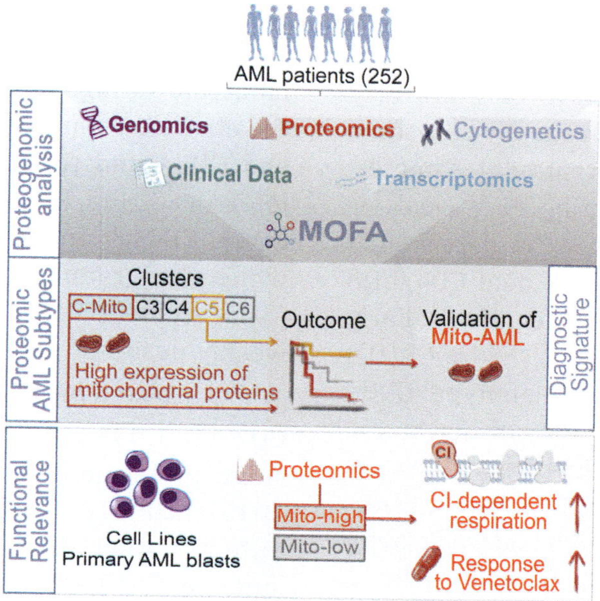

Figure 4.9. *The proteogenomic subtypes of acute myeloid leukemia.*

Source: https://www.ncbi.nlm.nih.gov/books/NBK586209/figure/Ch4-f0003/.

4.7.2.2. Assignment of Blast Lineage

Accurate and rapid classification of acute leukemia as AML, B-ALL or T-ALL is very important for the timely selection of appropriate treatment (Spector et al., 2005). Leukemic blasts often have an antigen expression profile that resembles a specific cell type and can therefore be assigned to this lineage by FCM analysis. As shown in Figure 4.9, lymphoblasts of ALL usually have a low SSC and the phenotype of progenitor B cells or progenitor T cells. Leukemic blasts of de novo B-ALL are almost always positive for CD19, cytoplasmic CD22, and cytoplasmic CD79a, and negative for surface Ig.

Most B-ALL cases are positive for surface CD22, CD10, CD38, TdT, and CD24. CD34 is frequently expressed, but its expression is quite variable and often weak or partial. CD45 is usually weakly expressed and may be completely negative (Stumpel et al., 2015), whereas CD20 is usually negative or partially positive. B-ALL cases can be subdivided based on the stage of development detected by immunophenotyping, which is of little clinical significance nowadays and need not be mentioned in pathology reports. For example, the majority of B-ALL cases express CD10 and are referred to as common ALL (intermediate stage of development); the CD10-negative B-ALL cases are classified as pro-B ALL (early stage); the B-ALL cases expressing a cytoplastic μ-chain are classified as pre-B ALL (late stage). Leukemic blasts of B-ALL may abnormally express myeloid antigens (usually CD13 and CD33, occasionally CD15) and often show abnormal expression patterns of some nonspecific markers such as CD58 and CD9 (Figure 4.9(A)), which are commonly included in the FCM panel for MRD detection of B-ALL. Leukemic blasts of T-ALL are always positive for cytoplasmic CD3, usually positive for TdT, CD7, CD38, CD45 (dim) and variably positive for other pan-T-cell antigens (surface CD3, CD2, CD4, CD5, CD8), T-cell receptor, CD10 and other immature markers (CD1a, CD34 and CD99) (Figure 4.9(C)). In some T-ALL cases, CD56, CD79a, CD117, or myeloid markers such as CD13 or CD33 may be expressed in an aberrant manner. In some cases, especially in post-treatment samples, the immature markers may be very weak or absent, and immaturity must be determined by the absence of surface CD3, dual CD4/CD8 positivity, or dual CD4/CD8 negativity. Early T-cell precursor T-ALL (ETP-ALL, Figure 4.9(D)) is defined by a characteristic phenotype: CD8-, CD1a-, CD5- or dimly+ in <75% of blasts and positive for at least one of the myeloid or stem cell markers (CD11b, CD13, CD33, CD34, CD65, CD117, HLA-DR). ETP-ALL is considered a high-risk T-ALL subtype, especially in adult patients, and is listed as a separate entity in the WHO classification (Stumpel et al., 2009).

The morphology and phenotype of AML cases vary greatly depending on the direction of differentiation and the degree of maturity of the blasts. Leukemic blasts of AML with minimal differentiation (FAB-M0) or AML without maturation (FAB-M1, Figure 4.10(A)) usually have low SSC, express early hematopoietic progenitor antigens (CD34, CD38, and HLA-DR), and lack antigens associated with myeloid and monocytic maturation, such as CD11b, CD14, CD15, and CD65. Blasts express at least two myeloid-associated antigens, such as CD13, CD33 and CD117. The expression of CD38 and/or HLA-DR may be reduced. Rare cases may show asynchronous expression of CD11b or CD15. Myeloperoxidase (MPO) is usually positive in AML-M1 and negative or slightly positive in AML-M0 by FCM. Blasts can express CD7 or rarely other lymphoid markers differently. The leukemic blasts of AML with maturation (FAB M2) usually express several myeloid antigens associated with granulocytic differentiation, such as MPO, CD11b, CD13, CD15, CD33, and CD65. HLA-DR, CD34, CD38, and CD117 are usually positive, but can also be partially negative. The hypergranular variant of APL (FAB-M3) (Figure 4.10(B)) usually has moderate to high SSC and is characterized by the absence or minimal expression of HLA-DR and CD34 and the absence of the leukocyte integrins CD11a, CD11b and CD18. CD13, CD33, CD64, CD117, and MPO are usually positive, while the granulocytic maturation markers CD15 and CD65 are usually negative or only weakly positive.

In cases with microgranular morphology, CD2 and CD34 are often expressed by at least some of the leukemic cells (Stumpel et al., 2013). Leukemic blasts of AML with monocytic differentiation variably express the myeloid antigens CD13, CD15, CD33 (often bright), and CD65; they always express some monocytic markers such as CD14, CD64, CD4, CD163, CD11b, CD11c, CD36, and lysozyme. Most cases have HLA-DR, CD38, and CD123. CD34 and CD117 are positive in a subset of cases, whereas MPO is often negative in acute monoblastic leukemia, but may be partially positive in acute monocytic leukemia and acute myelomonocytic leukemia. Glycophorin A is the lineage-specific marker for acute erythroid leukemia (FAB M6), which is usually also positive for CD71, CD36, and CD117 and negative for CD34 and HLA-DR. CD41, CD61, and CD42b are specific markers for acute megakaryoblastic leukemia (FAB M7), which is often negative for CD34 and HLA-DR. The abnormal megakaryoblasts are usually positive for CD36, frequently express CD13, CD33, and CD117, and may variably express CD7, CD4, or CD56. The surface staining of CD41 and CD61 is less specific than their cytoplasmic staining because platelets can adhere to blasts, leading to a false positive interpretation (Takachi et al., 2021).

Blastic plasmacytoid dendritic cell neoplasms (BPDCN) express CD4, CD56 (light), CD36, CD38, CD43, CD45, CD71, HLA-DR, and markers associated with plasmacytoid dendritic cells (PDC) (CD123, CD303, CD304, TCF4, TCL1). CD45 expression can be weak to moderate. The SSC of tumor cells is usually low. CD7 and CD33 are expressed relatively frequently. TdT is positive in about one-third of cases, and in some cases, CD117 can be expressed. Based on the WHO diagnostic criteria, BPDCN can be diagnosed in the presence of CD123 and one other PDC-associated marker in addition to CD4 and/or CD56, or three PDC-associated markers. It can also be diagnosed by the absence of CD34 and other cell type-specific markers such as CD3, CD14, CD19, lysozyme, and MPO. Given the presence of other hematologic malignancies with similar phenotypes, correlation with histomorphology, clinical information, and IHC, studies are always required to make a definitive diagnosis of BPDCN (Taketani et al., 2004).

Lineage classification can be difficult in some cases. There are approximately 4% of cases of acute leukemia where there is no obvious evidence of differentiation along a single lineage. These cases can be categorized into two groups: acute undifferentiated leukemias and mixed phenotype acute leukemias (MPALs, Figure 4.10). MPALs may have a population of blasts expressing antigens belonging to two lineages (biphenotypic, Figure 4.10) or two distinct blast populations (bilineal, Figure 4.11(C)). There are defined criteria for the assignment of more than one lineage to a leukemic cell population for WHO classification (Figure 4.10(A)). To qualify for a B-cell lineage, the leukemic blasts with strong CD19 expression should have strong expression of at least one of the following features: CD10, CD79a, and cytoplasmic CD22, or the leukemic blasts with weak CD19 expression should have at least two of these three other B-cell markers. For CD19 expression to be considered strong, the intensity of CD19 must reach 50 of the hematogonal level in at least some of the leukemic blasts. CD3 (cytoplasmic or surface) is the only marker defining the T cell lineage, and its presence in high intensity (at least partially >50% of mature T cells) is sufficient to assign the blasts to the T cell lineage. Myeloid lineage is determined by the expression of cytoplasmic MPO, which can be detected by FCM, IHC staining, or cytochemical staining. Monocytic lineage is determined by the diffuse expression of at least two of the following: non-specific esterase, CD11c, CD14, CD64, and lysozyme.

The most common combination is a myeloid lineage with a T-cell or B-cell lineage. Other combinations are also possible. There are no clear cut-off values for the percentage of positive blast cells for these stemness-defining markers. MPO may be present at low levels in a small proportion of leukemic lymphoblasts (Tomizawa, 2023). In the absence of other myeloid markers, this type of MPO expression should not be interpreted as myeloid and lymphoid MPAL. Acute undifferentiated leukemias do not have antigens specific for any of the cell lines mentioned above, but frequently express HLA-DR, CD34, and CD38 and may express TdT (Tomizawa et al., 2020).

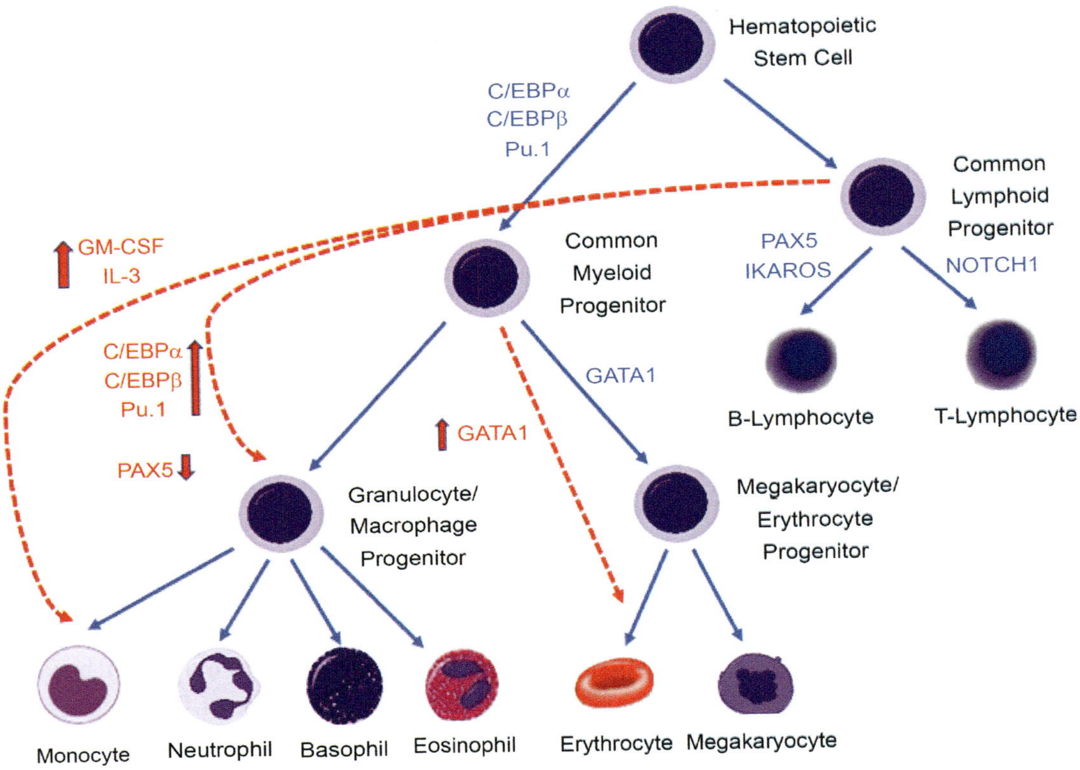

Figure 4.10. *Mixed-phenotype acute leukemia (MPAL).*

Source: Batra, S., & Ross, A. J., (2021). Pediatric mixed-phenotype acute leukemia: What's new? Cancers, 13, 4658. https://doi.org/10.3390/cancers13184658.

4.7.2.3. Enumeration of Blasts

The FCM study can determine the exact percentage of blasts in the samples. However, the percentage of blasts determined by FCM often differs from that determined by the gold standard method — manual differential counting of aspirate smears. There are several possible explanations for this discrepancy. First, BM aspirate samples submitted for FCM analysis are often not the first collection and contain fewer bone marrow spicules with greater dilution with PB. Secondly, the sample is likely to contain non-lysed red cells which will increase the denominator for calculating the blast percentage (van der Linden et al., 2009). Third, some blasts may be phenotypically difficult to detect and may not belong to the blast population. These are all possible reasons why the blast percentage is lower with FCM than with manual differential counting. The proportion of blasts in FCM analysis may also be higher because the denominator is lower due to the loss of nucleated erythroid progenitor cells during erythrocyte lysis. In addition, FCM analysis can identify neoplastic cells that may be missed by manual counting due to atypical morphology or suboptimal smears. In addition, some normal immature progenitor cells, such as hematogones, may be detected as leukemic blasts during manual counting. Therefore, it is necessary to perform both FCM and manual counting for blast enumeration and investigate the cause of significant discrepancies (Van der Sluis et al., 2023).

4.7.2.4. Predicting Cytogenetic Abnormality and Prognosis

Currently, cytogenetic/molecular tests are crucial for further WHO classification and risk stratification of acute leukemias. The prognostic value of FCM immunophenotyping is most likely due to the prediction of certain cytogenetic/molecular subtypes. For example, CD10-B-ALL is frequently observed in B-ALL with KMT2A rearrangement, which is also frequently positive for CD15 and has a very poor prognosis. Detection of CRLF2 expression (Figure 4.8(B)) is associated with CRLF2 gene alteration, which is common in Philadelphia-like ALL and is associated with a poor prognosis. AML with t(8; 21)(q22;q22) frequently expresses B-cell markers such as CD19 and is associated with a favorable prognosis. Aberrant expression of CD2 in APL is associated with FLT3–ITD. However, FCM immunophenotyping should not be considered a replacement tool for the detection of these subtypes due to its lack of specificity and sensitivity (Van der Velden et al., 2009). As previously mentioned, ETP-ALL (Figure 4.8(D)) is defined by the typical early T-precursor immunophenotype and is associated with poor clinical outcomes in adult patients. AML with RAM phenotype (Figure 4.9(D)) is defined by the characteristic phenotype (strong CD56 expression, weak to absent CD38, weak to absent CD45, and absent HLA-DR) and is associated with a very poor prognosis.

FCM can be used to measure the DNA content and assess the DNA ploidy of a cell population. In this procedure, the cells are stained with a DNA-binding fluorescent dye and then the fluorescence signals of the cells in question are analyzed. A histogram is displayed with different ploidy patterns based on the DNA content of the cells in the sample (Figure 4.11). DNA ploidy is used for further classification of B-ALL and provides important prognostic information. High hyperdiploidy in B-ALL (usually DNA index ≥1.16, Figure 4.11(B)) is associated with a very favorable prognosis, while hypodiploidy (DNA index <1, Figure 4.12(C)) is associated with a poor prognosis.

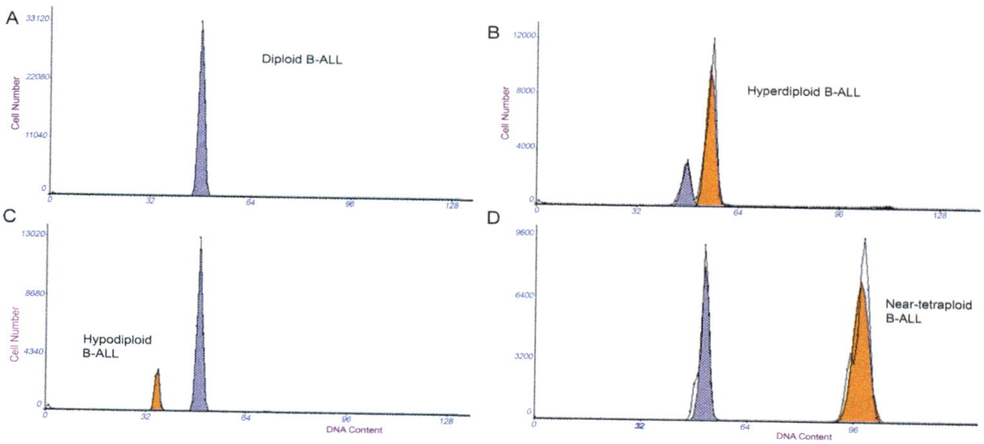

Figure 4.11. *DNA ploidy histogram of precursor B-cell acute lymphoblastic leukemia (B-ALL). (A) DNA diploid B-ALL (leukemic cells not separated from normal blood cells). (B) DNA hyperdiploid B-ALL (orange color peak, DNA Index = 1.16). And (C) DNA hypodiploid B-ALL (orange).*

Source: NCBI, Creative Commons License.

4.7.3. Flow Cytometry in the Diagnosis of Mature B-Cell Leukemias

Mature B-cell neoplasms are a heterogeneous group of lymphoid neoplastic diseases that are derived from B cells and can be briefly divided into two groups: Hodgkin lymphomas (HL) and non-Hodgkin lymphomas/leukemia/lymphoproliferative disorders (non-HL). Although many of the non-HLs may have a leukemic phase with significant BM and/or PB involvement, the term "leukemia" is only used in the names of a very limited number of non-HLs, i.e., chronic lymphocytic leukemia (CLL), hairy cell leukemia (HCL), and splenic B-cell lymphoma/leukemia with prominent nucleoli. FCM is a very powerful tool for the diagnosis of non-HLs. FCM analysis can efficiently identify an atypical lymphoid population, distinguish neoplastic proliferation from reactive proliferation, characterize the phenotype of the neoplastic cell population, and aid in WHO classification. Neoplastic B cells can be distinguished from normal/reactive B cells by identifying two major types of phenotypic abnormalities: Immunoglobulin light chain restriction and aberrant antigen expression. These two types of abnormalities are present in most non-HL cases and can be efficiently identified by FCM analysis. Due to the large size, low proportion of tumor cells, and T-cell conversion to tumor cells in HL, FCM is not suitable for the diagnosis of HL (Viardot et al., 2016).

4.7.3.1. Immunoglobulin Light Chain Restriction/ B-Cell Clonality Assessment

Neoplastic B cells express only one class of light chains (i.e., kappa or lambda) (Figure 4.12(A)–(D)), whereas normal or reactive B cells always consist of a mixture of kappa-expressing B cells and lambda-expressing B cells (Figure 4.12(E)). The detection of only one light chain class (light chain restriction) indicates monoclonal B cell proliferation. Light chain restriction can occasionally occur in non-neoplastic reactive B-cell populations; therefore, it should not be considered equivalent to monoclonality or the sole diagnosis of neoplasia. It should always be interpreted in combination with clinical information, morphology, and sometimes cytogenetic or molecular test results. The identification of a large population of light chain-restricted B cells is usually straightforward and is reflected by an abnormal kappa-to-lambda ratio (Figure 4.12(A)–(D)). However, in samples with many mixed reactive B cells, evaluation of the kappa-to-lambda ratio may not be sufficient to identify a small clonal population.

To increase sensitivity, separate evaluations of B cell subsets with different phenotypes and/or light scattering characteristics should be performed. Caution should be exercised when testing small B cell populations for light chain restriction, as reactive B cells may comprise small subsets of phenotypically identical cells. Some germinal center B (GCB) B cells may show the absence of both light chain classes or an excess of one light chain class and should not be interpreted as an abnormal CD10+ B cell population (Figure 4.12(F)).

It is important to include a pre-wash step to avoid false-negative results due to soluble antibodies in the samples that interfere with the binding of fluorochrome-conjugated antibodies. It should be noted that B lymphoblasts, plasma cells, and thymic B cells are negative for surface Ig, as are their neoplastic counterparts: B-ALL, plasma cell neoplasms, and primary mediastinal large B-cell lymphoma.

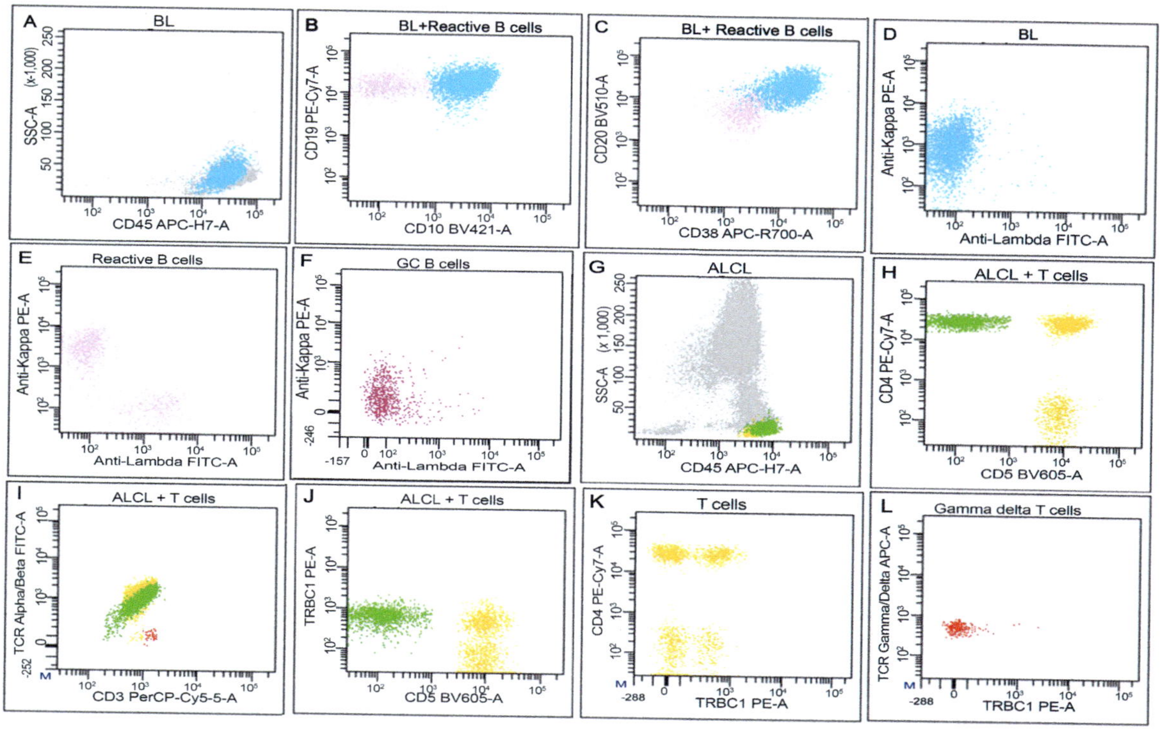

Figure 4.12. *Assessment of clonality of B-cells and T-cells by flow cytometry. Burkitt leukemia (BL, blue) expressing CD45 (A), CD19 and CD10 (B), CD20 and CD38 (C), and showing kappa restriction (D). Reactive B cells (light pink) being polytypic (E). Germinal center B cells (magenta) showing kappa predominance and partial double-negativity for both kappa and lambda in a thyroid FNA sample from a patient with autoimmune thyroiditis. (F). Anaplastic large cell lymphoma (ALCL, green) being CD45+ (G), CD4+ and CD5-(H), TCR alpha beta+ and CD3+ (I), and expressing TRBC1 only (monotypic, J). Reactive CD4+ and CD4- T cells (golden) containing mixed TRBC1+ and TRBC1- populations (polytypic, K). Gamma delta T cells (red) always negative for TRBC1 (L).*

Source: NCBI, Creative Commons License.

4.7.3.2. Aberrant B-Cell Antigen Expression

FCM analysis can detect phenotypic deviations of mature B-cell neoplasms from normal B-cell antigen expression patterns. The most easily recognizable phenotypic deviation is the presence of antigens that are not normally expressed by B cells. For example, CD5, a T-cell antigen, may be abnormally expressed in CLL and mantle cell lymphoma (MCL). It should be noted that a small population of mature B cells normally express CD5. These mature CD5+ B cells are often found in PB but can also be detected in lymph nodes or other tissue samples, especially in pediatric patients or patients with autoimmune diseases. Therefore, the interpretation of CD5 expression of B cells must be correlated with other phenotypic features. Another type of phenotypic abnormality is the abnormal expression of antigens that are not normally present in the B cells of a particular subset. For example, normal GCB cells are Bcl-2-deficient, whereas Bcl-2 is positive in most other B cell subsets (von Stackelberg et al., 2016). Abnormal Bcl-2 expression is found in most cases of follicular lymphoma (FL) derived from GCB cells expressing the GCB markers CD10 and BCL6.

Other phenotypic abnormalities include changes in the expression of B-cell-associated antigens. For example, CLL often has a reduced CD20, a significantly reduced or absent FMC7, and a detectable CD23 (17).

4.7.3.3. Classification of Mature B-Cell Leukemias/Lymphomas

FCM immunophenotyping plays an important role in the classification of mature B-cell neoplasms. Each of these disease types has some unique or relatively specific phenotypic features, and the FCM findings in combination with histomorphologic features can establish the definitive diagnosis in most cases. Most mature non-plasma cell B-cell neoplasms are positive for the B-cell markers CD19, CD20, CD22, CD79a, and surface Ig (sIg), but the expression levels of these markers vary between neoplasms. CLL is the most common leukemia in the Western world and is characterized by clonal proliferation of abnormal mature CD5+ B cells in BM, PB, spleen, and lymph nodes. CLL has a characteristic phenotype: CD20+ (weak), CD22+ (weak), CD23+ (often moderate to bright), FMC-7-, and sIg+ (weak with light chain restriction). This phenotype in combination with the typical morphology is sufficient to make the diagnosis in most cases. CD200 is consistently expressed in CLL, but not in MCL. The inclusion of CD200 in the panel has increased the sensitivity in the identification of CLL, even in the atypical cases. Lymphoid enhancer-binding factor 1 (LEF1) is highly expressed in CLL but not detected in most other B-cell neoplasms, which is why it is considered a highly specific marker for CLL. The inclusion of LEF1 in the FCM panel will increase the sensitivity and specificity of CLL diagnosis. MCL, another CD5+ small lymphocytic neoplasm, may also show significant PB involvement and should be differentiated from CLL. MCL usually shows a phenotype that can be easily distinguished from CLL by FCM: CD20+ (moderate to bright), sIg+ (moderate to bright), CD23- or only weak+, FMC-7+, CD200-, LEF1-. The phenotype of MCL is more variable than that of CLL; therefore, additional tests are usually required to confirm the diagnosis. These tests include IHC staining for cyclin-D1 in kerosene sections, cytogenetic testing to identify the translocation t(11; 14)(q13;q32) or fluorescence in situ hybridization (FISH) analysis for CCND1 gene rearrangement.

HCL is a rare indolent neoplasm of small mature B cells with characteristic hairy projections. It usually affects the PB and diffusely infiltrates the BM and the red pulp of the spleen. HCL has a very distinct phenotype: CD20+ (bright), CD11c+ (bright), CD25+, CD103+, CD22+ (bright), sIg+ (intermediate to bright and with light chain restriction), FMC-7+, CD23-, CD5-, and CD10-. This phenotype together with the characteristic morphology is sufficient to make the diagnosis of HCL. Occasionally, classical HCL may show some deviations from this characteristic phenotype, e.g., CD10+, CD23+, CD103- or CD25-. The presence of phenotypic variations does not necessarily qualify the case as variant HCL (vHCL) (29). The term vHCL, which was included in the new entity of splenic B-cell lymphoma/leukemia with prominent nucleoli in the 5th edition of the WHO classification, is used to describe cases with an unusual combination of morphologic, clinical, and phenotypic findings (1). vHCL usually presents with leukocytosis without monocytopenia and shows tumor cells with a more variable morphology, often without TRAP staining and negative for CD25, annexin A1 and CD200. Marginal zone lymphomas (MZL) are usually distinguished from HCL by the lack of combined positivity for CD11c, CD25, and CD103 and the absence of bright staining for CD20 and CD22. Diffuse large B-cell lymphoma (DLBCL) is a heterogeneous group of B-cell lymphomas that are variably positive for B-cell markers with light chain restriction. A high FSC value is usually present in DLBCL reflects the size of the tumor cells and can serve as a distinguishing feature between DLBCL and small mature B-cell neoplasms. It should be remembered that there may be occasional cases with an atypical phenotype in each subtype of these B-cell neoplasms. Correlation with morphologic features, clinical information, and sometimes cytogenetic/molecular findings is always necessary for accurate interpretation of FCM results (Xie et al., 2020).

4.7.3.4. Enumeration of Clonal B-Cells

FCM counting of clonal B cells, either on one platform using quantification beads or on two platforms using the leukocyte count from the hematology analyzer, is important to differentiate monoclonal B-cell lymphocytosis (MBL) from CLL. For the diagnosis of CLL, a number of monoclonal B cells ≥ 5 x109/L with the characteristic morphology and phenotype of CLL must be present in the PB. Individuals with a clonal CLL-like cell count < 5 x109/L and without lymphadenopathy, organomegaly, or other extramedullary disease are considered to have MBL. MBL is defined as the presence of a clonal B-cell population of less than 5 × 109/L in the PB with no other evidence of lymphoma or lymphoproliferative disorder. Most MBL cases have the immunophenotype of CLL. Depending on the number of B cells, MBL can be classified as low-cell (<0.5 × 109/L) or high-cell (>0.5 × 109/L). Low-cell MBL can be detected in up to 5% of adults over the age of 40. Low-grade MBL and high-grade MBL have different prognoses and some different biological and genetic features. High-grade MBL progresses to CLL at a rate of 1% to 2% per year, while low-grade MBL rarely progresses to CLL.

4.7.3.5. Diagnosing Plasma Cell Leukemia

Plasma cell neoplasm (PCN) results from the proliferation of a clone of abnormal, terminally differentiated B cells – plasma cells. Plasma cell leukemia (PCL) is a rare form of PCN in which clonal plasma cells account for >20% of the total leukocytes in the PB. The detection of a large clonal plasma cell population with restricted cytoplasmic light chain expression is the basis for the diagnosis of PCL. CD38 and CD138 are two commonly used markers for the identification of plasma cells. CD38 is expressed by a variety of cell types at a lower intensity than plasma cells, while CD138 is more specific for plasma cells but less sensitive. The neoplastic plasma cells often exhibit an abnormal CD19–CD20 phenotype, which is different from most normal CD19+ CD20 plasma cells and CD19+ CD20+ mature B-cell neoplasms. Aberrant CD56 expression is found in most cases of PCN. Decreased CD38 and/or CD138 expression, abnormal increase in CD28, and loss of CD27 are common in PCN, and some PCN cases express CD117. Although FCM is very useful in identifying abnormal plasma cell populations and distinguishing between plasma cell neoplasms and other mature B-cell malignancies, the diagnostic utility of FCM is limited by its difficulty in enumerating plasma cells. FCM generally identifies fewer plasma cells than manual enumeration on smears or IHC staining on biopsy sections. This discrepancy is likely due to differences in sampling, loss of plasma cells during sample processing, or a combination of both (Zhu et al., 2018).

4.7.4. FCM in the Diagnosis of Mature T/NK Cell Leukemias

Mature T-cell or NK-cell neoplasms are a heterogeneous group of neoplastic diseases originating from T-cells or NK-cells. Mature T-cell or NK-cell neoplasms with "leukemia" in their name include T-prolymphocytic leukemia (T-PLL), T-large granular lymphocytic leukemia (T-LGL), NK-large granular lymphocytic leukemia (NK-LGL), adult T-cell leukemia/lymphoma (ATLL) and aggressive NK-cell leukemia (A-NKL). Other T/NK cell neoplasms, such as Sezary syndrome (SS), also have a leukemic presentation or leukemic phase, even if they do not have "leukemia" in their name. FCM is very useful in the diagnosis and classification of mature T/NK cell neoplasms. However, it is often more difficult to identify phenotypically abnormal mature T or NK cells than abnormal mature B cells, and the immunophenotypic features of FCM are usually not specific or diagnostic for any subtype of T/NK cell neoplasms.

Abnormal mature T-cell or NK-cell populations can often be identified by FCM studies through the detection of abnormal antigen expression. With the recent availability of specific antibodies against TRBC1, the clonality of an alpha-beta T cell population can also be assessed using a single-tube FCM assay. The use of clonality assessment by TRBC1 expression has increased the sensitivity and specificity of FCM analysis in identifying an abnormal mature T cell population.

4.7.4.1. Identification of Restricted Populations of T-Cells or NK Cells/ Clonality Assessment

A change in the CD4/CD8 ratio in T cells is not a useful indicator of clonality or neoplasia, as it can be observed in many reactive or medical conditions. However, a significant deviation of the CD4/CD8 ratio from normal may raise concern about the presence of an abnormally restricted T cell population. For example, an elevated CD4/CD8 ratio in the PB may lead to further investigation of CD26 and CD7 expression on CD4+ T cells. Significant loss or absence of CD7 and/or CD26 in the CD4+ T cell population suggests a diagnosis of SS. The traditional FCM method for assessing T cell clonality is to evaluate the TCR-Vβ repertoire. Normal T cell populations consist of a mixture of cells expressing different subtypes of the Vβ family, whereas T cell neoplasm is the expansion of a clone of T cells with restricted Vβ expression. Since there are more than 20 functional Vβ families and many more subfamilies, this FCM assay for the TCR-Vββ repertoire is complex and labor-intensive, and it consumes a large amount of samples and reagents with limited sensitivity. Therefore, it is not commonly used in clinical FCM laboratories. FCM assessment of T-cell clonality has improved significantly with the recent introduction of the antibody specific for TRBC1, one of the two mutually exclusive constant regions of the TCR-β chain. Normal/reactive alpha-beta T cells contain a mixture of cells expressing TRBC1 or TRBC2 (TRBC1-) (Figure 4.12(K)), while the clonal T cell population is either TRBC1-positive (Figure 4.12(G)–(J)) or negative. This FCM assay has been tested in many mature alpha-beta T-cell neoplasms and has been shown to be very useful (4, 5). In addition to TRBC1, the panel should also include antibodies for TCR αβ and/or TCR γδ, as TRBC1 is usually negative in γδ T cells, which can serve as an internal negative control (Figure 4.12(L)). This assay is not suitable for γδ- or CD3-negative mature T-cell neoplasms due to the absence of the TCR-β chain (Xie et al., 2018).

NK cells do not have a TCR and therefore cannot be analyzed for clonality using the TCR Vβ / TRBC1 FCM assay or PCR for TCR gene rearrangement. FCM analysis of NK receptor (NKR) expression was developed to find evidence of NK cell clonality. Normal and reactive NK cell populations express a variety of NKRs, whereas neoplastic NK cell populations express a more restricted NKR repertoire.

4.7.4.2. Aberrant T-Cell Antigen Expression

T-cell neoplasms frequently exhibit altered expression of T-cell markers, often characterized by the complete loss of one or more pan-T-cell antigens. In rare extreme cases, several or all T cell-associated antigens may be absent, resulting in a "null" phenotype that can make cell lineage determination very difficult. CD5 and CD7 are the most frequently lost antigens in

T-cell neoplasms. It should be noted that a small population of non-neoplastic CD7 T cells is well recognized in PB, BM, and skin biopsy samples and that CD7 T cells can proliferate in some reactive conditions, such as benign dermatoses. In addition, small subsets of T cells may lack CD5, for example; CD3+CD5–γδ T cells. Some mature T cell neoplasms may be dual CD4/8- or dual CD4/8+, which is more common in T ALL/LBL and also occurs in some normal/reactive T cell subsets. Altered intensity of T-cell antigen staining is more common in T-cell and NK-cell neoplasms than their complete loss. However, these changes are more subtle and must be differentiated from the normal or reactive T/NK cell subsets that normally exhibit these changes. T/NK cell neoplasms can also express antigens of other cell types such as CD15, CD13, and CD33 in an aberrant manner. Again, it should be noted that small subsets of normal/reactive T/NK cells may have markers that are more specific for other cell types, for example, subsets of NK cells expressing CD19, CD33, or CD117.

4.7.4.3. Classification of Mature T-Cell or NK-Cell Leukemias/ Lymphomas

Although there is phenotypic heterogeneity in almost all T-cell neoplasms, the common or typical features can be identified by FCM in most cases. SS and mycosis fungoides (SS/MF) usually show a CD3+ CD4+ CD26–CD7–T-cell phenotype, which is not specific for these diseases and should therefore be interpreted in conjunction with the clinical presentation and morphological features. There is CD8+ MF, which is more common in the pediatric population and is hypopigmented. Although SS and MF share many similarities in morphology and phenotype, they have different cell origins and should be considered as two distinct diseases. The normal counterparts of SS tumor cells are circulating central memory T cells, whereas the counterparts of MF tumor cells are skin-resident memory T cells. ATLL can have a similar CD3+ CD4+ CD7 phenotype to SS/MF, but usually has strong CD25 expression and is positive for human T-cell leukemia virus-1 (HTLV-1), the causative agent of ATLL. Anaplastic large cell lymphoma (ALCL) primarily affects lymph nodes and the skin, but can also affect the bone marrow, CNS, and other sites with variable phenotype and morphology. ALCL is usually CD4+, CD2+, CD25+, and positive for cytotoxic granule-associated proteins and EMA, and often lacks several other T-cell antigens. IHC staining is typically required for a definitive diagnosis of ALCL. CD30 is always positive, diffuse, and strong with membrane and Golgi staining patterns. The diagnosis of ALK+ ALCL is based on the expression of the ALK-1 protein or the identification of an ALK gene rearrangement. T-LGL usually shows a CD8+ T-cell phenotype with a frequent decrease in CD5 and/or CD7 expression. Most T-LGL cases express CD57, CD16, the cytotoxic granule-associated proteins granzyme-B, perforin, and TIA-1, while expression of CD56 is rare. The diagnosis of T-LGL is often made by combining this phenotype with morphological and clinical features. Hepatosplenic T-cell lymphoma (HSTL) is often CD4-CD8- (occasionally CD4-CD8+) with expression of CD56 and no expression of CD57 and CD5. Most HSTL cases express TCR γδ, show a non-activated cytotoxic phenotype with expression of TIA-1 but lacking granzyme-B and perforin, and often have the cytogenetic abnormality of isochromosome 7q. T-PLL has a mature T-cell phenotype with expression of surface CD3 and most other T-cell antigens including CD2, CD5, and CD7. T-PLL is often CD4+ or dual CD4/8+, negative for CD25 and cytotoxic granule-associated proteins. The diagnosis of T-PLL can be made in most cases by correlating the immunophenotype with morphology, clinical features, and/or the detection of a TCL1A/B gene rearrangement. Enteropathy-associated T-cell lymphoma (EATL) is usually negative for CD4, CD5, and CD8, positive for CD3, CD7, CD103 and the cytotoxic granule-associated proteins TIA-1, granzyme-B, and perforin. EATL is often associated with coeliac disease. Monomorphic epitheliotropic intestinal T-cell lymphoma (MEITL) has some similarities in phenotype with EATL but is usually CD8+ and CD56+ and shows no clear association with celiac disease. As expected, the phenotype of PTCL, NOS is quite heterogeneous and often overlaps with other mature T-cell neoplasms. Other specified T-cell neoplasms must be excluded before a diagnosis of PTCL, or NOS can be made.

NK-cell neoplasms, including NK-LGL, A-NKL, extranodal NK/T-cell lymphomas (ENK/TCL), and EBV+ NK-cell lymphoproliferative disorders of childhood, have some overlapping phenotypic features and it is important to distinguish the more aggressive neoplasms (A-NKL and ENK/TCL) from those with a more indolent course. A-NKL and ENK/TCL share many common features, including an NK cell phenotype and the presence of EBV (Viardot et al., 2016). They are usually positive for CD2, CD56, EBV, and the cytotoxic granule-associated proteins TIA-1, granzyme-B, and perforin. CD3 is negative at the surface, but the cytoplasmic CD3-epsilon is usually positive. CD4, CD5, and CD57 are usually negative. Differentiation is usually based on the clinical course. A-NKL presents with BM involvement, circulating neoplastic cells, cytopenias, and constitutional symptoms, while ENK/TCL is a tissue-based mass lesion that often occurs in and around the nasal cavity and has an angiocentric and angiodestructive growth pattern. NK-LGL, formerly known as chronic lymphoproliferative disorder of NK cells, is characterized by a persistent proliferation of NK cells in the PB without an identifiable cause. NK-LGL is rare, not associated with EBV and usually shows a chronic clinical course with many similarities to T-LGL. On FCM examination, NK-LGL usually shows a mature NK cell phenotype with low or absent CD2, CD7 and CD57 and reduced or abnormal NK cell receptor expression.

4.7.5. Flow Cytometry in the Diagnosis of Mature or Maturing Myeloid Leukemias

Maturing myeloid neoplasms are a diverse group of neoplasms composed of neoplastic hematopoietic precursors at different stages of maturation. Most of these diseases occur as chronic leukemia. The diagnosis of these diseases is based on a combination of clinical information, blood cell counts, histomorphological examinations of the bone marrow, and cytogenetic/molecular test results. Although the aberrant phenotype of hematopoietic progenitor cells is frequently detected in these neoplasms, the diagnostic value of FCM immunophenotyping in these neoplasms is limited, and the importance of identifying phenotypic abnormalities in these diseases is not well characterized. In most myeloproliferative neoplasms, FCM testing is mainly used to quantify blasts to detect the accelerated phase or transformation to AML. The advantages and limitations of FCM blast quantification are the same as those mentioned above for acute leukemia, and FCM cannot replace manual blast counting (Zhu et al., 2016).

A Closer Look

Hairy Cell Leukemia

Hairy Cell Leukemia (HCL) is a rare, chronic lymphoproliferative disorder characterized by the proliferation of atypical B cells with a distinctive "hairy" appearance. The condition was first described in the 1950s and has been increasingly recognized for its unique clinical and biological features. HCL predominantly affects middle-aged men, with a male-to-female ratio of approximately 4:1. Patients often present with splenomegaly, cytopenias (such as anemia and thrombocytopenia), and recurrent infections due to immunosuppression. The diagnosis is typically established through peripheral blood smear analysis, bone marrow biopsy, and immunophenotyping, which reveals the characteristic hairy cells expressing CD11c, CD25, and CD103.

Recent research has focused on the molecular and genetic underpinnings of HCL, enhancing our understanding of its pathophysiology. Notably, mutations in the BRAF gene (specifically BRAF V600E) have been identified in approximately 90% of HCL cases. This mutation leads to constitutive activation of the MAPK signaling pathway, promoting the survival and proliferation of hairy cells. A study by Tiacci et al. (2011) provided groundbreaking insights by demonstrating that the presence of the BRAF V600E mutation is a hallmark of HCL and serves as a potential therapeutic target. These findings have prompted investigations into targeted therapies that could improve treatment outcomes for HCL patients.

Traditional treatment options for HCL include purine analogs such as cladribine and pentostatin, which have demonstrated high overall response rates. However, the development of resistance and relapsed cases remains a clinical challenge. Recent studies have explored novel therapeutic strategies, including the use of BRAF inhibitors, which have shown promising results in patients with BRAF V600E-positive HCL. A clinical trial by Pal et al. (2018) evaluated the efficacy of vemurafenib, a selective BRAF inhibitor, in HCL patients and reported a significant response rate, highlighting the potential for personalized medicine in this rare disease.

Despite advancements in understanding and treating HCL, challenges remain, particularly concerning long-term management and the potential for secondary malignancies. Ongoing research aims to elucidate the long-term outcomes of HCL patients, focusing on survival rates, quality of life, and the impact of novel therapies. Future studies will likely emphasize the integration of targeted therapies with traditional approaches to enhance patient outcomes while minimizing treatment-related complications. As our understanding of HCL continues to evolve, it is crucial to maintain a focus on developing effective and safe treatment options to improve the prognosis for affected individuals.

Summary

- Infant leukemia is a rare form of cancer that affects children under the age of one. It is characterized by the rapid production of abnormal white blood cells in the bone marrow, which interferes with the production of normal blood cells. There are two main types of infant leukemia: ALL and AML.
- Symptoms of infant leukemia can vary but may include fever, easy bruising or bleeding, pale skin, irritability, and poor feeding. Diagnosis is typically made through blood tests and a bone marrow biopsy.
- Treatment for infant leukemia usually involves chemotherapy, which is the use of powerful drugs to kill cancer cells. In some cases, a stem cell transplant may be necessary to replace diseased bone marrow with healthy stem cells. The outlook for infants with leukemia has improved significantly in recent years, with many infants achieving long-term remission or cure with appropriate treatment. However, the prognosis can vary depending on factors such as the type of leukemia and how early it is diagnosed.

References

1. Andersson, A. K., Ma, J., Wang, J., Chen, X., Gedman, A. L., Dang, J., Nakitandwe, J., Holmfeldt, L., Parker, M., Easton, J., et al. (2015). The landscape of somatic mutations in infant MLL-rearranged acute lymphoblastic leukemias. *Nature Genetics, 47*(3), 330–337.
2. Annesley, C., Summers, C., Pulsipher, M. A., Wayne, A. S., Rivers, J., Lamble, A. J., Wilson, A., Wu, Q. V., Brand, A., Mgebroff, S., et al. (2019). Clinical experience of CAR T cell immunotherapy for relapsed and refractory infant ALL demonstrates feasibility and favorable responses. *Blood, 134*(15), 3869.
3. Attarbaschi, A., Mann, G., König, M., Steiner, M., Strehl, S., Schreiberhuber, A., Schneider, B., Meyer, C., Marschalek, R., Borkhardt, A., et al. (2006). Mixed lineage leukemia-rearranged childhood pro-B and CD10-negative pre-B acute lymphoblastic leukemia constitute a distinct clinical entity. *Clinical Cancer Research, 12*(10), 2988–2994.
4. Boer, J. M., Valsecchi, M. G., Hormann, F. M., Antić, Ž., Zaliova, M., Schwab, C., Cazzaniga, G., Arfeuille, C., Cavé, H., Attarbaschi, A., et al. (2021). Favorable outcome of NUTM1-rearranged infant and pediatric B cell precursor acute lymphoblastic leukemia in a collaborative international study. *Leukemia, 35*(11), 2978–2982.
5. Bolouri, H., Farrar, J. E., Triche, T., Jr., Ries, R. E., Lim, E. L., Alonzo, T. A., Ma, Y., Moore, R., Mungall, A. J., Marra, M. A., et al. (2018). The molecular landscape of pediatric acute myeloid leukemia reveals recurrent structural alterations and age-specific mutational interactions. *Nature Medicine, 24*(1), 103–112.
6. Breese, E. H., Krupski, C., Nelson, A. S., Perentesis, J. P., & Phillips, C. L. (2021). Use of CD19-directed CAR T-cell therapy in an infant with refractory acute lymphoblastic leukemia. *Journal of Pediatric Hematology/Oncology, 43*(2), 152–154.
7. Brown, P. (2013). Treatment of infant leukemias: Challenge and promise. *Hematology American Society of Hematology Education Program, 2013*, 596–600.

8. Brown, P. A., Kairalla, J. A., Hilden, J. M., Dreyer, Z. E., Carroll, A. J., Heerema, N. A., Wang, C., Devidas, M., Gore, L., Salzer, W. L., et al. (2021). FLT3 inhibitor lestaurtinib plus chemotherapy for newly diagnosed KMT2A-rearranged infant acute lymphoblastic leukemia: Children's Oncology Group trial AALL0631. *Leukemia, 35*(5), 1279–1290.
9. Brown, P., Pieters, R., & Biondi, A. (2019). How I treat infant leukemia. *Blood, 133*(3), 205–214.
10. Caslini, C., Yang, Z., El-Osta, M., Milne, T. A., Slany, R. K., & Hess, J. L. (2007). Interaction of MLL amino terminal sequences with menin is required for transformation. *Cancer Research, 67*(15), 7275–7283.
11. Cheung, L. C., Aya-Bonilla, C., Cruickshank, M. N., Chiu, S. K., Kuek, V., Anderson, D., Chua, G. A., Singh, S., Oommen, J., Ferrari, E., et al. (2023). Preclinical efficacy of azacitidine and venetoclax for infant KMT2A-rearranged acute lymphoblastic leukemia reveals a new therapeutic strategy. *Leukemia, 37*(1), 61–71.
12. Clements, J. D., Zhu, M., Kuchimanchi, M., Terminello, B., & Doshi, S. (2020). Population pharmacokinetics of blinatumomab in pediatric and adult patients with hematological malignancies. *Clinical Pharmacokinetics, 59*(4), 463–474.
13. Clesham, K., Rao, V., Bartram, J., Ancliff, P., Ghorashian, S., O'Connor, D., Pavasovic, V., Rao, A., Samarasinghe, S., Cummins, M., et al. (2020). Blinatumomab for infant acute lymphoblastic leukemia. *Blood, 135*(12), 1501–1504.
14. Diaz-Flores, E., Comeaux, E. Q., Kim, K. L., Melnik, E., Beckman, K., Davis, K. L., Wu, K., Akutagawa, J., Bridges, O., Marino, R., et al. (2019). Bcl-2 is a therapeutic target for hypodiploid B-lineage acute lymphoblastic leukemia. *Cancer Research, 79*(9), 2339–2351.
15. Dreyer, Z. E., Hilden, J. M., Jones, T. L., Devidas, M., Winick, N. J., Willman, C. L., Harvey, R. C., Chen, I. M., Behm, F. G., Pullen, J., et al. (2015). Intensified chemotherapy without SCT in infant ALL: Results from COG P9407 (Cohort 3). *Pediatric Blood & Cancer, 62*(3), 419–426.
16. Du, J., Chisholm, K. M., Tsuchiya, K., Leger, K., Lee, B. M., Rutledge, J. C., Paschal, C. R., Summers, C., & Xu, M. (2021). Lineage switch in an infant B-lymphoblastic leukemia with t (1;11) (p32; q23); KMT2A/EPS15, following blinatumomab therapy. *Pediatric Developmental Pathology, 24*(4), 378–382.
17. El Chaer, F., Keng, M., & Ballen, K. K. (2020). MLL-rearranged acute lymphoblastic leukemia. *Current Hematology and Malignancy Reports, 15*(3), 83–89.
18. Fazio, G., Bardini, M., De Lorenzo, P., Grioni, A., Quadri, M., Pedace, L., Corral Abascal, L., Palamini, S., Palmi, C., Buldini, B., et al. (2021). Recurrent genetic fusions redefine MLL germ line acute lymphoblastic leukemia in infants. *Blood, 137*(14), 1980–1984.
19. Ford, A. M., Ridge, S. A., Cabrera, M. E., Mahmoud, H., Steel, C. M., Chan, L. C., & Greaves, M. (1993). In utero rearrangements in the trithorax-related oncogene in infant leukaemias. *Nature, 363*(6433), 358–360.
20. Forgione, M. O., McClure, B. J., Eadie, L. N., Yeung, D. T., & White, D. L. (2020). KMT2A rearranged acute lymphoblastic leukaemia: Unravelling the genomic complexity and heterogeneity of this high-risk disease. *Cancer Letters, 469*, 410–418.
21. George, S. L., Fernbach, D. J., Vietti, T. J., Sullivan, M. P., Lane, D. M., Haggard, M. E., Berry, D. H., Lonsdale, D., & Komp, D. (1973). Factors influencing survival in pediatric acute leukemia. The SWCCSG experience, 1958–1970. *Cancer, 32*(6), 1542–1553.

22. Gore, L., Locatelli, F., Zugmaier, G., Handgretinger, R., O'Brien, M. M., Bader, P., Bhojwani, D., Schlegel, P. G., Tuglus, C. A., & von Stackelberg, A. (2018). Survival after blinatumomab treatment in pediatric patients with relapsed/refractory B-cell precursor acute lymphoblastic leukemia. *Blood Cancer Journal, 8*(1), 80.

23. Gruber, T. A., Pei, D., Choi, J., Cheng, C., Coustan-Smith, E., Campana, D., Swanson, H. D., Pauley, J. L., Inaba, H., Metzger, M. L., et al. (2022). Clofarabine treatment of KMT2A-rearranged infantile patients with acute lymphoblastic leukemia in St. Jude Total Therapy Study 16. *Blood Advances, 6*(22), 6131–6134.

24. Guenther, M. G., Jenner, R. G., Chevalier, B., Nakamura, T., Croce, C. M., Canaani, E., & Young, R. A. (2005). Global and Hox-specific roles for the MLL1 methyltransferase. *Proceedings of the National Academy of Sciences USA, 102*(24), 8603–8608.

25. Guest, E. M., Kairalla, J. A., Hilden, J. M., Dreyer, Z. E., Carroll, A. J., Heerema, N. A., Wang, C. Y., Devidas, M., Gore, L., Salzer, W. L., et al. (2022). Outstanding outcomes in infants with KMT2A-germline acute lymphoblastic leukemia treated with chemotherapy alone: Results of the Children's Oncology Group AALL0631 trial. *Haematologica, 107*(5), 1205–1208.

26. Guest, E., Kairalla, J., Devidas, M., Hibbitts, E., Carroll, A. J., Heerema, N. A., Kubaney, H., August, A., Pauly, M., Wechsler, D., et al. (2022). A pilot study of azacitidine as epigenetic priming for chemotherapy in infants less than 1 year of age with KMT2A-rearranged acute lymphoblastic leukemia (ALL); Results from the Children's Oncology Group (COG) Trial AALL15P1. *Blood, 140*(13), 3256–3257.

27. Hilden, J. M., Dinndorf, P. A., Meerbaum, S. O., Sather, H., Villaluna, D., Heerema, N. A., McGlennen, R., Smith, F. O., Woods, W. G., Salzer, W. L., et al. (2006). Analysis of prognostic factors of acute lymphoblastic leukemia in infants: Report on CCG 1953 from the Children's Oncology Group. *Blood, 108*(2), 441–451.

28. Ibrahimova, A., Pommert, L., & Breese, E. H. (2021). Acute leukemia in infants. *Current Oncology Reports, 23*(3), 27.

29. Isoyama, K., Eguchi, M., Hibi, S., Kinukawa, N., Ohkawa, H., Kawasaki, H., Kosaka, Y., Oda, T., Oda, M., Okamura, T., et al. (2002). Risk-directed treatment of infant acute lymphoblastic leukaemia based on early assessment of MLL gene status: Results of the Japan Infant Leukaemia Study (MLL96). *British Journal of Haematology, 118*(4), 999–1010.

30. Issa, G. C., Aldoss, I., DiPersio, J., Cuglievan, B., Stone, R., Arellano, M., Thirman, M. J., Patel, M. R., Dickens, D. S., Shenoy, S., et al. (2023). The menin inhibitor revumenib in KMT2A-rearranged or NPM1-mutant leukaemia. *Nature, 615*(7951), 920–924.

31. Karol, S. E., Cooper, T. M., Bittencourt, H., Gore, L., O'Brien, M. M., Fraser, C., Gambart, M., Cario, G., Zwaan, C. M., Bourquin, J. P., et al. (2019). Safety, efficacy, and PK of the BCL2 inhibitor venetoclax in combination with chemotherapy in pediatric and young adult patients with relapsed/refractory acute myeloid leukemia and acute lymphoblastic leukemia: Phase 1 study. *Blood, 134*(24), 2649.

32. Keating, A. K., Gossai, N., Phillips, C. L., Maloney, K., Campbell, K., Doan, A., Bhojwani, D., Burke, M. J., & Verneris, M. R. (2019). Reducing minimal residual disease with blinatumomab prior to HCT for pediatric patients with acute lymphoblastic leukemia. *Blood Advances, 3*(13), 1926–1929.

33. Khaw, S. L., Suryani, S., Evans, K., Richmond, J., Robbins, A., Kurmasheva, R. T., Billups, C. A., Erickson, S. W., Guo, Y., Houghton, P. J., et al. (2016). Venetoclax responses of pediatric ALL xenografts reveal sensitivity of MLL-rearranged leukemia. *Blood, 128*(11), 1382–1395.

34. Koh, K., Tomizawa, D., Moriya Saito, A., Watanabe, T., Miyamura, T., Hirayama, M., Takahashi, Y., Ogawa, A., Kato, K., Sugita, K., et al. (2015). Early use of allogeneic hematopoietic stem cell transplantation for infants with MLL gene-rearrangement-positive acute lymphoblastic leukemia. *Leukemia, 29*(1), 290–296.

35. Kosaka, Y., Koh, K., Kinukawa, N., Wakazono, Y., Isoyama, K., Oda, T., Hayashi, Y., Ohta, S., Moritake, H., Oda, M., et al. (2004). Infant acute lymphoblastic leukemia with MLL gene rearrangements: Outcome following intensive chemotherapy and hematopoietic stem cell transplantation. *Blood, 104*(11), 3527–3534.

36. Kotecha, R. S., Gottardo, N. G., Kees, U. R., & Cole, C. H. (2014). The evolution of clinical trials for infant acute lymphoblastic leukemia. *Blood Cancer Journal, 4*(8), e200.

37. Krivtsov, A. V., Evans, K., Gadrey, J. Y., Eschle, B. K., Hatton, C., Uckelmann, H. J., Ross, K. N., Perner, F., Olsen, S. N., Pritchard, T., et al. (2019). A menin-MLL inhibitor induces specific chromatin changes and eradicates disease in models of MLL-rearranged leukemia. *Cancer Cell, 36*(6), 660–673.

38. Leahy, A. B., Devine, K. J., Li, Y., Liu, H., Myers, R., DiNofia, A., Wray, L., Rheingold, S. R., Callahan, C., Baniewicz, D., et al. (2022). Impact of high-risk cytogenetics on outcomes for children and young adults receiving CD19-directed CAR T-cell therapy. *Blood, 139*(16), 2173–2185.

39. Lee, B. J., Griffin, S. P., Doh, J., Chan, A., O'Brien, S., Jeyakumar, D., Ciurea, S. O., Becker, P. S., & Kongtim, P. (2022). CD19-directed immunotherapy use in KMT2A-rearranged acute leukemia: A case report and literature review of increased lymphoid to myeloid lineage switch. *American Journal of Hematology, 97*(4), E439–E443.

40. Li, K. L., Xiong, H., Li, H., Wang, Z., Chen, Z., Yang, L., Lu, W. J., Qi, S. S., & Sun, M. (2023). Clinical analysis of infants with acute lymphoblastic leukemia (18 cases). *Zhongguo Shi Yan Xue Ye Xue Za Zhi, 31*(4), 1670–1675. (In Chinese)

41. Mann, G., Attarbaschi, A., Schrappe, M., De Lorenzo, P., Peters, C., Hann, I., De Rossi, G., Felice, M., Lausen, B., Leblanc, T., et al. (2010). Improved outcome with hematopoietic stem cell transplantation in a poor prognostic subgroup of infants with mixed-lineage-leukemia (MLL)-rearranged acute lymphoblastic leukemia: Results from the Interfant-99 Study. *Blood, 116*(13), 2644–2650.

42. Maude, S. L., Laetsch, T. W., Buechner, J., Rives, S., Boyer, M., Bittencourt, H., Bader, P., Verneris, M. R., Stefanski, H. E., Myers, G. D., et al. (2018). Tisagenlecleucel in children and young adults with B-cell lymphoblastic leukemia. *New England Journal of Medicine, 378*(5), 439–448.

43. Meyer, C., Burmeister, T., Gröger, D., Tsaur, G., Fechina, L., Renneville, A., Sutton, R., Venn, N. C., Emerenciano, M., Pombo-de-Oliveira, M. S., et al. (2018). The MLL recombinome of acute leukemias in 2017. *Leukemia, 32*(2), 273–284.

44. Meyer, C., Larghero, P., Almeida Lopes, B., Burmeister, T., Gröger, D., Sutton, R., Venn, N. C., Cazzaniga, G., Corral Abascal, L., Tsaur, G., et al. (2023). The KMT2A recombinome of acute leukemias in 2023. *Leukemia, 37*(4), 988–1005.

45. Moskop, A., Pommert, L., Baggott, C., Prabhu, S., Pacenta, H. L., Phillips, C. L., Rossoff, J., Stefanski, H. E., Talano, J. A., Margossian, S. P., et al. (2022). Real-world use of tisagenlecleucel in infant acute lymphoblastic leukemia. *Blood Advances, 6*(15), 4251–4255.

46. Myers, R. M., Jacoby, E., Pulsipher, M. A., Pasquini, M. C., Grupp, S. A., Shah, N. N., Laetsch, T. W., Curran, K. J., & Schultz, L. M. (2023). INSPIRED Symposium Part 1: Clinical variables associated with improved outcomes for children and young adults treated with chimeric antigen receptor T cells for B cell acute lymphoblastic leukemia. *Transplantation and Cellular Therapy, 29*(6), 598–607.

47. Pieters, R., De Lorenzo, P., Ancliffe, P., Aversa, L. A., Brethon, B., Biondi, A., Campbell, M., Escherich, G., Ferster, A., Gardner, R. A., et al. (2019). Outcome of infants younger than 1 year with acute lymphoblastic leukemia treated with the Interfant-06 protocol: Results from an international phase III randomized study. *Journal of Clinical Oncology, 37*(25), 2246–2256.

48. Pieters, R., Schrappe, M., De Lorenzo, P., Hann, I., De Rossi, G., Felice, M., Hovi, L., LeBlanc, T., Szczepanski, T., Ferster, A., et al. (2007). A treatment protocol for infants younger than 1 year with acute lymphoblastic leukaemia (Interfant-99): An observational study and a multicenter randomized trial. *Lancet, 370*(9583), 240–250.

49. Pilheden, M., Ahlgren, L., Hyrenius-Wittsten, A., Gonzalez-Pena, V., Sturesson, H., Hansen Marquart, H. V., Lausen, B., Castor, A., & Pronk, C. J. (2022). Duplex sequencing uncovers recurrent low-frequency cancer-associated mutations in infant and childhood KMT2A-rearranged acute leukemia. *Hemasphere, 6*(7), e785.

50. Place, A. E., Goldsmith, K., Bourquin, J. P., Loh, M. L., Gore, L., Morgenstern, D. A., Sanzgiri, Y., Hoffman, D., Zhou, Y., Ross, J. A., et al. (2018). Accelerating drug development in pediatric cancer: A novel phase I study design of venetoclax in relapsed/refractory malignancies. *Future Oncology, 14*(21), 2115–2129.

51. Qasim, W., Ciocarlie, O., Adams, S., Inglott, S., Murphy, C., Rivat, C., Wright, G., Lucchini, G., Silva, J., Rao, K., et al. (2017). Preliminary results of UCART19, an allogeneic anti-CD19 CAR T-cell product in a first-in-human trial (PALL) in pediatric patients with CD19+ relapsed/refractory B-cell acute lymphoblastic leukemia. *Blood, 130*(10), 1271.

52. Qasim, W., Zhan, H., Samarasinghe, S., Adams, S., Amrolia, P., Stafford, S., Butler, K., Rivat, C., Wright, G., Somana, K., et al. (2017). Molecular remission of infant B-ALL after infusion of universal TALEN gene-edited CAR T cells. *Science Translational Medicine, 9*(380), eaaj2013.

53. Roberts, I., Fordham, N. J., Rao, A., & Bain, B. J. (2018). Neonatal leukaemia. *British Journal of Haematology, 182*(2), 170–184.

54. Schneider, P., Wander, P., Arentsen-Peters, S. T. C. J. M., Vrenken, K. S., Rockx-Brouwer, D., Adriaanse, F. R. S., Hoeve, V., Paassen, I., Drost, J., Pieters, R., et al. (2023). CRISPR-Cas9 library screening identifies novel molecular vulnerabilities in KMT2A-rearranged acute lymphoblastic leukemia. *International Journal of Molecular Sciences, 24*(22), 13207.

55. Shi, Y., Lu, Y., Zhang, R. D., Zhang, Y. Y., Lin, W., Yu, J. J., Wu, Y., Fan, J., Qi, P. J., Huang, P. L., et al. (2024). Clinical characteristics and prognosis of 28 cases of infant acute lymphoblastic leukemia. *Zhonghua Er Ke Za Zhi, 62*(1), 49–54. (In Chinese)

56. Silverman, L. B., McLean, T. W., Gelber, R. D., Donnelly, M. J., Gilliland, D. G., Tarbell, N. J., & Sallan, S. E. (1997). Intensified therapy for infants with acute lymphoblastic leukemia: Results from the Dana-Farber Cancer Institute Consortium. *Cancer, 80*(11), 2285–2295.

57. Spector, L. G., Xie, Y., Robison, L. L., Heerema, N. A., Hilden, J. M., Lange, B., Felix, C. A., Davies, S. M., Slavin, J., Potter, J. D., et al. (2005). Maternal diet and infant leukemia: The DNA topoisomerase II inhibitor hypothesis: A report from the Children's Oncology Group. *Cancer Epidemiology, Biomarkers & Prevention, 14*(3), 651–655.

58. Stumpel, D. J., Schneider, P., Pieters, R., & Stam, R. W. (2015). The potential of clofarabine in MLL-rearranged infant acute lymphoblastic leukaemia. *European Journal of Cancer, 51*(15), 2008–2021.

59. Stumpel, D. J., Schneider, P., van Roon, E. H., Boer, J. M., de Lorenzo, P., Valsecchi, M. G., de Menezes, R. X., Pieters, R., & Stam, R. W. (2009). Specific promoter methylation identifies different subgroups of MLL-rearranged infant acute lymphoblastic leukemia, influences clinical outcome, and provides therapeutic options. *Blood, 114*(24), 5490–5498.

60. Stumpel, D. J., Schneider, P., van Roon, E. H., Pieters, R., & Stam, R. W. (2013). Absence of global hypomethylation in promoter hypermethylated Mixed Lineage Leukaemia-rearranged infant acute lymphoblastic leukaemia. *European Journal of Cancer, 49*(1), 175–184.

61. Takachi, T., Watanabe, T., Miyamura, T., Moriya Saito, A., Deguchi, T., Hori, T., Yamada, T., Ohmori, S., Haba, M., Aoki, Y., et al. (2021). Hematopoietic stem cell transplantation for infants with high-risk KMT2A gene-rearranged acute lymphoblastic leukemia. *Blood Advances, 5*(16), 3891–3899.

62. Taketani, T., Taki, T., Sugita, K., Furuichi, Y., Ishii, E., Hanada, R., Tsuchida, M., Sugita, K., Ida, K., Hayashi, Y., et al. (2004). FLT3 mutations in the activation loop of tyrosine kinase domain are frequently found in infant ALL with MLL rearrangements and pediatric ALL with hyperdiploidy. *Blood, 103*(3), 1085–1088.

63. Tomizawa, D. (2023). Evolution and optimization of therapies for acute lymphoblastic leukemia in infants. *International Journal of Hematology, 117*(2), 162–172.

64. Tomizawa, D., Miyamura, T., Imamura, T., Watanabe, T., Moriya Saito, A., Ogawa, A., Takahashi, Y., Hirayama, M., Taki, T., Deguchi, T., et al. (2020). A risk-stratified therapy for infants with acute lymphoblastic leukemia: A report from the JPLSG MLL-10 trial. *Blood, 136*(15), 1813–1823.

65. van der Linden, M. H., Valsecchi, M. G., De Lorenzo, P., Möricke, A., Janka, G., Leblanc, T. M., Felice, M., Biondi, A., Campbell, M., & Hann, I. (2009). Outcome of congenital acute lymphoblastic leukemia treated on the Interfant-99 protocol. *Blood, 114*(18), 3764–3768.

66. Van der Sluis, I. M., de Lorenzo, P., Kotecha, R. S., Attarbaschi, A., Escherich, G., Nysom, K., Stary, J., Ferster, A., Brethon, B., Locatelli, F., et al. (2023). Blinatumomab added to chemotherapy in infant lymphoblastic leukemia. *New England Journal of Medicine, 388*(16), 1572–1581.

67. Van der Velden, V. H., Corral, L., Valsecchi, M. G., Jansen, M. W., De Lorenzo, P., Cazzaniga, G., Panzer-Grümayer, E. R., Schrappe, M., Schrauder, A., Meyer, C., et al. (2009). Prognostic significance of minimal residual disease in infants with acute lymphoblastic leukemia treated within the Interfant-99 protocol. *Leukemia, 23*(6), 1073–1079.

68. Viardot, A., Goebeler, M. E., Hess, G., Neumann, S., Pfreundschuh, M., Adrian, N., Zettl, F., Libicher, M., Sayehli, C., Stieglmaier, J., et al. (2016). Phase 2 study of the bispecific T-cell engager (BiTE) antibody blinatumomab in relapsed/refractory diffuse large B-cell lymphoma. *Blood, 127*(12), 1410–1416.

69. von Stackelberg, A., Locatelli, F., Zugmaier, G., Handgretinger, R., Trippett, T. M., Rizzari, C., Bader, P., O'Brien, M. M., Brethon, B., Bhojwani, D., et al. (2016). Phase I/Phase II study of blinatumomab in pediatric patients with relapsed/refractory acute lymphoblastic leukemia. *Journal of Clinical Oncology, 34*(37), 4381–4389.

70. Xie, J., Span, M., van Maarseveen, E., Langenhorst, J., Boddy, A. V., Sia, K. C., Sutton, R., Venn, N., Punt, A. M., Tyrrel, V., et al. (2020). Optimization of a clofarabine-based drug combination regimen for the preclinical evaluation of pediatric acute lymphoblastic leukemia. *Pediatric Blood & Cancer, 67*(3), e28133.

71. Zhu, M., Kratzer, A., Johnson, J., Holland, C., Brandl, C., Singh, I., Wolf, A., & Doshi, S. (2018). Blinatumomab pharmacodynamics and exposure-response relationships in relapsed/refractory acute lymphoblastic leukemia. *Journal of Clinical Pharmacology, 58*(2), 168–179.

72. Zhu, M., Wu, B., Brandl, C., Johnson, J., Wolf, A., Chow, A., & Doshi, S. (2016). Blinatumomab, a bispecific T-cell engager (BiTE®) for CD-19 targeted cancer immunotherapy: Clinical pharmacology and its implications. *Clinical Pharmacokinetics, 55*(10), 1271–1288.

Chapter

RARE TUMORS OF THE COLON AND RECTUM

5

Contents

Introduction

Rare tumors of the colon and rectum present a unique challenge in oncology due to their low incidence and diverse histological subtypes. These tumors, comprising only a small fraction of colorectal malignancies, are defined by their occurrence rates of less than 2% of all cases (Bach et al., 2018). Despite their rarity, they pose significant clinical and diagnostic dilemmas, necessitating a comprehensive understanding of their epidemiology, clinical behavior, and treatment outcomes.

Adenocarcinomas are the most common histological subtype, accounting for 95–97% of malignant tumors in the colon and rectum. Other rare subtypes include carcinoids, lymphomas, gastrointestinal stromal tumors (GISTs), squamous cell carcinomas, melanomas, and a variety of extremely rare forms such as teratomas, plasmacytomas, schwannomas, and metastatic tumors. These tumors exhibit unique clinical features and often require tailored treatment approaches (Bjørnland et al., 2005).

The incidence of rare tumors of the colon and rectum varies widely among different subtypes. Carcinoids, for example, represent approximately 1.8% of all colorectal tumors, while primary lymphomas account for 0.1–1%. GISTs and melanomas have incidence rates of 0.9% and 0.5–1%, respectively, while squamous cell carcinomas are rare, comprising only 0.1% of cases excluding those in the anal canal. The remaining extremely rare forms collectively represent less than 0.1% of colorectal malignancies (Cai et al., 2012).

Recent studies have shown a significant increase in the annual percentage change in incidence for each rare tumor subtype over the past decade, with the exception of squamous cell carcinoma. This trend highlights the importance of recognizing and addressing these rare malignancies, which may require specialized diagnostic and therapeutic approaches (Cappellen et al., 2007).

Despite advancements in surgical techniques and the introduction of novel treatment modalities such as targeted therapies and immunotherapy, the prognosis for rare tumors of the colon and rectum remains serious. The study of rare tumors of the colon and rectum aims to determine their population incidence, characterize their clinical features, compare treatment outcomes across different gastrointestinal sites, and evaluate overall and five-year survival rates (Carreira et al., 2014). However, due to the rarity of these tumors, conducting large-scale randomized trials or meta-analyses remains challenging.

Orientation and Directional Terms

Term	Definition	Illustration
Carcinoids	A type of slow-growing neuroendocrine tumor that typically occurs in the gastrointestinal tract, lungs, or other organs. They can secrete hormones causing symptoms.	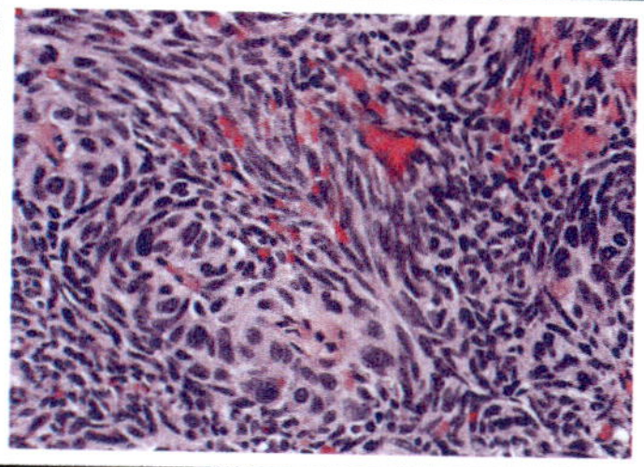
Laparotomy	A surgical procedure involving a large incision through the abdominal wall to gain access to the abdominal cavity, often used for diagnosis or surgery.	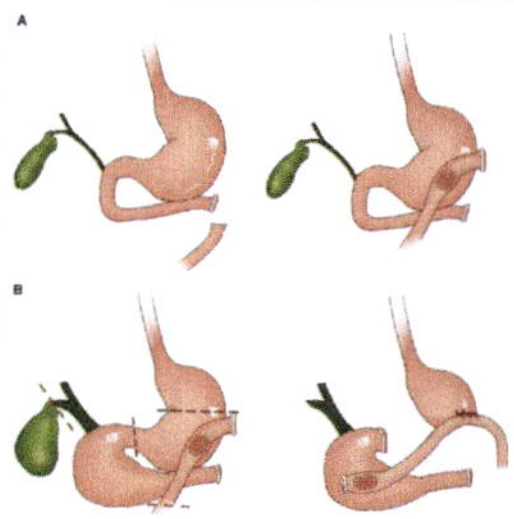
Gastrointestinal Stromal Tumors (GIST)	A rare type of tumor that forms in the digestive tract, most commonly in the stomach or small intestine, arising from specialized cells in the GI wall.	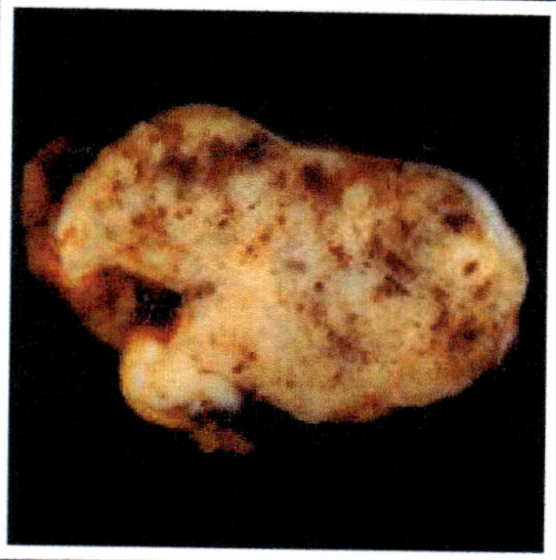
Squamous Cell Carcinoma	A type of skin cancer that arises from squamous cells, the flat cells found in the outer layer of the skin and other areas like the lungs or esophagus.	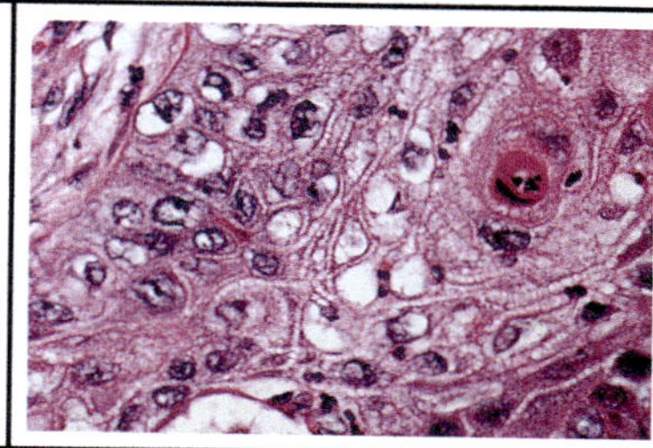
Melanoma	A dangerous type of skin cancer that develops from melanocytes, the cells responsible for producing the pigment melanin, often triggered by UV radiation exposure.	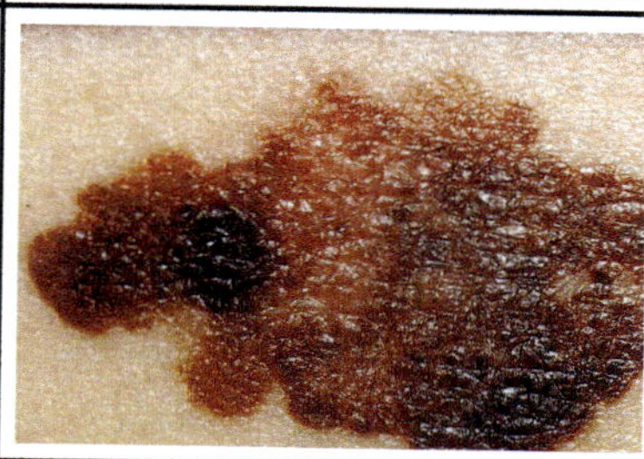

5.1. An Overview of Malignant Tumors

Malignant tumors of the colon and rectum represent a distinct entity due to their early clinical presentation, specific diagnostic approaches, and treatment strategies focused on preserving sphincter function while ensuring oncological surgical principles and radicality. Despite advancements in surgical techniques and improvements in radiotherapy and chemotherapy, the prognosis for these tumors remains serious (Chan et al., 2005).

In terms of histological types, these tumors can be categorized as adenocarcinomas, carcinoids, lymphomas, gastrointestinal stromal tumors (GISTs), squamous cell carcinomas, melanomas, and other extremely rare forms of malignant tumors. Adenocarcinomas comprise 95–97% of all malignant tumors, with the remaining 3–5% classified as rare tumors of the colon and rectum (Cheng et al., 2014). The annual incidence change for each rare tumor type has significantly increased over the past decade, except for squamous cell carcinoma.

Rare colon and rectal tumors can be further divided into two groups based on their incidence rates: tumors with an incidence of 0.1–2% and those with an incidence of <0.1%. The more common tumors in the first group include carcinoids (1.8%), primary lymphomas (0.1–1%), GISTs (0.9%), melanomas (0.5–1%), and squamous cell carcinomas (0.1%, excluding anal canal). The second group comprises extremely rare forms such as teratomas, plasmacytomas, schwannomas, and metastatic tumors (Chomczynski, 1987).

Data on rare colon and rectal tumors are limited, primarily consisting of case series from specific institutions or national studies. There is a lack of randomized trials or meta-analyses due to the rarity of these tumors (Choong et al., 2014).

The objectives of studying rare colon and rectal tumors include determining their population incidence, understanding their clinical characteristics, comparing treatment outcomes across different gastrointestinal sites, and evaluating overall and five-year survival rates among patients (Cong et al., 2018).

5.2. Carcinoids

Carcinoid tumors are rare, slow-growing tumors and account for 1.8% of all malignant tumors of the colon. There is no clear gender predominance, and, in most cases, patients are in their 60s or 70s. They arise from the enterochromaffin cells (argentafil, Kulchitsky) as part of the diffuse endocrine system and belong to the group of neuroendocrine tumors, the so-called well-differentiated "NETs." They are also known as APUDomas, an abbreviation for "amine precursor uptake and decarboxylation," due to their ability to take up and decarboxylate amines, which was originally described by Pearse in 1969. They can occur in all parts of the gastrointestinal tract and also outside the tract (Cyr-DePauw et al., 2016). Therefore, carcinoids are classified according to their site of occurrence and the division of the primitive gut during embryologic development:

- Anterior intestinal carcinoid tumors begin in the lungs, bronchi, or stomach;
- Midgut carcinoid tumors begin in the small intestine, cecum, or proximal colon;
- Carcinoid tumors in the hindgut begin in the distal colon or rectum.

Data from the literature suggest that the incidence of carcinoids varies in specific locations, although they are thought to be most commonly localized in the vermiform appendix, accounting for about 40% of cases, the ileum about 25%, the rectum 15–20%, and the respiratory tract about 10%. On the other hand, the Japanese National Study identified 345 cases of carcinoids in the small and large intestine in 90,057 operated patients over a 15-year period, of which 0.9% were localized in the ileum, 2.3% in the appendix, 8.2% in the colon and 88.6% in the rectum. Their secretion is active, and they secrete about 30 vasoactive substances, the most important of which are serotonin, histamine, and substance P. In 1867, Langhans first described a carcinoid intestinal tumor, but the first detailed description of the carcinoid-like tumor was made by Lubrasch in 1888 after he had performed autopsies on two individuals who had previously been treated for multiple tumors of the ileum. A German pathologist, Oberndorfer, first mentioned the term "carcinoid" in 1907, while Siburg published the first data on rectal carcinoid in 1929. The term "carcinoid" indicates that the tumor resembles a carcinoma according to some histological features but behaves more benignly and less aggressively (Davis et al., 2008). They are often discovered by chance during colonoscopy or by examining clinical symptoms such as rectagia or diarrhea. At initial diagnosis, 60–90% of carcinoids are less than 1 cm in size. These tumors have variable malignant potential depending on the size, location, depth of invasion, and the nature of growth of the tumor itself (Dong et al., 2016) (Figure 5.1).

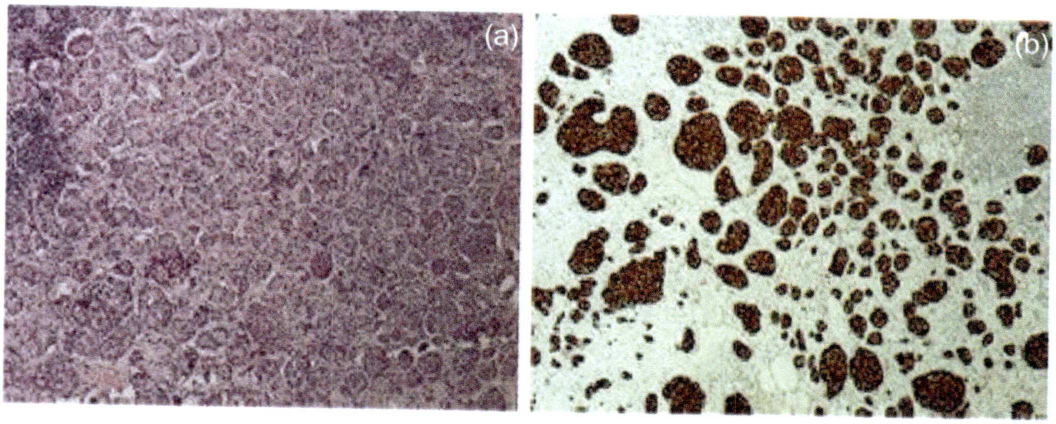

Figure 5.1. *(a) Colon carcinoid (H&E 10x); and (b) colon carcinoid (chromogranin A 10x).*

Source: Image by Goran Stanojević; https://www.researchgate.net/figure/a-colon-carcinoid-H-E-10x-b-colon-carcinoid-chromogranin-A-10x_fig1_298786874.

5.2.1. Clinical Presentation and Diagnosis

The clinical presentation is characterized by the presence of symptoms due to the secretion of various biochemical substances and the growth of the tumor itself. Occasional abdominal pain, followed by facial flushing, diarrhea, bronchospasm, cardiac arrhythmias, hyperthermia, blood pressure fluctuations, and vasomotor collapse, which, depending on the intensity, can lead to a life-threatening condition or a so-called "carcinoid crisis." Various everyday activities and psychological conditions such as alcohol consumption, emotional stress, increased body temperature, and difficult defecation increase the intensity of the symptoms (Dong et al., 2016).

The diagnosis of colonic carcinoids was usually made by a detailed history and clinical examination of the abdomen and a digital rectal examination. Very often it is an unclear finding due to the intact mucosa, so a biopsy is required from both the part of the tumor surface and the deeper structures. It is also necessary to include a colonoscopy in the clinical examination, as a synchronous lesion may be present, as well as magnetic resonance imaging or endoluminal ultrasound of the pelvis for preoperative staging (Ejarque et al., 2017). The examination of the liver metastases should be supplemented by an ultrasound and CT scan. Modern diagnosis of carcinoids also includes so-called functional or biochemical examinations, which are based on the uptake of certain substances by the tumor cells that distinguish them from normal tissue. The biochemical properties of carcinoid tumors reflect the presence of neurosecretory granules. They are classified as biochemically typical or atypical based on the presence of high levels of serotonin in so-called typical tumors (Fehr et al., 2000). The best-known metabolite of serotonin in carcinoid tumors is 5-HIAA (hydroxylindoleacetic acid). The urine level of 5-HIAA in a 24-hour sample is the most commonly used test in the endocrine work-up of carcinoid tumors (Fromigué et al., 2008). Despite its popularity, it is not sufficiently sensitive and specific for the diagnosis of carcinoid tumors, as 5-HIAA may not be elevated in atypical carcinoids and may be elevated in other conditions such as tropical sprue, celiac disease, Whipple's disease, and small bowel obstruction, and may be caused by the ingestion of foods high in serotonin or certain medications (Geng et al., 2014).

Although a number of other tumor markers for carcinoid tumor overproduction have been investigated, serum analysis of chromogranin A, a glycoprotein secreted along with other hormones by neuroendocrine tumors, appears to be the most promising, with a specificity approaching 95% and a sensitivity for carcinoid tumors approaching 80%. In patients with multiple myeloma, a false-positive rate of 40% was found (Guan et al., 2015).

For this purpose, scintigraphy of somatostin receptors on the surface of tumor cells or SRS and PET scan using metabolic uptake of FDG fluorin-18 fluorodeoxyglucose by tumor cells is used. The results of the study show that octreoscan is best suited for identifying the primary tumor and positive lymph nodes, while CT or NMR are used in the case of distant metastases (Guo et al., 1999). As part of the biochemical analysis, the content of 5-hydroxyindoleacetic acid in the urine must be determined if there is any doubt about the presence of a carcinoid.

5.2.2. Treatment

The treatment of the colon carcinoid can be divided into two groups:

i. Minimally invasive procedure; and
ii. Laparotomy.

Minimally invasive procedure includes several types of interventions:

i. endoscopic mucosectomy or submucosectomy;
ii. transanal tumor extirpation;
iii. TEM (transanal endoscopic microsurgery);
iv. laparoscopic resections of colon and rectum.

Endoscopic mucosectomy or submucosectomy is one of the possible methods in the early stages of the disease, without penetrating the muscularis mucosae and up to a size of 1 cm (Hamam et al., 2014). The literature data show that endoscopic mucosetomy or submucosetomy is performed in 54% of patients with rectal carcinoid, transanal tumor extirpation/TEM in 27% of operated patients on the one hand and in 6% of patients treated with the invasive procedure on the other.

The results of the treatment show that of the 83 patients treated with the endoscopic method had positive margins (R1 status), 16% had residual tumor (R2 status) with 2% acute complications in terms of the occurrence of postoperative bleeding. Submucosectomy was performed in 12 patients (14%), with 42% of positive margins (Han et al., 2012).

The advantages of the endoscopic approach are a minimally invasive procedure, faster recovery of the patient, and less surgical trauma, but there are also disadvantages in terms of the high percentage of R1 or R2 procedures (positive margins or residual tumor).

Transanal extirpation/TEM is indicated for rectal carcinoid invasion into the submucosa and muscularis propria. They are mainly performed after an unsuccessful, previously performed mucosectomy, i.e., a submucosectomy. The results of the treatment show that an R0 resection was performed in 43% of the operated patients, while an R1, that is R2 resection was performed in 52 of the cases. Postoperative complications occurred in about 9% of patients. The disadvantage of the procedure is still a high percentage of R1 and R2 operations (Haudenschild et al., 2004).

Laparoscopic resections of the colon and rectum represent a trend in modern colorectal surgery, with all the characteristics of the minimally invasive procedure. It is indicated for tumors that spread to structures deeper than the lamina muscularis mucosa (T2 stage), most commonly in the upper third of the rectum but also in the other parts of the rectum where performing the endoscopic procedure, would result in a high percentage of R1 and R2 operations (He et al., 2014).

5.2.3. Laparatomy

Laparotomy is indicated for carcinoids of larger median size, so-called bulky tumors, with infiltration of the surrounding organs and potential risk of intestinal obstruction (Hu et al., 2014):

1. Resection of colon (according to the type of segmental or right/left hemicolectomies).
2. Resections of the rectum with different forms of reconstructions (T-T anastomosis, L-T anastomosis, colonic J pouch, etc.).
3. Incontinence operations (abdominoperineal amputation of the rectum, etc.).
4. In case of inoperability of the tumor, the performance of colostomy is conducted.

In terms of treatment outcome, resection procedures are associated with a higher percentage of local recurrence, which is explained by the existence of more invasive and larger tumors treated in this way. (Hua et al., 2017).

Systemic therapy in carcinoid treatment has two aims:

- To reduce the intensity of the systemic effects of disease; and
- Treatment of metastasis.

To reduce the intensity of the systemic effects, various medications are used, such as H2 blockers, phenothiazine, corticosteroids, serotonin blockers, bronchodilators, and many more. The analogs of somatostatin have a significant effect which, by blocking the receptors, reduces the production and systemic effects, especially the intensity of flushing and diarrhea, in 80% of patients (Huang et al., 2018).

In the treatment of metastases, the effect of chemotherapy (5-fluorouracil, streptozotocin, doxorubicin, etoposide, cisplatin, carboplatin, etc.) is insignificant, with a clinical response (response rate (RR)) of 0 to 30%. In some cases, interferon is used with a duration of up to 2.5 years, but due to the numerous unfavorable effects, its use is limited (Huang et al., 2020).

The prognosis of the disease depends on the TNM stage. A search of 15,983 patients with carcinoid tumors from the National Cancer Institute's SEER (Surveillance Epidemiology and End Results) database identified 2,459 patients with colon tumors and 4,701 patients with rectal carcinoid tumors from 1973 to 2004. Patients were analyzed according to various clinicopathological factors and a staging system for tumor (T1, T2, T3), lymph nodes (N0, N1), and metastases (M0, M1) was established according to these parameters (Huang et al., 2022). The results are shown in Table 5.1.

Table 5.1. *Staging System and 5-Year Survival Rate*

Staging System	Colon Carcinoids% Patien. 5-year surv.%		Rectal Carcinoids% Patient. 5-Year surv.%	
I	13	97	83	97
II	32	69	6.5	84
III	12	21	2.8	27
IV	43	17	7.4	20
N 0	52		96	
1	48		4	
M 0	76		97.6	
1	24		2.4	

5.3. Primary Non-Hodgkin Lymphomas

Lymphomas of the colon and rectum are the rare tumors that account for 1.4% of human lymphomas, 10–20% of gastrointestinal lymphomas, 0.2–0.6% of all malignant tumors of the colon, i.e., 0.1–1% of all tumors of the colon (Huang et al., 2015). In terms of incidence in the gastrointestinal system in adults, they occupy third place after the stomach and small intestine, in contrast to the age of up to 17 years, where intestinal localization is predominant. In terms of the frequency of all malignant diseases of the colon and rectum, they are in third place, after adenocarcinoma and carcinoids. The preferred sites of occurrence are the cecum and rectum, as there is a large amount of lymphatic tissue in these regions of the colon (Ji et al., 2018) (Figure 5.2).

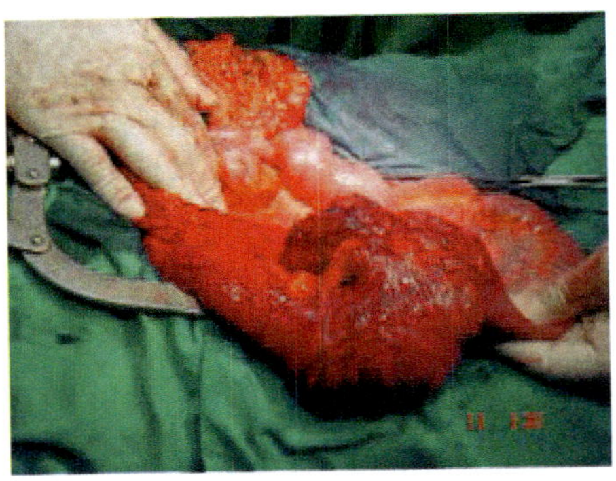

Figure 5.2. *Primary non-Hodgkin lymphoma of the cecum.*

Source: Image by Goran Stanojević; https://www.wjgnet.com/1948-5204/full/v3/i1/14.htm.

It occurs more frequently in male patients older than 50 years. Regarding the degree of spread, a distinction can be made between primary (localized) and secondary (diffuse) disease (Jiang et al., 2012). Primary lymphomas of the colon are characterized by the presence of the so-called Dawson criteria:

- no palpable, superficial lymph nodes at presentation;
- no enlarged mediastinal lymph nodes on chest x-ray;
- normal range for white blood cell count including total and differential;
- at surgery, only the regional lymph nodes are involved;
- the liver and spleen are without disease.

Primary lymphoma of the colon is a predominantly extranodal form of non-Hodgkin's lymphoma, whereas Hodgkin's lymphoma is much rarer, occurring in less than 5% of all patients who undergo autopsy for this disease. Devin and his colleagues at the Mayo Clinic have published the largest study of patients with rectal lymphoma, showing that of 61 patients treated over a 27-year period, 49 had a diffuse form and only 12 had localized disease. The tumors usually take the form of a polypoid and ulcerative mass, and sometimes they form excretions on the mucosa, similar to multiple adenomatous polyposis.

The etiologic factors for the development of colonic lymphoma are not known, as they are for other types of malignancies. However, a higher incidence has been found in conditions of immunosuppression, such as the inflammatory disease – ulcerative colitis, HIV infection, and after organ transplantation, although there is no clear scientific evidence of the links between these diseases (Kaczorowska et al., 2020).

More than two-thirds of intestinal lymphomas could constitute of B-cell lymphomas, while T-cell lymphomas in the intestine are rather rare and often multifocal and are most frequently localized in the small intestine. In terms of B-cell histologic type, non-Hodgkin's lymphomas can be diffuse B-cell type, MALT lymphoma, mantle type, Burkitt's type, and follicular lymphoma. The frequency of some histopathological forms differs from study to study. For example, Anderson and his colleagues presented data from the International Study Group on Lymphomas, which included 1,378 patients from 8 different cities on 4 continents (Kansara et al., 2014). Of the total number of histopathologic findings, B-cell lymphoma was diagnosed in 80% of cases, with the most common form being large cell, while the other forms such as mantle, Burkitt's, and MALT types were significantly less common. In terms of histological grades, moderate and intermediate types of diffuse large cell lymphoma were found in 75 of the tumors (Figure 5.3).

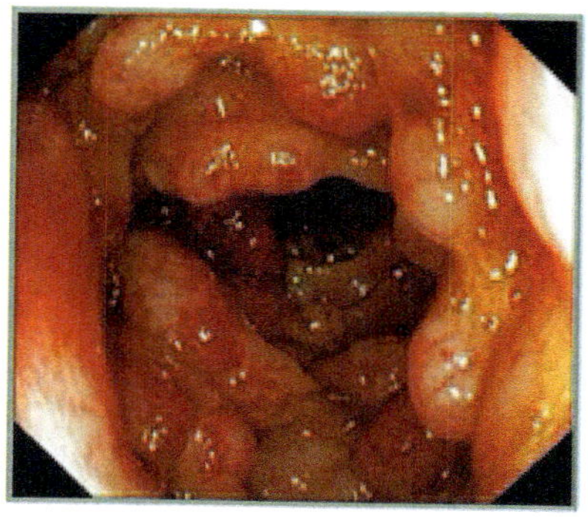

Figure 5.3. *Mantle type of primary non-Hodgkin lymphoma.*

Source: Image by Goran Stanojević; https://www.researchgate.net/figure/Mantle-type-of-primary-non-Hodgkin-lymphoma_fig3_298786874.

The degree of spread of the disease to the surrounding structures was best visualized by the so-called Ann Arbor staging, a modification according to Musshoffu. The aim of successful treatment is early detection of the disease at stage IE or IIE, when curative resection is still possible (Katagiri & Watabe, 2016). The data from the literature differ considerably with regard to the stage of disease of the treated patients, which is a consequence of the different criteria according to which the patients were included in the study, as well as the different methods of implementation and the level of health culture in the population studied (Table 5.2).

Table 5.2. *Ann-Arbor Staging–Musshoff Modifications of Primary Colorectal Lymphoma*

Stage	Characteristics
IE	Limited to the colonic/rectal wall.
IIE 1	Involvement of paracolic lymph nodes.
IIE 2	Involvement of intermedial lymph nodes.
III	Involvement of the large bowel and lymph nodes on both sides of diaphragm.
IV	Involvement of distant organs (large bowel and one or more extralymphatic organs or tissue).

5.3.1. Clinical Presentation and Diagnosis

The clinical presentation is characterized by the presence of rectagia and altered bowel habits (Kochanowska et al., 2002). In analyzing the symptoms of the disease, Cho and his associates presented study data showing that of 23 patients, 56% had nonspecific symptoms, abdominal pain, and weight loss or anorexia, i.e., 35% of the patients studied underwent surgery in the advanced stage of the disease. Data from the study by Fan and coworkers showed that of 37 patients studied, 59% had only abdominal pain and 75.7% were operated on at the stage of the disease when positive lymph nodes were present in the mesentery of the colon and mesorectum (Kochanowska et al., 2002).

Specific symptoms, such as bleeding from the rectum, occurred in only 12.5% of patients. The non-specificity of symptoms often delays timely medical consultation and diagnosis, leading to a much higher incidence of the advanced stages of the disease. Primary colorectal lymphomas, which present as surgical emergencies and are caused by stage IIIE and IVE tumors, pose a particular problem. Surgical emergencies caused by colonic obstruction or perforation require urgent surgical intervention, resulting in a significantly higher mortality rate of 58% and more frequent recurrence of the disease. The diagnosis can be made on the basis of anamnestic data and clinical examination, including rectal examination and colonoscopy with biopsy.

There are data from the literature that show that it is not always possible to make the diagnosis by endoscopic procedures, as the biopsy of the tumor is insufficiently performed and adequate immunohistochemical staining must be performed in a timely manner during the histopathological examination performed by a pathologist (Kundu et al., 2019). This very often leads to the fact that the pathological findings cannot be interpreted correctly.

5.3.2. Treatment

Modern treatment of primary lymphoma of the colon and rectum involves a multimodal approach, which is surgery, chemotherapy and radiotherapy in selected cases. Despite the undoubted improvements in surgical technique, anesthesiology and chemotherapy over the last three decades, the five-year survival rate of patients undergoing surgery is still low at 42%. There are different views on the treatment of colorectal non-Hodgkin's lymphoma, ranging from the exclusive use of chemotherapy and radiotherapy on the one hand to the performance of surgical interventions on the other. In 2005, Bilsel and his colleagues published a report on a case in which the primary rectal lymphoma responded completely clinically after treatment with chemotherapy and radiotherapy. The other authors also presented similar data. In their analysis of the 2002 case presentation, Pricolo and coworkers describe treatment of rectal lymphoma with resection procedures followed by chemotherapy and radiotherapy, while Shimono from Japan recommends preoperative radiotherapy followed by surgery. Regarding the type of surgery, there are recommendations that limited resection or transanal extirpation of the tumor is sufficient for small primary rectal lymphoma and low malignant potential – MALT or mantle lymphoma (Lauvrak et al., 2013).

The differences in attitude are the consequence of the results obtained based on case reports or studies on a small number of patients and a heterogeneous group of treated tumors, at different stages of the disease and histopathological diagnoses. Nevertheless, based on the authors' modest experience, resection of the colon is recommended whenever possible, together with neo- or adjuvant therapy.

5.4. Gastrointestinal Stromal Tumors

Gastrointestinal stromal tumors, or GISTs for short, are the most common mesenchymal tumors characterized by positive c-KIT, which is CD117 and CD 34 antigens, and account for 0.1–1% of all tumors of the gastrointestinal tract. They occur most frequently in the stomach (60–70%) and small intestine (20–25%), while they are least common in the colon (about 5%) and account for 0.9% of all tumors in the rectum. As far as the frequency of occurrence in the colon is concerned, they occur in the rectum in 80% of all patients, while they only occur in the colon in 20% of cases. They occur equally in middle-aged people between 40 and 60 years of age and in both sexes, with an incidence of 6.8 / 1,000,000 (Laxman et al., 2016).

At the beginning of the 20th century, Theodor Bilroth provided the first descriptions of stromal tumors. However, the term "stromal tumor" was not introduced until 1983 by Mazur and Clark, after the development of immunohistochemistry. A year later, in 1984, Henry Appelman introduced the term "GIST-gastrointestinal stromal tumors" for the first time, while Kindblom and his colleagues demonstrated that GIST originates from the interstitial Cajal cells, which are the so-called pacemaker cells of the gastrointestinal tract. Due to the similar structural and immunohistochemical characteristics of GISTs and Cajal cells, many authors believe that they originate from the same mesenchymal cell (Li et al., 2015). The invasiveness or metastatic risk assessment of GISTs at different sites is determined by tumor size and mitotic index, as shown in Table 5.3.

Table 5.3. *Metastasis Risk Assessment of GISTs in Different Parts of GI Tract*

Mitotic Count	Size	Gastric GIST	Duodenal GIST	Jejunal and Ileal GIST	Rectal GIST
≤5/50	<2 cm	0%	0%	0%	0%
	>2 ≤5	1.9%	8.3%	4.3%	8.5%
	>5 ≤10	3.6%	34%	24%	57%
	>10	12%		52%	
>5/50	≤2	0%	N/A	50%	54%
	>2 ≤5	16%	50%	73%	52%
	>5 ≤10	55%	86%	85%	71%
	>10	86%		90%	

5.4.1. Clinical Presentation and Diagnosis

GISTs are symptomatic in about 70% and asymptomatic in about 10%, and is discovered at autopsy in 20% of cases, which shows that 1/3 of colonic stromal tumors are clinically completely silent. The symptoms are very similar to other colon tumors and are characterized by hematochezia, abdominal or rectal pain, the appearance of complete rectal prolapse, and many more. Depending on the size of the tumor, obstruction or ileus may occur due to the growth of GISTs. The diagnosis can be made based on anamnestic data, clinical examination including a digital rectal examination supplemented with rectoscopy, colonoscopy, endorectal ultrasound, and magnetic resonance imaging. It is necessary to perform a tumor biopsy with immunohistochemical analysis to definitively confirm the presence of GIST in the colon. If there is any doubt about metastasis in the liver, an ultrasound and CT scan must also be performed as part of the complete staging of the tumor. A PET scan is indicated for follow-up in patients who have undergone surgery (Li et al., 2016).

5.4.2. Treatment

Surgical intervention is the method of choice in the treatment of colonic GISTs and is used in the following cases:

- Primary disease;
- Metastatic disease;
- Recurrence.

The main goals of surgical treatment of primary disease are complete resection, so-called R0 resection, and preservation of the tumor pseudocapsule without wide resection margins and lymphadenectomy (Lin et al., 2021). This is very important in the treatment of rectal GISTs, as the aim is to preserve the sphincter muscle and improve the patient's quality of life. Depending on the size and location of the colonic stromal tumors, different surgical procedures can be used: segmental resection and local excision, as well as anterior and abdominoperineal resection. Performing anterior resection (high or low) means adhering to the principles of partial or total mesorectal excision to avoid sacral nerve injury, bleeding, or local recurrence (Figure 5.4).

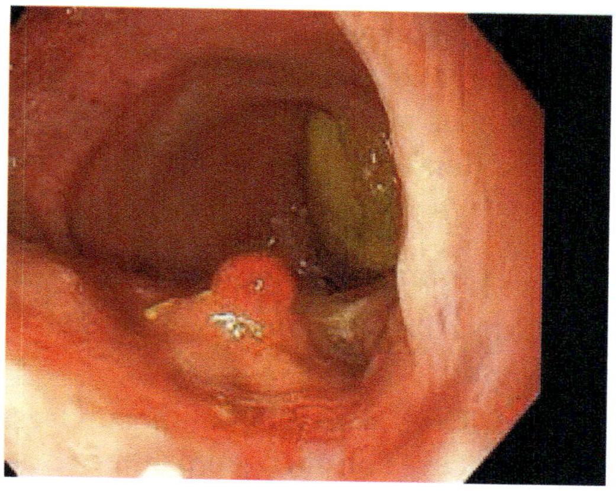

Figure 5.4. *Rectal GIST.*

Source: https://encrypted-tbn0.gstatic.com/images?q=tbn:ANd9GcR8NVfF-dXLOChMJcLhrBz6Mwv7P9EyG4XMJeRvjKv0pA&s.

If GIST adheres to adjacent organs, en bloc resection should be considered. Modern aspects of GIST treatment include the use of imatinib, a drug that has made a revolutionary contribution to significantly improved treatment outcomes in GIST. Joensuua, Heinrick van Oosterona, and Tuveson first reported on the use of imatinib in 2001. An immediate impetus for the invention of this drug was the discovery by Hirot of abnormal activation of the KIT oncoprotein or transmembrane receptor tyrosine kinase and the subsequent mutation of the C-kit gene leading to abnormal cell proliferation. Imatinib selectively inhibits the transmembrane tyrosine kinase receptors and thus blocks the abnormal growth of the tumor (Liu et al., 2014). Van Oosteron and colleagues published the results of 70% of clinical responses in KIT-positive metastatic GISTs. Primary unresectable GISTs of the colon are initially treated with imatinib to reduce the tumor size – "downsizing." If metastatic disease is present, non-adjuvant use of imatinib is indicated to achieve a good clinical response, that is disease without progression, with the possibility of R0 resection. In the case of small-volume metastases in the liver, some authors recommend simultaneous resection of the colon and liver and subsequent use of imatinib (Liu et al., 2015). Distant metastases in the liver occur in over 50% of cases and are treated with the initial use of imatinib, followed by various resection procedures.

Treatment of GIST with chemotherapy has a minimal effect, RR<10%, and has no impact on overall survival, nor does the use of radiotherapy, as the tumor is radioresistant (Long et al., 2013).

5.4.3. Treatment Outcomes

The outcome of colorectal GIST treatment is associated with a high percentage of local and distant recurrences, such that after R0 resection these occur in 45–50% of cases 20–25 months after surgery. The average five-year survival rate is 50%, 73% after R0 resection, and 26% after R1 and R2 resections. In an advanced of the disease with local recurrence and metastasis, the five-year survival rate is 28–35%.

5.5. Squamous Cell Carcinoma

Squamous cell carcinoma of the colon is a very rare disease, in contrast to its localizations in the esophagus and anal canal. The data from the literature are based on a review of clinical cases and series with a small number of patients. Schmidtmann first described squamous cell carcinoma of the colon, more specifically the cecum, in 1919, and Reiford described the same disease in the rectum in 1933. Currently, about 100 cases of squamous cell carcinoma of the colon have been described in the literature, and the incidence of the disease is 0.1–0.25 per 1,000 patients suffering from colorectal carcinoma (Lucero et al., 2013).

Due to the very rare occurrence of the tumor, there is a lack of prospective studies or meta-analyzes that would provide data on patient demographics, risk factors, disease progression, and optimal treatment. Colorectal squamous cell carcinoma mainly occurs in patients with an average age of 60 years and is more common in women (66%) than in men (34%). The etiology of colorectal squamous cell carcinoma is still unknown, as is that of other malignancies, although there are several theories that attempt to explain the development of this neoplasm:

- The influence of stem cell differentiation.
- Squamous metaplasia at the site where a colorectal adenoma has arisen.
- Proliferation of uncommitted basal cells of the mucosa into squamous epithelial cells, which subsequently undergo malignant transformation.
- Oncogenic influence of chronic renal insufficiency, as well as the use of immunosuppressive therapy in relation to the development of some cancer viruses or oncogenic differentiation of stem cells.
- Special influences of radiation, colocutaneous fistula, ulcerative colitis, Entamoeba histolityca colitis, homosexuality, immunosuppression, schistosomiasis, and the still unclear influence of HIV (human papillomavirus types 16, 18, 31, 33).

5.5.1. Clinical Presentation and Diagnosis

The symptoms of the disease are very similar to the symptoms of colon carcinoma, such as bleeding, abdominal pain, change in bowel habits with episodes of diarrhea and constipation, and weight loss (Luo et al., 2018). The diagnosis is made based on anamnestic data, clinical examination including digital rectal examination, and should be supplemented by rectoscopy, colonoscopy, MSCT, endorectal ultrasound, and NMR. Williams and his associates published the following criteria for the diagnosis of squamous cell carcinoma of the colon in 1979:

- Absence of squamous cell carcinoma and its metastases to other sites (especially the skin).
- Careful anoscopy and rectoscopy to exclude proximal extension of anal squamous cell carcinoma.
- Absence of a fistulous tract lined with squamous cells.

These criteria should be supplemented by excisional biopsy of the tumor and PH or immunohistochemical confirmation (presence of cytokeratin CAM 5.2, AE1/AE3 i 34B12). Submucosal localizations of squamous cell carcinoma pose a special problem, as they are difficult to detect with standard examinations (Lv et al., 2016).

Therefore, an endoluminal, ultrasound-guided needle biopsy of the tumor is recommended in these cases. The determination of tumor marker values is one of the possible auxiliary diagnostic procedures for determining the disease, provided that the marker is specific for a particular tumor. In the case of squamous cell carcinoma of the colon and rectum, there are no specific tumor markers, so those commonly used for anal squamous cell carcinoma or the so-called squamous cell carcinoma antigen (squamous cell carcinoma antigen "-SCC Ag)" are used. According to some authors, SCC Ag is not specific for initial diagnosis, but for tracking the occurrence of local and distant recurrences after treatment.

5.5.2. Treatment

Surgical intervention is the method of choice to treat squamous cell carcinoma of the colon. The type of surgical intervention depends on the size of the tumor, its location, the depth of invasion into the intestinal wall, the presence of local and distant metastases, the BMI (body mass index), the general condition of the patient, and the presence of comorbidities. The types of surgical intervention are similar to those for colon cancer: endoscopic mucosal/submucosal resection, segmental or hemicolectomy, local excision, resection of the rectum, and abdominoperineal amputation of the rectum. Endoscopic mucosal/submucosal resection is used based on experience gained in the treatment of adenocarcinomas and is indicated for patients with superficial tumors – T1 stage and with a pronounced comorbidity (Melnik et al., 2019). Endoscopic mucosal/submucosal resection, local excision (transanal or transanal endoscopic microsurgery (TEM)) is the method of choice for a T1 stage of the disease, i.e., a tumor that spreads to the mucosa/submucosa. There are some dilemmas in the treatment of stage T2 (spread to the muscularis proprie), as recurrence occurs in 20% of operated patients after local excision. In these cases, good preoperative staging of the tumor in terms of the presence of positive lymph nodes and the extent of spread to the colon wall is necessary. In cases where there is transmural spread to the wall, extending up to the pericolic or perirectal fat tissue (T3 stage), or infiltration into surrounding organs (T4 stage), there are ongoing debates regarding the optimal sequence of treatment. Specifically, there is uncertainty about whether it is more effective to perform surgery first followed by chemotherapy, or to administer chemotherapy before proceeding with surgery. Studies based on the application of the identical treatment protocol for anal squamous cell carcinoma – (combination of chemotherapy and radiotherapy 5-FU + mitomycin-C and radio 45 Gy) – have not yielded the expected results in the localization of the proximal parts of the rectum and colon.

There is data in the literature that only recommend the use of chemotherapy and radiotherapy and concurrent chemoradiation. However, most authors agree that the optimal therapy at present and based on the experience gained in the treatment of a small number of patients is surgical intervention and adjuvant chemoradiation. Surgical treatment of advanced disease consists of the use of resection procedures (colectomy, high and low resection of the rectum) and abdominoperineal amputations of the rectum. The resection of the rectum as a sphincter-preserving operation enables a better quality of life for the patient on the one hand and compliance with oncological principles on the other (Mukhametov et al., 2022).

Notwithstanding the advantages of resection procedures over rectal amputation surgery, data from the literature show that Miles surgery was performed twice as frequently in the treatment of rectal squamous cell carcinoma, which is explained by a large number of advanced tumors at the time of diagnosis.

Disease prognosis is based on the determination of the TNM stage, the most important prognostic factor, which is identical to that of anal squamous cell carcinoma (Nakka et al., 2017). The TNM stage is listed in Table 5.4.

Table 5.4. *TNM Staging System of Squamous Cell Carcinoma of the Large Bowel*

Stadium	T	N	M
0	Tis	N0	M0
I	T1	N0	M0
–	T2	N0	M0
IIA	T3	N0	M0
IIB	T4	N0	M0
IIIA	T1-T2	N1	M0
IIIB	T3-T4	N1	M0
IIIC	Any T	N2	M0
IV	Any T	Any N	M1

When comparing the disease prognosis of adenocarcinomas of the colon and rectum at the same stage, it was found that disease stages I and II have a similar prognosis, in contrast to the advanced stages (stages III and IV), where squamous cell carcinomas have a poorer prognosis (Namlos et al., 2012). The average five-year survival rate is 32%, with variations related to the individual stages: Dukes B 50%, Dukes C 33% and Dukes D 0%. The use of adjuvant therapy improves a patient's overall survival while preoperative radiotherapy increases the percentage of sphincter-preserving surgery.

5.6. Melanoma

Melanoma of the gastrointestinal tract is a rare melanoma of the mucous membranes with a particularly aggressive biology compared to cutaneous melanomas at the same stage. These tumors most commonly present as metastatic lesions, with primary tumors being rare. When they do occur as primary tumors, they are most likely to be found in areas where melanocytes are normally present, such as the esophagus, stomach, small intestine, and anorectum (Pan et al., 2017). There are several theories that describe the development of colonic melanoma: relationship to neural crest cells, model of tumor regression, and ectodermal differentiation, but none of these have been fully proven to date. Localization in the anorectum ranks third in frequency of location, behind the rest of the skin and ocular surfaces, and accounts for 1–1.5% of all melanomas in the human body and 3–15% of all tumors of the colon and rectum. Moore first described it in 1857 and to date, a total of 500 cases have been described in the literature. It occurs most frequently on the skin, under the dentate line, and rarely at the level of the cuboidal epithelium of the transition zone and the mucosa of the distal rectum. It occurs more frequently in women (twice as often as in men) between the ages of 60 and 70. Melanoma is a disease of neuroectodermal origin, most frequently originating from melanocytes and nevus cells of the basal layer of the epidermis and much less frequently from the mucosa (Paula et al., 2015). It has an extremely poor long-term prognosis, as the disease is detected at an advanced stage, mainly with metastases in the inguinal nodes. In addition to lymphogenous spread, spread is possible through local ingrowth and by hematogenous means. Local spread takes the form of radial (horizontal) and vertical growth. Radial growth means a circular spread around the primary tumor, through the epithelium of the mucosa and the superficial layers of the submucosa, without a tendency to metastasize (Pautke et al., 2004).

Vertical growth means penetration into the deeper layers of the colon wall with simultaneous metastasis. Determining the extent of vertical tumor growth, which is the involvement of the wall layers of the colon and rectum, is crucial for the choice of surgical intervention. MSCT (multi-slice scanner), NMR (magnetic resonance), and endoluminal ultrasound play the most important role here. Hematogenous dissemination occurs when melanoma cells enter the blood vessels and spread throughout the body. About 30% of patients are considered to have a disseminated process at the time of diagnosis, while only 17% of operated patients have a five-year survival rate (Punzo et al., 2020). It differs from cutaneous melanoma in that 25% of tumors contain no pigment of the so-called "colored" tumor and that ultraviolet radiation is a protective factor and not a risk. In the presence of a pigmented tumor of the rectum, the macroscopic appearance is very similar to thrombosed external and prolapsing internal hemorrhoids (*see* Figure 5.5), which can mislead a physician in making a diagnosis.

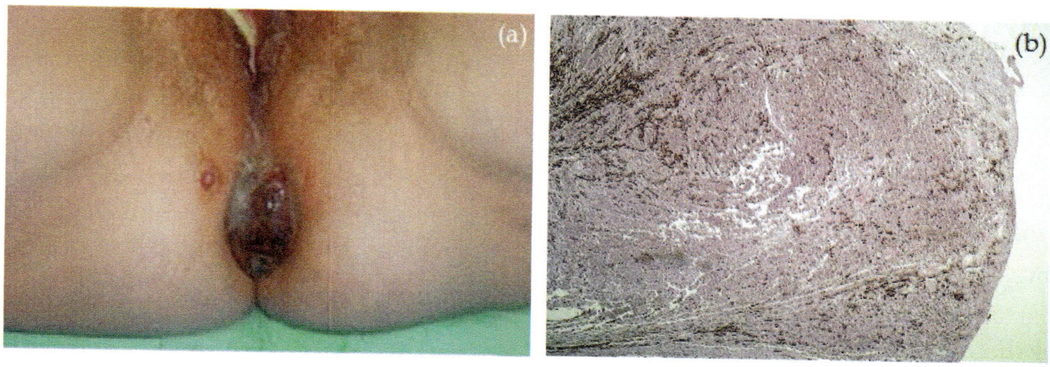

Figure 5.5. *(a) Prolapsed melanoma recti; and (b) histopathological finding of melanoma recti (H&E 40x).*

Source: https://www.researchgate.net/profile/Goran-Stanojevic-3/publication/298786874/figure/fig5/AS:613514976694275@1523284777020/a-Prolapsed-melanoma-recti-b-Histopathological-finding-of-melanoma-recti-H-E-40x.png.

The symptoms of the disease vary, but the most common are abdominal pain, weight loss, and bleeding. Diagnosis of the disease requires a detailed history, physical examination with special attention to the inspection of all skin areas and the eyes as the most common primary localizations. It is also necessary to perform biochemical laboratory analyzes, digito-rectal examination, colonoscopy, barium enema, multi-slice scanner (MSCT), magnetic resonance imaging (NMR), endoluminal ultrasound, and tumor biopsy with pathohistological and immunohistochemical processing (Schleinitz et al., 2011). Particular attention should be paid to the examination of certain groups of lymph nodes, depending on the location of the primary tumor. Taking into account the findings of Kalid and his co-workers, the most common localization of primary colonic melanoma is the ascending and transverse cecum, while in metastatic melanoma it is the ascending and descending parts of the colon. The curative treatment of colon melanoma is exclusively surgical (Sekar et al., 2019). The main goal of treatment is to find a compromise between the need for radical oncologic treatment and the need to preserve the patient's quality of life. The modern approach to the treatment of primary melanoma of the colon and rectum involves performing surgical procedures such as:

- Colectomy with wide excision margins (partial, hemicolectomy, subtotal, and total);
- Transanal wide local excision with preservation of the anal sphincter (in the case of the initial stage of the rectal tumor);
- Extensive surgery depending on the type of rectal resection or abdominoperineal amputation.

There are numerous dilemmas about which type of surgical intervention should be used at certain stages of the disease (Seweryn et al., 2020). Proponents of radical treatment recommend resection or abdominoperineal amputation of the rectum with dissection of both inguinal regions, depending on the location, citing the following advantages:

- Possibility of detailed exploration of the abdomen and possible detection of distant metastases;
- Lower percentage of local recurrence.

On the other hand, some authors recommend a wide local tumor excision with preservation of the sphincter mechanism for the following reasons:

- Absence of definitive stoma; and
- Similar five-year survival rate.

The authors from MD Anderson Cancer Center present their 20-year experience with the treatment of 54 patients with localized anorectal melanoma and show that the combination of surgical-wide local excision and adjuvant radiotherapy provides good local disease control with acceptable side effects. The existence of such different opinions in the literature is primarily a consequence of inconsistent criteria of the examinations performed, the comparison of different localizations of anorectal melanoma, and the stage of the disease (Sheng et al., 2022). The most important parameter driving the decision on the type of surgical intervention to be made is the thickness of the tumor. According to Weynadt and his associates, melanomas up to 4 mm thick are indicated for wide local excision, with the limits of excision up to 2 cm from the primary tumor without involving the sphincter, while extensive rectal surgery is recommended for melanomas thicker than 4 mm. As for adjuvant therapy, melanomas are considered semi-resistant tumors, so certain cytostatic drugs work in 10–25% of treated melanomas. The most commonly used drugs are Dacarbazine, Temozolamide, Cisplatin, Carboplatin, and Nitrosoureas. Recent research has shown that the determination of the biological markers RAS/RAF/MEK/ERK is an important indicator of the intensity of cell growth, invasion, and survival (Shi & Zhang, 2017). Adjuvant therapy of anorectal melanoma is not very successful however, as all these tumors are radioresistant and hardly respond to chemotherapy.

5.7. Extremely Rare Tumors

Other tumors include extremely rare malignant diseases of the colon: primary teratomas, extramedullary plasmacytomas, schwannomas, and metastases of distant tumors.

Primary teratomas of the colon are very rare diseases and only about 50 cases have been published in the literature so far, mainly located in the rectum and in the form of clinical presentation. They occur more frequently in women with an average age of 42.5 years. They are thought to arise as a result of the ectopic development of so-called "trapped" ectodermal tissue, although some structures of mesodermal endodermal origin are possible in their composition (Shi et al., 2018). Histologically, it is composed of stratified squamous epithelia, fat cells, hair follicles, cartilage, and some glandular tissue. They are usually benign tumors, but some malignant transformations are also possible, requiring the complete removal of the tumor to comply with oncological principles. Data from the literature indicate that teratomas usually occur in the ovaries, testes, mediastinum, and midlines such as the sacrococcygeal region, while they are less common in the gastrointestinal tract (rectum, sigmoid part of the colon, appendix, and terminal ileum). The rectal teratomas usually have a polypoid cystic form with a protrusion into the lumen area. They are usually solitary cysts filled with a whitish sebaceous fluid in which the sebaceous glands, hair follicles, and teeth are immersed. In addition to the cystic form, the presence of solid tumors is also possible, which indicates a mature form of teratoma (Sikora et al., 2019).

The clinical picture is characterized by pain during bowel movements, bleeding, and a change in bowel habits. The diagnosis is made by history and digital rectal examination, which confirms the presence of the polypoid tumor mass with predominantly smooth edges and a pedicle. Cases are described in which the ovarian teratoma has invaded the rectal lumen, which presents similar difficulties. The additional diagnostic procedures such as endoluminal ultrasound, multi-slice scanner, and magnetic resonance imaging provide additional information about the extent of the tumor itself as well as the assessment of operability (Simpson et al., 2017). Some malignant transformations of teratomas with a tendency to form squamous cell carcinomas are possible, and therefore it is not advisable to perform transanal puncture, firstly because of the risk of spreading malignant cells and secondly because of the possible infection. The method of choice for treatment is the complete elimination of the cystic tumor.

The most common form of plasma cell neoplasia is multiple myeloma. Of the total number of multiple myelomas, only 2% are so-called extramedullary plasmacytomas. More than 75% of extramedullary plasmacytomas occur in the upper part of the respiratory system, while the most common sites of occurrence in the gastrointestinal tract are the stomach and small intestine. To date, 22 cases of extramedullary plasmacytoma in the colon have been reported, with the average age of the patients being 52.3 years. The most common localizations in the colon are the cecum with 36.4% and the rectum with 22.7%. In the differential diagnosis, it is essential to distinguish between primary and secondary plasmacytoma, i.e., the metastasis of multiple myeloma (Smieszek et al., 2019). It is achieved by determining the Bence-Jones proteins in the urine, performing serum electrophoresis, and conducting immunohistochemical detection of accumulations of monoclonal plasma cells.

The treatment involves the application of:

- Surgical intervention in 81.8% of cases;
- Radiotherapy in 9% of cases;
- Combined application of surgical intervention and radiotherapy in 4.5% of cases.

Schwannomas originate from Schwann cells, which form the nerve sheath and belong to the group of stromal tumors. In the gastrointestinal tract, they occur most frequently in the stomach, while primary schwannomas of the colon are extremely rare and only 39 clinical cases have been reported to date. They occur mainly in older patients around the age of 65, equally in both sexes. They grow slowly and there are a large number of patients who have no symptoms at the time of diagnosis. Symptoms depend on the size and location of the tumor, but vague abdominal pain, bleeding, and changes in bowel habitus are the most common signs (Smieszek et al., 2020). Preoperative diagnosis using standard procedures such as medical history, physical examination, colonoscopy, MSCT, NMR, and endoluminal ultrasound allows determination of the tumor mass, but not the nature and type of the tumor, as it is similar to GIST tumors of the colon. The most accurate diagnosis implies the elimination of the tumor as a whole with pathohistological and immunohistochemical analysis. Even with immunohistochemical analysis, it is difficult to distinguish it from GISTs, and some authors classify it as a subset of GISTs, such as GANT tumors, which is gastrointestinal autonomic nerve tumors.

5.8. Metastases in the Colon and Rectum from the Distant Tumors

Metastasis of distant primary tumors rarely spreads to the colon and is usually related to carcinomas of the surrounding organs (stomach, pancreas, ovaries, etc.), which, due to their growth and size, spread to the surrounding parts of the colon or "fall" on the intraperitoneal rectum with secondary infiltration (Son et al., 2014). The extent of tumor spread depends on the length of existence of the primary tumor and the histologic type, although literature data indicate that the serosa is infiltrated in 28%, the muscular layer in 31%, and the mucosa in 14% of patients. Spread of prostate cancer is possible, with perforation of the Denonvilliers fascia and secondary spread to the rectum, depending on the type of circumferential, that is annular, stenosis, without spread to the mucosa in men, as is carcinoma portie vaginalis uteri in women (Sulzbacher et al., 2002). The pouch of Douglas as the lowest point of the abdomen and in the immediate vicinity of the rectum is a site of intraperitoneal spread of carcinomas of all intra-abdominal or retroperitoneal organs, with the stomach and ovary predominating. Carcinoma metastases from retroperitoneal and extra-abdominal organs, the pancreas, the kidneys, and the breast are described in the literature (Tang et al., 2019). The clinical picture is similar to that of other colon tumors (including bleeding, change in bowel habits, and pain in the anus area), and supplemented by the symptoms of the primary localization of the malignant process. Diagnosis includes medical history, digital rectal examination, colonoscopy, endoanal ultrasound, multi-slice scanner, NMR, and biopsy with pathohistological confirmation (Tang et al., 2015).

The strategy of treatment depends on:

- Localization of the primary malignant process;
- Advancement of the disease;
- Histological type of the primary tumor.

If the primary tumor is located in the immediate vicinity of the colon and rectum (pancreas, sigmoid, prostate, cervix, and vagina), it is recommended to perform the so-called en bloc resections to achieve the oncological principle of radicality or the R0 procedure (Tian et al., 2019). Sometimes it is necessary to carry out non-adjuvant therapy to reduce the tumor volume, known as "downsizing," and the biological aggressiveness of the tumor, known as "downstaging," or even to supplement the surgical procedure with adjuvant therapy. In the case of extra-abdominal localization of the primary tumor, it is necessary to evaluate the success of the surgical procedure with regard to R0 resection or the use of neoadjuvant therapy (Tian et al., 2015).

A Closer Look

Carcinoids

A Closer Look at Carcinoids are neuroendocrine tumors (NETs) that originate from neuroendocrine cells, primarily found in the gastrointestinal tract and lungs. These tumors are typically slow-growing and may produce a variety of hormones, leading to distinct clinical syndromes depending on their location and secretory activity. The classification of carcinoids includes typical and atypical carcinoids, with atypical carcinoids often exhibiting more aggressive behavior and a higher rate of metastasis. Studies suggest that carcinoid tumors can often be asymptomatic in early stages, complicating diagnosis and potentially delaying treatment.

Recent research has focused on the epidemiology of carcinoid tumors, revealing a rising incidence over the past few decades. A population-based study published in the *Journal of Clinical Oncology* reported that the incidence of carcinoid tumors has increased from 1.0 per 100,000 in the 1970s to 5.0 per 100,000 by the early 2000s, with a significant increase noted among women. This rise is partially attributed to enhanced awareness and improved diagnostic techniques, including advanced imaging and endoscopic methods that allow for earlier detection of these tumors.

Therapeutic strategies for carcinoids have evolved, with a shift towards personalized medicine approaches. A pivotal study published in *The New England Journal of Medicine* demonstrated the efficacy of somatostatin analogs (e.g., octreotide and lanreotide) in controlling symptoms and stabilizing tumor growth in patients with advanced carcinoid syndrome. Additionally, the introduction of peptide receptor radionuclide therapy (PRRT) has provided a novel treatment option, as shown in a clinical trial published in *Lancet Oncology*, which highlighted significant tumor response rates and symptom improvement in patients with inoperable NETs.

Ongoing research continues to explore the molecular mechanisms underlying carcinoid tumors to identify novel therapeutic targets. Recent studies using genomic sequencing techniques have revealed specific mutations and molecular pathways associated with carcinoid tumorigenesis, such as alterations in the MEN1 and DAXX genes. These findings could pave the way for targeted therapies and personalized treatment strategies. Furthermore, the potential role of immunotherapy in carcinoid treatment is being investigated, with early-phase clinical trials assessing the efficacy of checkpoint inhibitors in patients with advanced neuroendocrine tumors. As our understanding of carcinoids deepens, it is crucial to continue to develop innovative diagnostic and therapeutic strategies to improve patient outcomes.

Summary

Rare tumors of the colon and rectum represent an important group of neoplasms, as they have a special prognosis due to their late diagnosis and do not respond to conventional cancer therapies. Over the last 20 years, their overall incidence has increased due to the introduction of new imaging techniques, in particular the development of more sophisticated diagnostic tools such as high-resolution CT and MRI, capsule endoscopy, and somatostatin scintigraphy for NETs. Although the development of specific targeted therapies such as tyrosine kinase inhibitors for GISTs and somatostatin analogs for NETs have improved prognosis, early detection remains the critical variable in determining outcome. Promising therapeutic data in some subgroups are encouraging; however, the majority of patients are still diagnosed at a late stage and lack targeted, effective therapies. The variability in survival rates among different tumor types results from several factors, including the biological aggressiveness of the tumor, its pattern of spread, and its tendency to metastasize, as well as the frequency of occurrence and symptomatology. Carcinoid tumors are considered indolent and have the best prognosis. In contrast, non-Hodgkin's lymphoma and squamous cell carcinoma of the colon generally show significantly poorer overall survival rates compared to adenocarcinoma, while melanoma is associated with the shortest survival time. This chapter aims to highlight the challenges and considerations of dealing with rare tumors in everyday clinical practice.

References

1. Bach, D. H., Park, H. J., & Lee, S. K. (2018). The dual role of bone morphogenetic proteins in cancer. *Molecular Therapy Oncolytics, 8*, 1–13.
2. Bjørnland, K., Flatmark, K., Pettersen, S., Aaasen, A. O., Fodstad, O., & Maelandsmo, G. M. (2005). Matrix metalloproteinases participate in osteosarcoma invasion. *Journal of Surgical Research, 127*(2), 151–156.
3. Cai, C. K., Zhao, G. Y., Tian, L. Y., Liu, L., Yan, K., Ma, Y. L., Ji, Z. W., Li, X. X., Han, K., Gao, J., et al. (2012). MiR-15a and MiR-16-1 downregulate CCND1 and induce apoptosis and cell cycle arrest in osteosarcoma. *Oncology Reports, 28*(5), 1764–1770.
4. Cappellen, D., Schlange, T., Bauer, M., Maurer, F., & Hynes, N. E. (2007). Novel C-MYC target genes mediate differential effects on cell proliferation and migration. *EMBO Reports, 8*(1), 70–76.
5. Carreira, A. C., Lojudice, F. H., Halcsik, E., Navarro, R. D., Sogayar, M. C., & Granjeiro, J. M. (2014). Bone morphogenetic proteins: Facts, challenges, and future perspectives. *Journal of Dental Research, 93*(4), 335–345.
6. Chan, J. A., Krichevsky, A. M., & Kosik, K. S. (2005). MicroRNA-21 is an antiapoptotic factor in human glioblastoma cells. *Cancer Research, 65*(14), 6029–6033.
7. Cheng, C., Chen, Z. Q., & Shi, X. T. (2014). MicroRNA-320 inhibits osteosarcoma cell proliferation by directly targeting fatty acid synthase. *Tumor Biology, 35*(4), 4177–4183.
8. Chomczynski, P. (1987). Single-step method of RNA isolation by acid guanidinium thiocyanate-phenol-chloroform extraction. *Analytical Biochemistry, 162*(1), 156–159.
9. Choong, P. F., Teh, H. X., Teoh, H. K., Ong, H. K., Choo, K. B., Sugii, S., Cheong, S. K., & Kamarul, T. (2014). Heterogeneity of osteosarcoma cell lines led to variable responses in reprogramming. *International Journal of Medical Sciences, 11*(11), 1154–1160.

10. Cong, C., Wang, W., Tian, J., Gao, T., Zheng, W., & Zhou, C. (2018). Identification of serum MiR-124 as a biomarker for diagnosis and prognosis in osteosarcoma. *Cancer Biomarkers, 21*(3), 449–454.

11. Cyr-Depauw, C., Northey, J. J., Tabariès, S., Annis, M. G., Dong, Z., Cory, S., Hallett, M., Rennhack, J. P., Andrechek, E. R., & Siegel, P. M. (2016). Chordin-like 1 suppresses bone morphogenetic protein 4-induced breast cancer cell migration and invasion. *Molecular and Cellular Biology, 36*(8), 1509–1525.

12. Davis, B. N., Hilyard, A. C., Lagna, G., & Hata, A. (2008). SMAD proteins control DROSHA-mediated microRNA maturation. *Nature, 454*(7200), 56–61.

13. Dong, J., Liu, Y., Liao, W., Liu, R., Shi, P., & Wang, L. (2016). MiRNA-223 is a potential diagnostic and prognostic marker for osteosarcoma. *Journal of Bone Oncology, 5*(2), 74–79.

14. Dong, P., Xiong, Y., Watari, H., Hanley, S. J., Konno, Y., Ihira, K., Suzuki, F., Yamada, T., Kudo, M., Yue, J., et al. (2016). Suppression of IASPP-dependent aggressiveness in cervical cancer through reversal of methylation silencing of microRNA-124. *Scientific Reports, 6*, 35480.

15. Ejarque, M., Ceperuelo-Mallafré, V., Serena, C., Pachón, G., Núñez-Álvarez, Y., Terrón-Puig, M., Calvo, E., Núñez-Roa, C., Oliva-Olivera, W., Tinahones, F. J., et al. (2017). Survivin, a key player in cancer progression, increases in obesity and protects adipose tissue stem cells from apoptosis. *Cell Death & Disease, 8*(4), e2802.

16. Fehr, J. E., Trotter, G. W., Oxford, J. T., & Hart, D. A. (2000). Comparison of Northern blot hybridization and a reverse transcriptase-polymerase chain reaction technique for measurement of mRNA expression of metalloproteinases and matrix components in articular cartilage and synovial membrane from horses with osteoarthritis. *American Journal of Veterinary Research, 61*(8), 900–905.

17. Fromigué, O., Hamidouche, Z., & Marie, P. J. (2008). Blockade of the RhoA-JNK-c-Jun-MMP2 cascade by atorvastatin reduces osteosarcoma cell invasion. *Journal of Biological Chemistry, 283*(46), 30549–30556.

18. Geng, S., Zhang, X., Chen, J., Liu, X., Zhang, H., Xu, X., Ma, Y., Li, B., Zhang, Y., Bi, Z., et al. (2014). The tumor suppressor role of MiR-124 in osteosarcoma. *PLoS ONE, 9*(10), e91566.

19. Guan, X., Gao, Y., Zhou, J., Wang, J., Zheng, F., Guo, F., Chang, A., Li, X., & Wang, B. (2015). MiR-223 regulates adipogenic and osteogenic differentiation of mesenchymal stem cells through a C/EBPs/MiR-223/FGFR2 regulatory feedback loop. *STEM CELLS, 33*(5), 1589–1600.

20. Guo, W., Gorlick, R., Ladanyi, M., Meyers, P. A., Huvos, A. G., Bertino, J. R., & Healey, J. H. (1999). Expression of bone morphogenetic proteins and receptors in sarcomas. *Clinical Orthopaedics and Related Research, 359*, 175–183.

21. Hamam, D., Ali, D., Vishnubalaji, R., Hamam, R., Al-Nbaheen, M., Chen, L., Kassem, M., Aldahmash, A., & Alajez, N. M. (2014). MicroRNA-320/RUNX2 axis regulates adipocytic differentiation of human mesenchymal (skeletal) stem cells. *Cell Death & Disease, 5*, e1499.

22. Han, G., Wang, Y., & Bi, W. (2012). C-Myc overexpression promotes osteosarcoma cell invasion via activation of MEK-ERK pathway. *Oncology Research Featuring Preclinical and Clinical Cancer Therapeutics, 20*(2), 149–156.

23. Haudenschild, D. R., Palmer, S. M., Moseley, T. A., You, Z., & Reddi, A. H. (2004). Bone morphogenetic protein (BMP)-6 signaling and BMP antagonist Noggin in prostate cancer. *Cancer Research, 64*(23), 8276–8284.
24. He, H., Ni, J., & Huang, J. (2014). Molecular mechanisms of chemoresistance in osteosarcoma (review). *Oncology Letters, 7*(4), 1352–1362.
25. Hu, X., Li, L., Lu, Y., Yu, X., Chen, H., Yin, Q., & Zhang, Y. (2018). MiRNA-21 inhibition inhibits osteosarcoma cell proliferation by targeting PTEN and regulating the TGF-β1 signaling pathway. *Oncology Letters, 16*(4), 4337–4342.
26. Hua, Y., Jin, Z., Zhou, F., Zhang, Y. Q., & Zhuang, Y. (2017). The expression significance of serum MiR-21 in patients with osteosarcoma and its relationship with chemosensitivity. *European Review for Medical and Pharmacological Sciences, 21*(13), 2989–2994.
27. Huang, J., Liang, Y., Xu, M., Xiong, J., Wang, D., & Ding, Q. (2018). MicroRNA-124 acts as a tumor-suppressive miRNA by inhibiting the expression of Snail2 in osteosarcoma. *Oncology Letters, 15*(4), 4979–4987.
28. Huang, T., Zhang, X., & Wang, H. (2020). Punicalagin inhibited proliferation, invasion and angiogenesis of osteosarcoma through suppression of NF-κB signaling. *Molecular Medicine Reports, 22*(5), 2386–2394.
29. Huang, X., Wu, W., Jing, D., Yang, L., Guo, H., Wang, L., Zhang, W., Pu, F., & Shao, Z. (2022). Engineered exosome as targeted LncRNA MEG3 delivery vehicles for osteosarcoma therapy. *Journal of Controlled Release, 343*, 107–117.
30. Huang, Y. Z., Zhang, J., Shao, H. Y., Chen, J. P., & Zhao, H. Y. (2015). MicroRNA-191 promotes osteosarcoma cells proliferation by targeting checkpoint kinase 2. *Tumor Biology, 36*(8), 6095–6101.
31. Ji, Q., Xu, X., Song, Q., Xu, Y., Tai, Y., Goodman, S. B., Bi, W., Xu, M., Jiao, S., Maloney, W. J., et al. (2018). MiR-223-3p inhibits human osteosarcoma metastasis and progression by directly targeting CDH6. *Molecular Therapy, 26*(5), 1299–1312.
32. Jiang, L., Liu, T., & Song, K. (2012). Growth characteristics of human adipose-derived stem cells during long time culture regulated by cyclin A and cyclin D1. *Applied Biochemistry and Biotechnology, 168*(9), 2230–2244.
33. Kaczorowska, A., Miękus, N., Stefanowicz, J., & Adamkiewicz-Drożyńska, E. (2020). Selected matrix metalloproteinases (MMP-2, MMP-7) and their inhibitor (TIMP-2) in adult and pediatric cancer. *Diagnostics, 10*(8), 547.
34. Kansara, M., Teng, M. W., Smyth, M. J., & Thomas, D. M. (2014). Translational biology of osteosarcoma. *Nature Reviews Cancer, 14*(11), 722–735.
35. Katagiri, T., & Watabe, T. (2016). Bone morphogenetic proteins. *Cold Spring Harbor Perspectives in Biology, 8*(12), a021835.
36. Kochanowska, I. E., Wlodarski, K., Wojtowicz, A., Kinsner, A., & Ostrowski, K. (2002). BMP-4 and BMP-6 involvement in the osteogenic properties of the HeLa cell line. *Experimental Biology and Medicine, 227*(1), 57–62.
37. Kochanowska, I. E., Wlodarski, K., Wojtowicz, A., Niemira, K., & Ostrowski, K. (2002). Osteogenic properties of various HeLa cell lines and the BMP family genes expression. *Annals of Transplantation, 7*(1), 58–62.

38. Kundu, B., Bastos, A. R. F., Brancato, V., Cerqueira, M. T., Oliveira, J. M., Correlo, V. M., Reis, R. L., & Kundu, S. C. (2019). Mechanical property of hydrogels and the presence of adipose stem cells in tumor stroma affect spheroid formation in the 3D osteosarcoma model. *ACS Applied Materials & Interfaces, 11*(14), 14548–14559.

39. Lauvrak, S. U., Munthe, E., Kresse, S. H., Stratford, E. W., Namløs, H. M., Meza-Zepeda, L. A., & Myklebost, O. (2013). Functional characterisation of osteosarcoma cell lines and identification of mRNAs and miRNAs associated with aggressive cancer phenotypes. *British Journal of Cancer, 109*(8), 2228–2236.

40. Laxman, N., Mallmin, H., Nilsson, O., & Kindmark, A. (2016). MiR-203 and MiR-320 regulate bone morphogenetic protein-2-induced osteoblast differentiation by targeting distal-less homeobox 5 (Dlx5). *Genes, 8*(1), 4.

41. Li, H., Yang, F., Wang, Z., Fu, Q., & Liang, A. (2015). MicroRNA-21 promotes osteogenic differentiation by targeting small mothers against decapentaplegic 7. *Molecular Medicine Reports, 12*(2), 1561–1567.

42. Li, J., Yang, Z., Li, Y., Xia, J., Li, D., Li, H., Ren, M., Liao, Y., Yu, S., Chen, Y., et al. (2016). Cell apoptosis, autophagy and necroptosis in osteosarcoma treatment. *Oncotarget, 7*(31), 44763–44778.

43. Lin, L., Liu, X., & Lv, B. (2021). Long non-coding RNA MEG3 promotes autophagy and apoptosis of nasopharyngeal carcinoma cells via PTEN up-regulation by binding to microRNA-21. *Journal of Cellular and Molecular Medicine, 25*(1), 61–72.

44. Liu, B., Li, G., Wang, X., & Liu, Y. (2014). A Furin inhibitor downregulates osteosarcoma cell migration by downregulating the expression levels of MT1-MMP via the Wnt signaling pathway. *Oncology Letters, 7*(3), 1033–1038.

45. Liu, Y., Teng, Z., Wang, Y., Gao, P., & Chen, J. (2015). Prognostic significance of survivin expression in osteosarcoma patients: A meta-analysis. *Medical Science Monitor, 21*, 2877–2885.

46. Long, J., Badal, S. S., Wang, Y., Chang, B. H. J., Rodriguez, A., & Danesh, F. R. (2013). MicroRNA-22 is a master regulator of bone morphogenetic protein-7/6 homeostasis in the kidney. *Journal of Biological Chemistry, 288*(51), 36202–36214.

47. Lucero, C. M. J., Vega, O. A., Osorio, M. M., Tapia, J. C., Antonelli, M., Stein, G. S., Van Wijnen, A. J., & Galindo, M. A. (2013). The cancer-related transcription factor Runx2 modulates cell proliferation in human osteosarcoma cell lines. *Journal of Cellular Physiology, 228*(3), 714–723.

48. Luo, L., Yang, R., Zhao, S., Chen, Y., Hong, S., Wang, K., Wang, T., Cheng, J., Zhang, T., & Chen, D. (2018). Decreased MiR-320 expression is associated with breast cancer progression, cell migration, and invasiveness via targeting aquaporin 1. *Acta Biochimica et Biophysica Sinica, 50*(5), 473–480.

49. Lv, C., Hao, Y., & Tu, G. (2016). MicroRNA-21 promotes proliferation, invasion and suppresses apoptosis in human osteosarcoma line MG63 through PTEN/Akt pathway. *Tumor Biology, 37*(7), 9333–9342.

50. Melnik, S., Werth, N., Boeuf, S., Hahn, E. M., Gotterbarm, T., Anton, M., & Richter, W. (2019). Impact of C-MYC expression on proliferation, differentiation, and risk of neoplastic transformation of human mesenchymal stromal cells. *Stem Cell Research & Therapy, 10*(1), 73.

51. Mukhametov, U., Lyulin, S., Borzunov, D., Sufianova, G., Shumadalova, A., Zhang, D., & Gareev, I. (2022). Functions of the bone morphogenetic protein signaling pathway through non-coding RNAs. *Noncoding RNA Research, 7*(4), 178–183.

52. Nakka, M., Allen-Rhoades, W., Li, Y., Kelly, A. J., Shen, J., Taylor, A. M., Barkauskas, D. A., Yustein, J. T., Andrulis, I. L., Wunder, J. S., et al. (2017). Biomarker significance of plasma and tumor MiR-21, MiR-221, and MiR-106a in osteosarcoma. *Oncotarget, 8*(62), 96738–96752.

53. Namløs, H. M., Meza-Zepeda, L. A., Barøy, T., Østensen, I. H. G., Kresse, S. H., Kuijjer, M. L., Serra, M., Bürger, H., Cleton-Jansen, A. M., & Myklebost, O. (2012). Modulation of the osteosarcoma expression phenotype by microRNAs. *PLoS ONE, 7*(7), e48086.

54. Pan, C., Gao, H., Zheng, N., Gao, Q., Si, Y., & Zhao, Y. (2017). MiR-320 inhibits the growth of glioma cells through downregulating PBX3. *Biological Research, 50*(1), 31.

55. Paula, A. C., Martins, T. M., Zonari, A., Frade, S. P., Angelo, P. C., Gomes, D. A., & Goes, A. M. (2015). Human adipose tissue-derived stem cells cultured in xeno-free culture condition enhance c-MYC expression increasing proliferation but bypassing spontaneous cell transformation. *Stem Cell Research & Therapy, 6*(1), 76.

56. Pautke, C., Schieker, M., Tischer, T., Kolk, A., Neth, P., Mutschler, W., & Milz, S. (2004). Characterization of osteosarcoma cell lines MG-63, Saos-2 and U-2 OS in comparison to human osteoblasts. *Anticancer Research, 24*(6), 3743–3748.

57. Punzo, F., Tortora, C., Argenziano, M., Pinto, D. D., Pota, E., Martino, M. D., Paola, A. D., & Rossi, F. (2020). Can denosumab be used in combination with doxorubicin in osteosarcoma? *Oncotarget, 11*(4), 2763–2773.

58. Schleinitz, D., Klöting, N., Böttcher, Y., Wolf, S., Dietrich, K., Tönjes, A., Breitfeld, J., Enigk, B., Halbritter, J., Körner, A., et al. (2011). Genetic and evolutionary analyses of the human bone morphogenetic protein receptor 2 (BMPR2) in the pathophysiology of obesity. *PLoS ONE, 6*(12), e28484.

59. Sekar, D., Mani, P., Biruntha, M., Sivagurunathan, P., & Karthigeyan, M. (2019). Dissecting the functional role of microRNA 21 in osteosarcoma. *Cancer Gene Therapy, 26*(5), 179–182.

60. Seweryn, A., Pielok, A., Lawniczak-Jablonska, K., Pietruszka, R., Marcinkowska, K., Sikora, M., Witkowski, B. S., Godlewski, M., Marycz, K., & Smieszek, A. (2020). Zirconium oxide thin films obtained by atomic layer deposition technology abolish the anti-osteogenic effect resulting from MiR-21 inhibition in the pre-osteoblastic MC3T3 cell line. *International Journal of Nanomedicine, 15*, 1595–1610.

61. Sheng, S., Su, W., Mao, D., Li, C., Hu, X., Deng, W., Yao, Y., & Ji, Y. (2022). MicroRNA-21 induces cisplatin resistance in head and neck squamous cell carcinoma. *PLoS ONE, 17*(8), e0267017.

62. Shi, C., & Zhang, Z. (2017). MicroRNA-320 suppresses cervical cancer cell viability, migration and invasion via directly targeting FOXM1. *Oncology Letters, 14*(4), 3809–3816.

63. Shi, Y., Lv, C., Shi, L., & Tu, G. (2018). MEG3 inhibits proliferation and invasion and promotes apoptosis of human osteosarcoma cells. *Oncology Letters, 15*(2), 1917–1923.

64. Sikora, M., Marcinkowska, K., Marycz, K., Wiglusz, R. J., & Śmieszek, A. (2019). The potential selective cytotoxicity of poly (L-lactic acid)-based scaffolds functionalized with nanohydroxyapatite and europium (III) ions toward osteosarcoma cells. *Materials, 12*(21), 3779.

65. Simpson, S., Dunning, M. D., de Brot, S., Grau-Roma, L., Mongan, N. P., & Rutland, C. S. (2017). Comparative review of human and canine osteosarcoma: Morphology, epidemiology, prognosis, treatment and genetics. *Acta Veterinaria Scandinavica, 59*(1), 71.

66. Smieszek, A., Kornicka, K., Szłapka-Kosarzewska, J., Androvic, P., Valihrach, L., Langerova, L., Rohlova, E., Kubista, M., & Marycz, K. (2019). Metformin increases proliferative activity and viability of multipotent stromal stem cells isolated from adipose tissue derived from horses with equine metabolic syndrome. *Cells, 8*(2), 80.

67. Smieszek, A., Marcinkowska, K., Pielok, A., Sikora, M., Valihrach, L., & Marycz, K. (2020). The role of miR-21 in osteoblasts–Osteoclasts coupling *in vitro*. *Cells, 9*(2), 479.

68. Son, Y. H., Ka, S., Kim, A. Y., & Kim, J. B. (2014). Regulation of adipocyte differentiation via microRNAs. *Endocrinology and Metabolism, 29*(2), 122–135.

69. Sulzbacher, I., Birner, P., Trieb, K., Pichlbauer, E., & Lang, S. (2002). The expression of bone morphogenetic proteins in osteosarcoma and its relevance as a prognostic parameter. *Journal of Clinical Pathology, 55*(5), 381–385.

70. Tang, J., Lin, X., Zhong, J., Xu, F., Wu, F., Liao, X., Cui, R. R., Li, F., & Yuan, L. (2019). MiR-124 regulates the osteogenic differentiation of bone marrow-derived mesenchymal stem cells by targeting Sp7. *Molecular Medicine Reports, 19*(5), 3807–3814.

71. Tang, Y., Wang, Y., Chen, Q., Qiu, N., Zhao, Y., & You, X. (2015). MiR-223 inhibited cell metastasis of human cervical cancer by modulating epithelial-mesenchymal transition. *International Journal of Clinical and Experimental Pathology, 8*(10), 11224–11229.

72. Tian, H., Zhou, T., Chen, H., Li, C., Jiang, Z., Lao, L., Kahn, S. A., Duarte, M. E. L., Zhao, J., Daubs, M. D., et al. (2019). Bone morphogenetic protein-2 promotes osteosarcoma growth by promoting epithelial-mesenchymal transition (EMT) through the Wnt/β-catenin signaling pathway. *Journal of Orthopedic Research, 37*(8), 1638–1648.

73. Tian, Z. Z., Guo, X. J., Zhao, Y. M., & Fang, Y. (2015). Decreased expression of long non-coding RNA MEG3 acts as a potential predictor biomarker in progression and poor prognosis of osteosarcoma. *International Journal of Clinical and Experimental Pathology, 8*(12), 15138–15142.

74. Trieb, K., Lehner, R., Stulnig, T., Sulzbacher, I., & Shroyer, K. R. (2003). Survivin expression in human osteosarcoma is a marker for survival. *European Journal of Surgical Oncology (EJSO), 29*(5), 379–382.

75. Vanas, V., Haigl, B., Stockhammer, V., & Sutterlüty-Fall, H. (2016). MicroRNA-21 increases proliferation and cisplatin sensitivity of osteosarcoma-derived cells. *PLoS ONE, 11*(1), e0161023.

76. Wang, L., Kang, F. B., Sun, N., Wang, J., Chen, W., Li, D., & Shan, B. E. (2016). The tumor suppressor MiR-124 inhibits cell proliferation and invasion by targeting B7-H3 in osteosarcoma. *Tumor Biology, 37*(11), 14939–14947.

77. Wang, R. N., Green, J., Wang, Z., Deng, Y., Qiao, M., Peabody, M., Zhang, Q., Ye, J., Yan, Z., Denduluri, S., et al. (2014). Bone morphogenetic protein (BMP) signaling in development and human diseases. *Genes & Diseases, 1*(1), 87–105.

78. Wang, X. N., Su, X. X., Cheng, S. Q., Sun, Z. Y., Huang, Z. S., & Ou, T. M. (2019). MYC modulators in cancer: A patent review. *Expert Opinion on Therapeutic Patents, 29*(5), 353–367.

79. Wang, X., Zhao, X., Yi, Z., Ma, B., Wang, H., Pu, Y., Wang, J., & Wang, S. (2018). WNT5A promotes migration and invasion of human osteosarcoma cells via SRC/ERK/MMP-14 pathway: WNT5A promotes migration and invasion. *Cell Biology International, 42*(5), 598–607.

80. Wang, Y., Chu, Y., Li, K., Zhang, G., Guo, Z., Wu, X., Qiu, C., Li, Y., Wan, X., & Sui, J. (2020). Exosomes secreted by adipose-derived mesenchymal stem cells foster metastasis and osteosarcoma proliferation by increasing COLGALT2 expression. *Frontiers in Cell and Developmental Biology, 8*, 353.

81. Wang, Y., Chu, Y., Yue, B., Ma, X., Zhang, G., Xiang, H., Liu, Y., Wang, T., Wu, X., & Chen, B. (2017). Adipose-derived mesenchymal stem cells promote osteosarcoma proliferation and metastasis by activating the STAT3 pathway. *Oncotarget, 8*(14), 23803–23816.

82. Wang, Y., Yang, J., Chen, P., Song, Y., An, W., Zhang, H., Butegeleqi, B., & Yan, J. (2020). MicroRNA-320a inhibits invasion and metastasis in osteosarcoma by targeting cytoplasmic polyadenylation element-binding protein 1. *Cancer Medicine, 9*(7), 2833–2845.

83. Włodarski, K. H., Kochanowska, I., Pieńikowski, M., & Ostrowski, K. (2004). Influence of osteoprotegerin (OPG) on experimentally induced ectopic bone. *Folia Biologica, 52*(3–4), 205–209.

84. Wu, H., Li, W., Zhang, M., Zhu, S., Zhang, D., & Wang, X. (2016). Inhibitory roles of miR-320 in osteosarcoma via regulating E2F1. *Journal of Cancer Research and Therapeutics, 12*(1), 68–71.

85. Wu, Z., Huang, W., Chen, B., Bai, P. D., Wang, X. G., & Xing, J. C. (2017). Up-regulation of miR-124 inhibits invasion and proliferation of prostate cancer cells through mediating JAK-STAT3 signaling pathway. *European Review for Medical and Pharmacological Sciences, 21*(10), 2338–2345.

86. Xu, J., Wu, S., & Shi, X. (2010). Expression of matrix metalloproteinase regulator, RECK, and its clinical significance in osteosarcoma. *Journal of Orthopaedic Research, 28*(12), 1621–1625.

87. Xu, N., Li, Z., Yu, Z., Yan, F., Liu, Y., Lu, X., & Yang, W. (2014). MicroRNA-33b suppresses migration and invasion by targeting c-Myc in osteosarcoma cells. *PLoS ONE, 9*(2), e115300.

88. Yadin, D., Knaus, P., & Mueller, T. D. (2016). Structural insights into BMP receptors: Specificity, activation and inhibition. *Cytokine & Growth Factor Reviews, 27*(1), 13–34.

89. Yang, S., Lim, M., Pham, L. K., Kendall, A. H., Altieri, D. C., & Roy-Burman, P. (2006). Bone morphogenetic protein 7 protects prostate cancer cells from stress-induced apoptosis via both Smad and c-Jun NH2-terminal kinase pathways. Retrieved from: https://pubmed.ncbi.nlm.nih.gov/16618753/ (accessed on 9 September 2024).

90. Zhang, X., Cai, D., Meng, L., & Wang, B. (2016). MicroRNA-124 inhibits proliferation, invasion, migration and epithelial-mesenchymal transition of cervical carcinoma cells by targeting astrocyte-elevated gene-1. *Oncology Reports, 36*(5), 2321–2328.

91. Zhang, X., Guo, J., Zhou, Y., & Wu, G. (2014). The roles of bone morphogenetic proteins and their signaling in the osteogenesis of adipose-derived stem cells. *Tissue Engineering Part B: Reviews, 20*(1), 84–92.

92. Zheng, Y., Wang, G., Chen, R., Hua, Y., & Cai, Z. (2018). Mesenchymal stem cells in the osteosarcoma microenvironment: Their biological properties, influence on tumor growth, and therapeutic implications. *Stem Cell Research & Therapy, 9*(1), 22.

Chapter 6

CYSTIC FIBROSIS

Contents

Introduction

Cystic fibrosis (CF) is a common life-shortening autosomal recessive genetic disorder, characterized by pulmonary manifestations, specifically chronic and progressive obstructive lung disease, sinusitis, malabsorption due to pancreatic exocrine insufficiency leading to malnutrition, liver disease (biliary cirrhosis), and CF-related diabetes mellitus (CFRD). Earlier diagnosis through newborn screening, improved therapies to optimize lung health and nutritional status, as well as aggressive treatment of chronic respiratory infections and lung transplantation for end-stage lung disease have led to significant improvements in survival. CF was a uniformly fatal disease in childhood at the time of its first description in 1938, but the predicted median survival time is currently 44.4 years. Currently, over 50% of people with CF are 18 years and older, which means that the disease has evolved from a purely pediatric disease to one in which sufferers transition to adulthood and adult providers. With the advent of newer therapies that target the underlying genetic defect that causes the disease and the expansion of the age and genetic variants for which these therapies are indicated, there is the prospect of continued improvement in quality of life and overall health, and survival. People with CF benefit from coordinated care from their primary care physician and their interdisciplinary team, in addition to routine visits to both. This review will address the current understanding of disease manifestations, diagnosis, and management, and complications commonly seen in people with CF (Aurora et al., 2005).

Orientation and Directional Terms

Term	Definition	Illustration
Airway Secretions	Fluids, mucus, and other substances produced by the respiratory tract, helping to moisten and protect the airways.	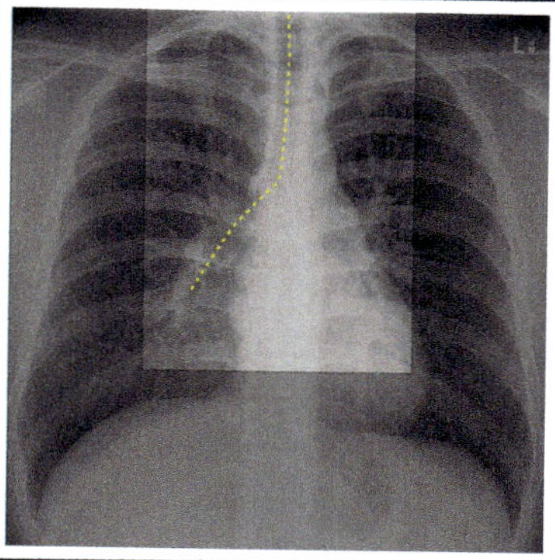
Hemoptysis	The coughing up of blood or blood-stained mucus from the lungs or airway, often a symptom of a respiratory condition.	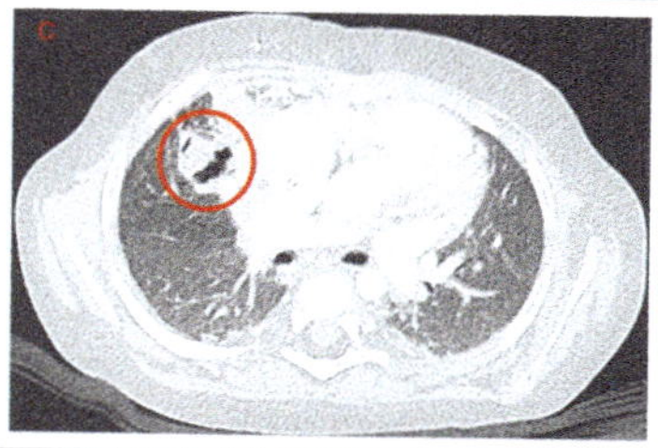
Pneumothorax	The presence of air or gas in the pleural space (between the lung and chest wall), causing lung collapse.	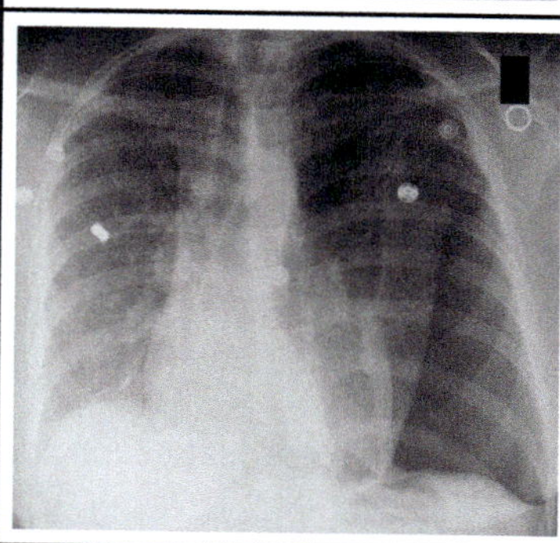
Chronic Rhinosinusitis	A long-term inflammation of the sinuses and nasal passages, leading to congestion, facial pain, and nasal discharge.	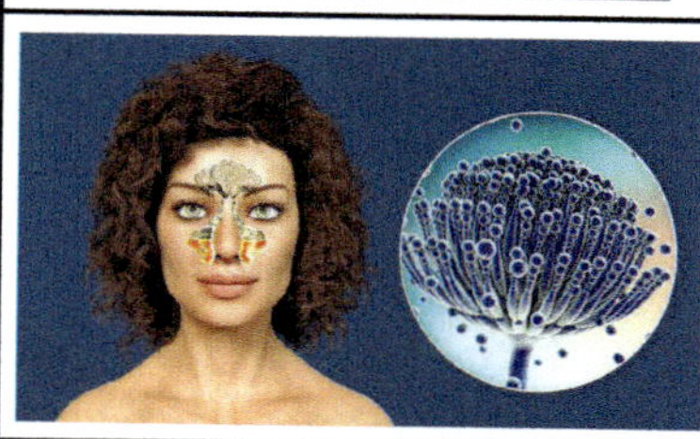
Nasal Polyposis	The formation of benign, soft growths (polyps) inside the nasal passages or sinuses, often associated with chronic inflammation.	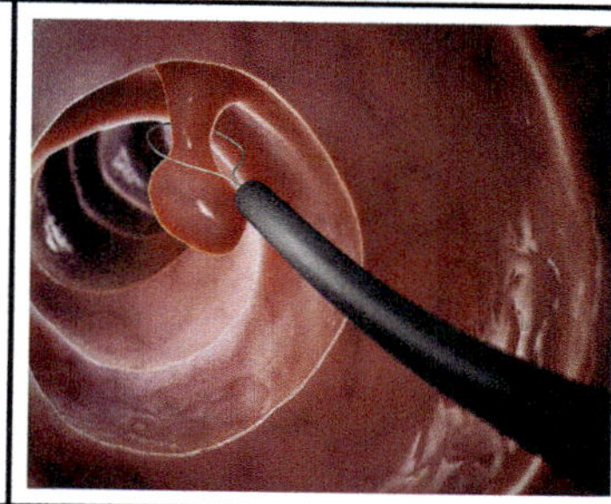

6.1. Epidemiology

CF is one of the most common genetic diseases in Caucasians, with an incidence of 1:3,200 individuals. However, the incidence varies significantly by race and ethnicity: 1:13,500 in people of Hispanic background, 1:15,000 in people of African descent and 1:35,000 in people of Asian descent. It is estimated that one in 35 Americans is a carrier of the genetic disease. According to statistics from the 2018

Annual Data Report published by the Cystic Fibrosis Foundation (CFF), there are an estimated 30,000 people living with CF in the United States (Aurora et al., 2004). Worldwide, there are an estimated 70,000 people, with the highest prevalence in North America, Europe, and Australia. Approximately 1,000 new cases are diagnosed in the United States every year (although the number of new cases may be decreasing due to prenatal screening), and the incidence is the same for men and women. Since 2010, newborns have been screened for CF in all 50 states, so 60% of new diagnoses are made through newborn screening.

6.2. Pathogenesis

CF is a multisystemic disease resulting from harmful genetic variants in the CFTR gene on chromosome 7q31.2, which codes for the CFTR protein (cystic fibrosis transmembrane conductance regulator). Defects in this protein lead to absent or poorly functioning chloride channels in the apical membranes of the lung surface or glandular epithelium, resulting in the formation of thick and sticky mucus, chronic lung infections, pancreatic and liver dysfunction, and reduced fertility (Bayfield et al., 2021). CF also leads to abnormal function of the chloride channels in the sweat glands, resulting in excessive salt loss in sweat.

This observation was first studied by Dr. Paul di Sant'Agnese after caring for infants with CF who were dehydrated during a heat wave in New York City in 1948. This clinical observation paved the way for the pilocarpine iontophoresis sweat test to diagnose the disease (Bell et al., 2020).

CF is an autosomal recessive disease, and its development requires the person to inherit 2 harmful CFTR variants. To date, more than 2,000 different CFTR variants are known, some of which have been shown to cause CF, while others are more likely to be associated with the disease. They are categorized into six distinct groups that reflect abnormalities in CFTR protein synthesis, structure and function (Figure 6.1).

The most common CF-causing variant is F508del (p.Phe508del), and it is a class II mutation, which means that the CFTR protein is produced but cannot reach the cell surface due to a misfolding ("trafficking defect"). Overall, 44.2% of people with CF are homozygous for F508del, with a further 40.5% having one copy of F508del and one other variant, and 15.3% having 2 non-F508del variants (Beydon et al., 2005). The specific CFTR variants carried by an individual determine the amount of functional CFTR protein present and correlate in part with the severity of the phenotype and organ involvement.

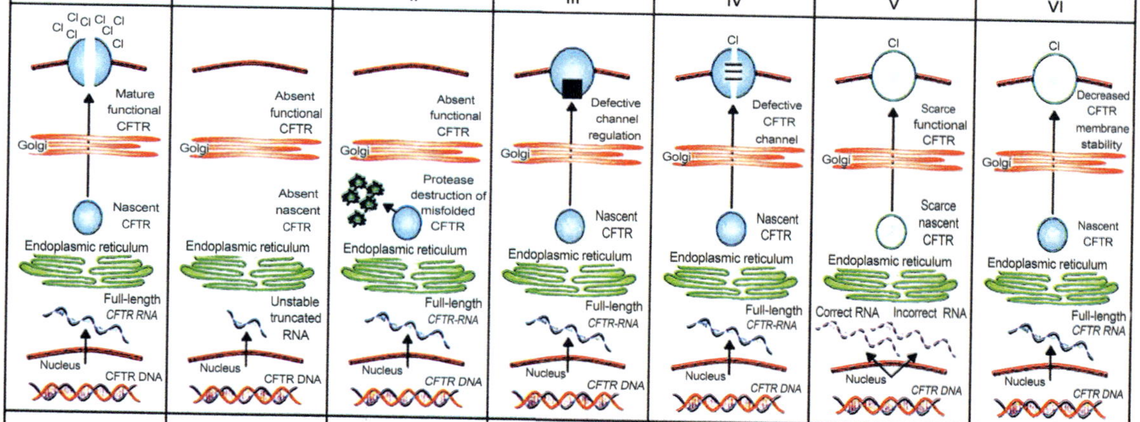

Normal	I	II	III	IV	V	VI
CFTR defect	No functional CFTR protein	CFTR trafficking defect	Defective channel regulation	Decrease channel conductance	Reduced synthesis of CFTR	Deceased CFTR stability
Type of mutations	Nonsense; frameshift; canonical splice	Missense; aminoacid deletion	Missense; aminoacid change	Missense; aminoacid change	Splicing defect; missense	Missense; aminoacid change
Specific mutation examples"	Gly542X Trp128X Arg553X 621+1G→T	Phe508del Asn130Lys Ile507del Arg560Thr	Gly551Asp Gly178Arg Gly551Ser Ser549Asn	Arg117His Arg347Pro Arg117Cys Arg334Trp	3849+10kbC→T 2789+5G→A 2789+5G→A 5T	4326delTC Gln142X 4279insA

Figure 6.1. *Cystic fibrosis transmembrane conductance regulator (CFTR) mutation classes. CFTR mutations have been grouped into 6 distinct classes based on abnormalities of CFTR synthesis, structure, and function.*

Source: Reprinted with from: Boyle, M. P., & DeBoeck, K., (2013). A new era in the treatment of cystic fibrosis: correction of the underlying CFTR defect. Lancet. Respir. Med., 1(2), 158–163.

6.3. Clinical Presentations

The classic manifestations of CF include (1) recurrent sinus and lung infections, (2) steatorrhea, and (3) malnutrition, which in its most severe form manifests as failure to thrive (Breuer et al., 2018). In the lungs, congestion of the mucous membranes by dehydrated thick secretions leads to inflammation, chronic infections, progressive obstruction of the small airways and the development of bronchiectasis observed as an abnormal and permanent enlargement of the bronchi (Figure 6.2). Bronchiectasis leads to a reduced ability to clear secretions, which results in an increased rate of infection and further dilates and damages the airways (Bush & Sly, 2015). In addition, the effects of reduced or absent chloride channel function can lead to dysfunction in various other organ systems (Figure 6.3).

Pancreatic involvement includes pancreatic exocrine insufficiency leading to fat, protein, and carbohydrate malabsorption and subsequent malnutrition, as well as insulin insufficiency and the development of CFRD (Castellani et al., 2018).

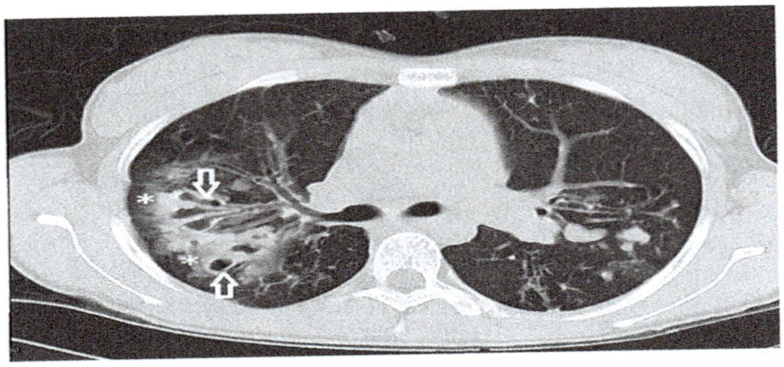

Figure 6.2. *Computed tomography of the chest of an adolescent girl with cystic fibrosis shows significant bronchiectasis (white open arrows) and mucus plugs (white asterisks).*

Source: Reprinted from: Paranjape, S. M., & Mogayzel, P. J., (2014). Cystic fibrosis. Pediatr. Rev., 35(5).

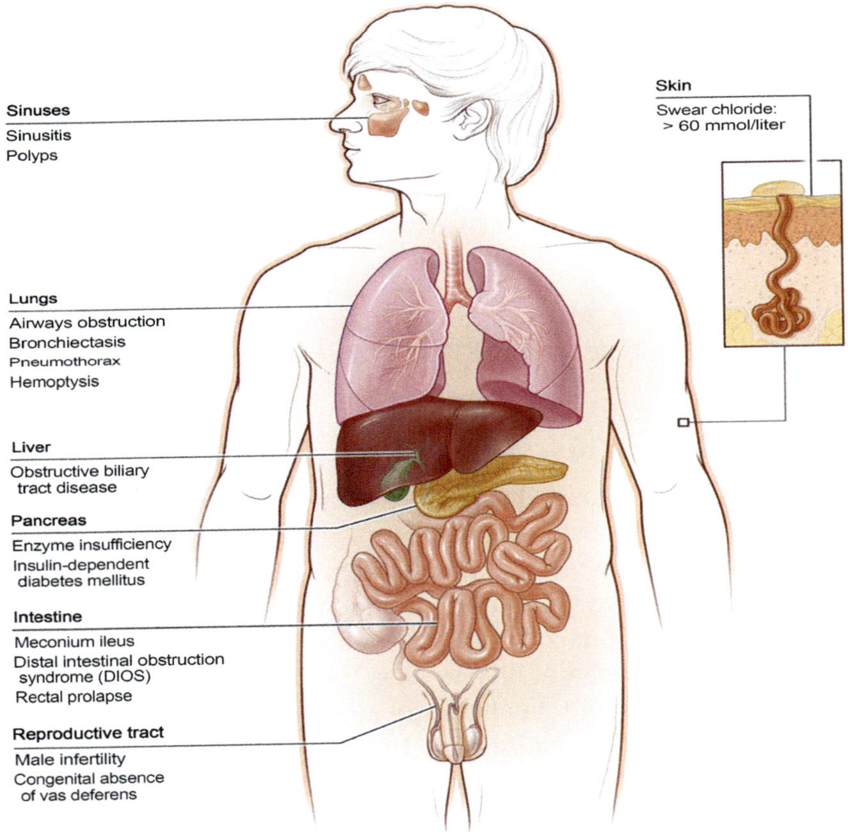

Figure 6.3. *Common clinical manifestations of cystic fibrosis.*

Source: Reprinted with permission from Link Studio LLC; Paranjape, S. M., & Mogayzel, P. J., (2014). Cystic fibrosis. Pediatr. Rev., 35(5).

In infants and young children, other signs may also indicate CF. In utero, ultrasonographic signs of hyperechogenic or dilated bowel indicate intestinal obstruction, which has been found in 50% to 78% of fetuses with CF (Cheney et al., 2020). Postnatally, 11.9% of infants of <1 years of age with CF have delayed meconium passage or meconium ileus caused by thick GI secretions that adhere to the intestinal mucosa and lead to intestinal obstruction. Meconium ileus is often associated with abdominal distension and dilated bowel loops on imaging. Intestinal perforation and peritonitis have been reported to occur in 30% of cases of meconium ileus (De Boeck et al., 2006). About 20% of untreated children (6 months to 3 years) have rectal prolapse, which is not due to constipation but to malabsorption, malnutrition, and bulky stools. Other clinical manifestations during the neonatal period may include prolonged jaundice due to biliary obstruction or biliary tract obstruction and neonatal hemorrhagic disease due to vitamin K deficiency (De Boer et al., 2011). In infancy and early childhood, salt wasting syndrome may also occur, characterized by hyponatremic, hypochloremic, hypokalemic metabolic alkalosis and edema/acrodermatitis due to hypoproteinemia from malabsorption (Desiraju & Agarwal, 2016).

Typical respiratory findings in older children, adolescents, and adults newly presenting with CF may include recurrent sinusitis, bronchitis or pneumonia, asthma that responds poorly to standard treatment, nasal polyposis or digital lumps on physical examination, and bronchiectasis on lung imaging studies (Esther et al., 2019). Common gastrointestinal symptoms may include malnutrition, poor growth, steatorrhea, intestinal obstruction, chronic constipation, rectal prolapse, and liver disease. In people with adequate pancreatic function (more likely to be diagnosed later in life due to adequate weight gain), pancreatitis can occur as a result of progressive pancreatitis, although the exact etiology is unclear. Finally, more than 98% of men with CF are infertile due to obstructive azotemia, which is due to a congenital bilateral absence of the vas deferens and can be diagnosed during an infertility workup. Newborn screening can be expected to reduce, but not eliminate, late clinical presentations due to the rate of false-negative screening results. Clinicians should also consider CF in cases of unexplained recurrent bacterial respiratory infections (pneumonia, bronchitis, persistent cough, and/or sinusitis) and/or failure to thrive.

6.3.1. Screening

Newborn screening (NBS) for CF was first introduced in the 1980s and is performed by measuring an immunoreactive trypsinogen level (IRT) in screening blood samples from newborns. In newborns, mucus plugs partially block the pancreatic ducts that lead into the small intestine (Evans et al., 2019). This prevents trypsinogen from entering the intestine and being converted into the pancreatic enzyme trypsin, even in infants who have an adequate pancreas. If an infant has an elevated IRT level, almost all state laboratories in the U.S. perform a confirmatory test of the CFTR variant (IRT/DNA), with one state laboratory currently repeating the IRT measurement (IRT/IRT). Screening is considered positive if the IRT value is persistently elevated between days 7 and 14 of life or if at least one harmful CFTR variant is identified in the genetic test. A positive NBS result triggers notification of either a neonatal intensivist or primary care physician, and the infant should be referred to a CFF-accredited center for definitive evaluation and sweat testing within 72 hours of a positive screening result (Farrell et al., 2008). Care centers can be found on the CFF website (www.cff.org/ccd/).

The benefits of diagnosing asymptomatic infants with CF include increased attention to lung health in the early stages to slow the progression of lung disease, optimization of nutritional status through early enzyme replacement and aggressive nutritional counseling, and psychosocial support for families to prevent or delay serious complications. Potential risks of NBS include an increased number of medical procedures, exposure to respiratory pathogens through CF clinic visits, financial hardships given the cost of CF-related therapies, potential iatrogenic complications (For example, early exposure to therapies with side effects), and caregiver anxiety or guilt due to false-positive screening results from perinatal asphyxia or other perinatal problems (Gangell et al., 2007). False-positive rates may also be higher in African–American children, as they have higher IRT scores than Caucasians but are at much lower risk for cystic fibrosis. NBS can also be false-negative, especially in newborns with meconium ileus or in children tested by IRT/DNA, as this test is less sensitive for detecting mutations in minorities. With current NBS practices, there is the possibility of positive NBS and identification of CFTR variants that do not meet clinical criteria for a CF diagnosis in individuals with normal or intermediate sweat chloride testing, a syndrome known as CFTR-Related Metabolic Syndrome/ Cystic Fibrosis Screen Positive, Inconclusive Diagnosis (CFSPID) (Heltshe et al., 2016).

6.3.2. Diagnosis

The CFF published consensus guidelines in 2017 stating that a diagnosis of CF can be made when an individual has clinical findings consistent with the disease, that is (1) a positive newborn screening, (2) clinical features consistent with CF, including the presence of characteristic phenotypes such as chronic, recurrent sinus and lung disease, nutritional and gastrointestinal abnormalities, and urogenital abnormalities in males, and (3) a positive family history of cystic fibrosis and evidence of CFTR dysfunction (for example chloride concentration in sweat ≥60 mmol/L).

While prenatal screening and NBS have allowed earlier detection of CF in asymptomatic individuals, the quantitative pilocarpine iontophoresis sweat test remains the gold standard for its diagnosis (Horsley et al., 2022). The sweat test, which was developed by Lewis Gibson and Robert Cooke in 1959, specifically measures the amount of chloride in a person's sweat. The sweat chloride test should be performed as soon as possible after a positive NBS result. It can be performed as early as 48 hours after birth (as sodium levels in sweat are temporarily elevated in the first 24 hours) but should be performed as soon as possible after 10 months of age and ideally by 4 weeks of age. Infants should weigh more than 2 kg or be corrected by 36 weeks gestation to increase the likelihood of adequate sweat collection. Infants with meconium ileus and any infant or child with symptoms suggestive of CF, such as recurrent bacterial respiratory infections and/or failure to thrive, should be tested for sweat chloride regardless of age or NBS results. Any abnormal sweat test result should be repeated at another time or confirmed by genetic testing (Kent et al., 2014).

Sweat chloride test results can be categorized as diagnostic, moderate, and unlikely. Diagnostic sweat chloride with levels of ≥60 mmol/L requires a confirmatory second sweat test or 2 identified CF-causing genetic variants to make the diagnosis. Mean values are between 30 and 59 mmol/L. In these individuals, the sweat chloride test should be repeated regularly and further testing at a CF center should be considered. CF can also be diagnosed in an individual with an intermediate value if the individual has 2 identified CF-causing genetic variants. Individuals with an intermediate sweat chloride level of 30–59 mmol/L and 0–1 CF-causing genetic variants may be diagnosed with a CFTR-related disorder depending on clinical presentation and family history. Individuals with sweat chloride levels of <30 mmol/L are unlikely to have CF, but if 2 CF-causing genetic variants are identified, they should still be diagnosed with the genetic disease (King et al., 2020).

In conjunction with sweat testing, genetic testing is now widely available to confirm the diagnosis of CF, particularly in cases with intermediate levels of chloride in sweat. Identification of an individual's specific CF-causing variants is necessary for the prescription of CFTR modulator therapies approved for specific CFTR variants. A diagnosis by genotype can be made by identifying 2 known pathogenic variants on separate chromosomes. Most people with CF can be diagnosed by commercial laboratories that test for the most common CFTR variants. However, the full sequencing of the CFTR gene may be necessary to confirm the diagnosis in people with clinically atypical presentations (Kraemer et al., 2006). Clinical information on specific CFTR variants can be found online (www.cftr2.org).

The era of genetic testing has expanded our understanding of CFTR dysfunction but has also increased the complexity of CF diagnosis, as there are individuals with CF phenotypes without known CF-causing mutations, as well as individuals with detected mutations who remain asymptomatic. The limitations of the sweat chloride test and the genetic test may make it necessary to perform both tests in selected patients in whom there is a strong clinical suspicion of CF (Lucy et al., 2023).

6.4. CF Management

In the United States, individuals with CF should be evaluated at least quarterly at a CFF-accredited care center that can provide interdisciplinary, patient- and family-centered care. Infants <6 months of age should be seen monthly and every 1 to 2 months during the second six months of life. These regular visits provide education on airway clearance methods, infection prevention, monitoring of age-appropriate growth and weight gain, and, in older children, assessment of lung function (Miller et al., 2005).

6.5. Therapies to Maintain Optimal Lung Health

CF is characterized by viscous secretions in the airways that lead to chronic mucus congestion, inflammation, and recurrent infections that cause long-term damage to the airways (bronchiectasis) and lung parenchyma. Chronic coughing and sputum production are characteristic symptoms. Treatment of respiratory symptoms focuses on maintaining lung function and preventing the development of bronchiectasis as well as the destruction of the lung parenchyma. In addition to promoting a smoke-free environment, children with CF are often prescribed several therapies that are likely to be lifelong and should be started shortly after diagnosis (Nguyen et al., 2014).

6.5.1. Clearance of Airway Secretions

Airway clearance therapy (ACT) is a crucial aspect of maintaining lung health. By clearing the mucus in the airways, ACT helps to reduce the bacterial load in the airways along with irritants, resulting in improved gas exchange and reduced airway obstruction (O'neill et al., 2016). The use of Twice-daily ACT as maintenance therapy is recommended for all patients with CF, regardless of symptoms or disease severity, and is more commonly performed during acute pulmonary exacerbations (PEx) of CF. Commonly used ACT modalities include manual percussion, positive expiratory pressure devices, and high-frequency oscillation of the chest wall (using an inflatable vest that delivers physical therapy to the chest through high-frequency oscillations). No one type of ACT has been shown to be better than another, and the choice of ACT should be individualized. Exercise should be encouraged as an adjunctive therapy but should not be used as a substitute for airway clearance. Nebulized agents that thin the viscous mucus of CF are often used in conjunction with ACT. These include recombinant human rhDNase (Dornase alfa/Pulmozyme) and hypertonic saline.

6.5.2. Chronic Airway Infections

In addition to patient education and infection control measures, aggressive management of chronic respiratory infections has been shown to prevent worsening lung function. Management includes frequent respiratory cultures (oropharyngeal or sputum), including surveillance for *Staphylococcus aureus* (especially methicillin-resistant *S. aureus*) and *Pseudomonas aeruginosa*. The receiving microbiology laboratories should be informed of the patient's CF diagnosis so that they can detect the respiratory pathogens commonly found in CF. The initial acquisition of *P. aeruginosa* is usually treated with antipseudomonal antibiotics such as nebulized tobramycin (TOBI nebs) to achieve eradication (Pattie et al., 2022). Nebulized antibiotics such as tobramycin or aztreonam (Cayston) can also be used as suppressive therapy for individuals with chronic infection or colonization with *P. aeruginosa* and/or other gram-negative organisms. This suppressive therapy is administered every two months to reduce the risk of antibiotic resistance. Other organisms such as *Burkholderia cepacia* complex, non-tuberculous mycobacteria (*Mycobacterium avium* complex and *Mycobacterium abscessus*), and fungal pathogens (Aspergillus fumigatus) are also monitored as they can have a significant impact on CF lung disease. People with CF also tend to develop a hypersensitivity reaction to Aspergillus known as allergic bronchopulmonary aspergillosis (ABPA), which can impair lung function and requires treatment with corticosteroids (Perrem et al., 2020).

6.5.3. Chronic Airway Inflammation

CF lung disease is caused by a combination of infection and inflammation. Routine use of oral or inhaled corticosteroids in CF is not indicated unless it is for another concomitant inflammatory disease such as asthma or ABPA. Chronic airway inflammation is treated with either high-dose ibuprofen or azithromycin. Although ibuprofen is beneficial in CF, its use is limited due to the risk of gastrointestinal bleeding and the need to monitor serum levels. Azithromycin has been shown to lead to improved lung function and reduced PEx and is usually administered orally three times a week. However, there is concern that individuals with undiagnosed mycobacterial infections who receive azithromycin over a prolonged period may develop resistance; screening with mycobacterial cultures is recommended before starting treatment (Perrem et al., 2020).

6.6. Therapies to Maintain Optimal Nutritional Status

The deterioration of lung condition is the hallmark of CF, but poor growth is one of the earliest manifestations. The combined effects of reduced nutritional intake, malabsorption, and increased metabolic demands contribute to the poor overall growth seen in infancy. Malnutrition is associated with increased morbidity and mortality in CF (Quittner et al., 2005). The CFF guidelines recommend that all children achieve a weight-to-length ratio at or above the 50th percentile by 2 years of age and that all children and adolescents aged 2 to 20 years have a body mass index at or above the 50th percentile. Caregivers and patients should receive lifelong education about the role of enteral tube feeding in optimizing nutritional status. Infants with CF should receive breast milk when possible and otherwise standard infant formula (and not formulas with hydrolyzed proteins). Infants <2 years of age should be given table salt, up to ¼ teaspoon per day until 6 months of age, as they are constantly losing salt. Infants with CF should have their fecal elastase measured after diagnosis to assess the functional status of the pancreas, as 85% of people with CF have exocrine pancreatic insufficiency (fecal elastase <200 ug/g). Pancreatic insufficiency leads to malabsorption, which manifests itself in the form of voluminous, foul-smelling stools, malnutrition, and ultimately failure to thrive (Quittner et al., 2009).

6.6.1. Pancreatic Enzyme Replacement Therapy

Pancreatic enzyme replacement therapy (PERT) should be initiated in individuals diagnosed with fecal elastase or two CFTR variants associated with pancreatic insufficiency and in individuals with clear signs or symptoms of malabsorption. Individuals with exocrine pancreatic insufficiency require enzyme replacement at each meal, snack, and enteral tube feeding, ranging from 2,000 to 2,500 units/kg of lipase per meal up to a maximum of 10,000 units/kg/day (Quittner et al., 2012). Immobilized lipase cartridges may be used in patients on continuous enteral tube feedings to assist in the hydrolysis of fats in enteral formulas. Exceeding the recommended dosage does not usually result in improved nutrient absorption, and supratherapeutic dosing is associated with fibrosing colonopathy, a rare complication characterized by shortening and strictures of the right colon. People with CF can achieve age-appropriate growth with optimized PERT (Ramsey et al., 2015).

6.6.2. Fat-Soluble Vitamin Replacement Therapy

Insufficiency of the pancreas leads to malabsorption of fat and the associated fat-soluble vitamins A, D, E, and K. A deficiency in vitamin A can lead to night blindness and dry eyes as well as dermatological symptoms such as follicular hyperkeratosis. A vitamin D deficiency can lead to rickets, osteopenia, and osteoporosis, which in turn can result in fractures. The recommended amount for people with CF is to aim for a serum level of 25-hydroxyvitamin D of at least 30 ng/ml. Vitamin E deficiency can lead to peripheral neuropathy, myopathy, and hemolysis, while vitamin K deficiency is associated with coagulopathy and can also contribute to bone disease. Supplemental vitamin therapy should begin after diagnosis, and it is recommended that vitamin A, vitamin D, and vitamin E serum levels be monitored annually by the CF physician (Ramsey et al., 2016).

6.7. CFTR Modulator Therapies

CFTR modulators are the first therapies that target the fundamental defect in CF by acting directly on the CFTR protein. They are categorized into 3 types: Potentiators, Correctors, and Amplifiers. Ivacaftor, the first approved modulator therapy, is a potentiator that improves chloride flux through the CFTR protein at the cell surface in patients with class III-V mutations. Correctors such as lumacaftor and tezacaftor help the CFTR protein to form correctly so that it can move to the cell surface. When added to potency agents, correctors such as lumacaftor/ivacaftor (Orkambi) or tezacaftor/ivacaftor (Symdeko) improve the amount of protein reaching the cell surface in patients with class II mutations. Kalydeco is currently approved by the Federal Drug Administration (FDA) for patients aged ≥6 months, while Orkambi is approved for patients aged ≥2 years with homozygous F508del variant and Symdeko is approved for patients aged ≥6 years with homozygous F508del or several other specific CF variants (Ranganathan et al., 2017).

In 2019, the FDA approved a triple combination therapy, elexacaftor/tezacaftor/ivacaftor (Trikafta), for people aged 12 years and older with at least one F508del variant. This new therapy will enable nearly 90% of people with CF to receive a highly effective treatment for the underlying cause of their disease. Trikafta has shown dramatic improvement in key disease characteristics in clinical trials, including improved lung function, decreased PEx, decreased sweat chloride levels, increased BMI, and improved quality of life according to patients. Enhancers are expected to increase the amount of CFTR protein a cell produces, but they are in development and are not currently clinically available (Rayment et al., 2018).

6.8. Diagnosis and Management of Common Pulmonary and Extrapulmonary Complications of CF

6.8.1. Pulmonary Exacerbation

One of the most common complications of CF lung disease is an episodic acute worsening of symptoms of PEx, which is characterized by increased respiratory symptoms, including cough, sputum production and/or wheezing, worsening lung function values (especially FEV1), fatigue, loss of appetite and weight loss (Robinson et al., 2013). Fever does not usually occur with PEx, and the incidence of PEx varies from person to person but contributes to the long-term decline in lung function in most people with CF. Treatment usually includes antibiotics and more frequent ACT to promote clearance of secretions from the airways. Antibiotic therapy and the route of administration (enteral, inhaled, and/or intravenous) depends on the severity of the exacerbation and the results of previous/current airway tests (Figure 6.4).

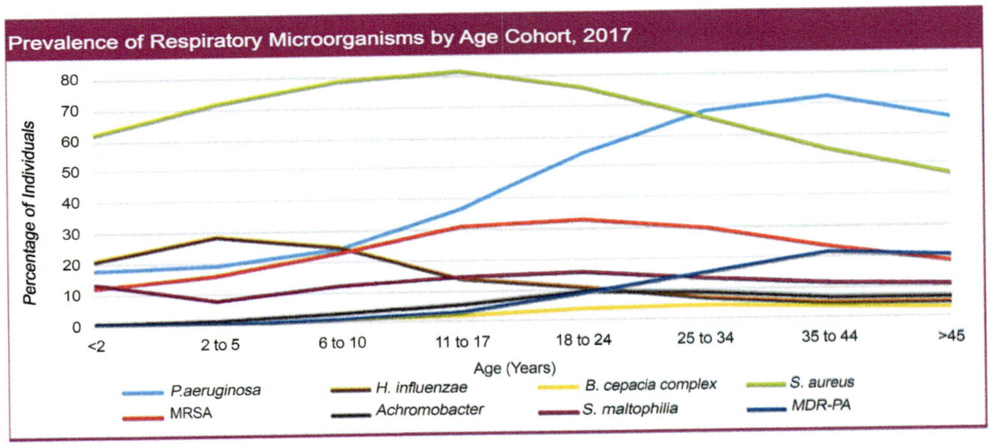

Figure 6.4. *Prevalence of bacterial pathogens in CF. MDR-PA = multidrug-resistant Pseudomonas aeruginosa, MRSA = methicillin-resistant Staphylococcus aureus.*

6.8.2. Hemoptysis

Hemoptysis is reported to occur in 3% of people with CF each year, and although it is often seen in severe lung disease, it can also be a manifestation of PEx. Hemoptysis associated with CF is most often the result of chronic infection and inflammation leading to erosion of hypertrophied bronchial arteries into the airways. Vitamin K deficiency, either due to malabsorption or liver disease, can contribute to hemoptysis. Treatment of mild to moderate hemoptysis (≤240 mL) includes evaluation, probable antibiotic therapy for PEx treatment, and consideration of limiting certain exacerbating therapies such as ibuprofen, hypertonic saline, DNAse, and ACT. Massive haemoptysis (>240 ml) is considered life-threatening, and management includes appropriate stabilization and discontinuation of anti-inflammatory and airway management measures. Treatment of massive haemoptysis or significant recurrent haemoptysis consists of bronchial artery embolization if the site of bleeding can be identified (Sakarya et al., 2016).

6.8.3. Pneumothorax

Pneumothoraces are secondary to air trapping. High alveolar pressure forces air into the lower-pressure interstitial spaces, leading to air leakage into the pleural space and causing symptoms such as acute chest pain and dyspnea. The prevalence of at least one pneumothorax is 3.4% of people with CF, and it is more likely observed in adults and people with advanced lung disease. The first diagnostic test is a chest X-ray, but in severe lung disease, a CT scan may be needed to determine the extent of a pneumothorax. Small pneumothoraces can be observed or treated with needle aspiration, but large pneumothoraces require placement of a chest tube and hospitalization. Pleurodesis is an option for recurrent pneumothoraces, but may complicate subsequent lung transplantation (Sanders et al., 2011). After developing a pneumothorax, patients should avoid devices that use positive pressure (including vest therapy) and pulmonary function tests for at least two weeks, as these may hinder the resolution of the pneumothorax or lead to recurrence (Sanders et al., 2010).

6.8.4. Chronic Rhinosinusitis and Nasal Polyposis

The epithelium of the paranasal sinuses also has a defective CFTR protein, so chronic paranasal sinus disease occurs almost universally in people with CF. In contrast, the prevalence of nasal polyposis is more variable and increases with age. Both rhinosinusitis and nasal polyposis are caused by a mucous obstruction of the paranasal sinus ostia. Clinical symptoms may include chronic headaches and facial pressure (Sanders et al., 2010). Long-term findings may include a widening of the nasal bridge and deformation of the nasal septum due to chronic nasal obstruction. Medical treatment includes nasal irrigation with saline to help loosen mucus and nasal steroids to reduce inflammation. Surgical treatment for severe and recurrent disease may improve mucus clearance, but not necessarily lung function.

6.8.5. Distal Intestinal Obstruction Syndrome

Distal intestinal obstruction syndrome (DIOS) is a common gastrointestinal complication of CF. It manifests as partial or complete obstruction of the small intestine due to viscous fecal impaction in the distal part of the bowel. Clinical manifestations include abdominal pain and bloating, vomiting, and a history of decreased bowel movements. The pathophysiology may be related to CFTR-dependent bile acid secretion and absorption in the distal ileum (Sands et al., 2009). Known risk factors for DIOS include dehydration, dietary changes, suboptimal fat absorption (that is, inadequate PERT dosing), immobilization, bacterial overgrowth, a previous episode of DIOS, and constipating medications. Differential diagnoses for DIOS include intussusception, constipation, bowel adhesions from previous abdominal surgery, volvulus, inflammatory bowel disease, and appendicitis. An abdominal radiograph, history, and physical examination are usually sufficient to make the diagnosis, but other causes of bowel obstruction should also be considered. Treatment usually involves rehydration and therapy with osmotic laxatives (Sawicki et al., 2010). More severe cases may require hospitalization, intravenous fluids, complete bowel evacuation, and the use of large volumes of polyethylene glycol. Near-complete obstruction may require sodium glumine diatrizoate enemas with retrograde irrigation and visualization of the terminal ileum by an experienced radiologist. With early diagnosis and appropriate medical treatment, surgical intervention is generally not required for DIOS.

6.8.6. CF-Related Diabetes Mellitus

CF leads to a disruption of both the exocrine and endocrine functions of the pancreas. CF-related diabetes mellitus (CFRD) is the result of persistent obstructive damage to the pancreas by thick secretions, which in turn leads to fatty infiltration of the pancreas and destruction of islet cells. CFRD typically occurs after the first decade and is found in up to 20% of adolescents and at least 50% of adults with CF. CFRD is typically diagnosed in patients with pancreatic insufficiency and is associated with increased morbidity and mortality due to poorer nutritional status and decreased lung function (Spano & Milla, 2021). CFRD is often asymptomatic, and unexplained deterioration in growth, weight, or lung function may be related to hidden CFRD. Annual screening using a 2-hour oral glucose tolerance test should be initiated at 10 years of age. Studies have shown that fasting levels of hyperglycemia or elevated levels of glycated hemoglobin are not sufficiently sensitive for the diagnosis of CFRD, therefore HbA1c levels should not be used to screen for CFRD. However, HbA1c levels can be used to monitor glycemic control in individuals with CFRD. While microvascular complications such as retinopathy, microalbuminuria, and neuropathy can occur in CFRD, ketoacidosis is rare, similar to other forms of diabetes. Treatment of CFRD focuses on glycemic control through insulin therapy as oral antihyperglycemic agents are not as effective as insulin in improving long-term outcomes (Stanojevic et al., 2021). Nutritional management continues to focus on maintaining a high-calorie diet while attempting to limit the intake of processed carbohydrates to avoid hyperglycemia.

6.8.7. CF Liver Disease

Liver disease accounts for 3.4% of all CF mortality. Approximately 3% of affected individuals develop CF-related cirrhosis (mainly in those with pancreatic insufficiency), with an average age at diagnosis of 10 years. Clinical manifestations include cholestasis, cholelithiasis, cirrhosis, portal hypertension, and, in severe cases, end-stage liver disease. The pathophysiology is thought to be related to the role of CFTR in promoting bile flow, with abnormal flow leading to cholestasis and biliary fibrosis. Males, as well as carriers of the alpha-1 antitrypsin Z allele, have an increased risk of developing advanced liver disease (Stanojevic et al., 2017). Annual screening for chronic liver disease should encompass a comprehensive assessment involving multiple diagnostic approaches. This includes evaluating liver function through blood tests that measure key enzymes such as AST (aspartate aminotransferase), ALT (alanine aminotransferase), and GGT (gamma-glutamyl transferase). Additionally, imaging techniques like ultrasound should be utilized to visually inspect the liver's structure. In some cases, further consultation with a gastroenterologist may be warranted to explore other potential causes of liver disease, particularly if initial screenings suggest abnormalities. The presence of CFLD should be considered when two of the following observations are present: (1) abnormal physical examination findings such as hepatosplenomegaly, (2) abnormal liver function test results above normal reference ranges on at least 3 consecutive determinations within a 12-month period, (3) ultrasound with Doppler evidence of abnormal liver echotexture or portal hypertension, or (4) a tissue biopsy has ruled out other causes of liver disease. Although there are currently no proven therapies to prevent the development or progression of CF-related cirrhosis, ursodiol is commonly used in the treatment of hyperbilirubinemia in CFLD (Tiddens et al., 2010).

6.8.8. Bone Disease

Another complication of CF is CF-related bone disease, which manifests itself in low bone density and an increased rate of bone fractures. Poor bone health is likely the result of a combination of factors, including malabsorption of fat-soluble vitamins such as vitamin D and K, in addition to poor nutritional status and chronic pneumonia. Prevention includes optimizing nutritional status and promoting physical activity, while dual X-ray absorptiometry is used to screen at-risk patients. Treatment includes aggressive management of potential pulmonary or endocrine comorbidities and may include bisphosphonates for patients with severe osteopenia (Van Horck et al., 2017).

6.8.9. Depression/Anxiety

Living with a chronic illness such as CF can be both challenging and isolating, putting people with CF at higher risk of mental health problems. About 15% of all people with CF report having either an anxiety disorder or depression, and 41% of people with CF report having both. It is recommended that all children with CF aged 7 to 11 years be clinically screened for depression and anxiety if a caregiver reports clinically elevated symptoms of depression or anxiety or if there is significant concern that the child is showing symptoms of depression or anxiety. Annual screening for depression and anxiety in people with CF should begin at age 12 using the PHQ-9 and GAD-7, respectively. Annual screening is also recommended for caregivers of children with CF (VanDevanter et al., 2021). Early identification of mental health problems is crucial to ensure that individuals are referred to appropriate mental health services to receive treatment and maintain their overall health and quality of life.

6.8.10. Preventative Care

Children with CF should receive routine preventive care, including all immunizations, according to the American Academy of Pediatrics guidelines. An annual influenza vaccination is recommended for children 6 months of age and older and for all household members. The use of palivizumab should be considered for all children with CF <2 years of age as prophylaxis against respiratory syncytial virus. Healthcare providers should encourage all children with CF to live in a smoke-free environment and caregivers should be informed about the health effects of secondhand smoke (Vermeulen et al., 2014).

6.8.11. Transition from Pediatric to Adult CF Care Centers

Since most people with CF live into adulthood, the issue of transitioning from pediatric care centers to adult care centers will continue to be important for patients and their families. One step that has been identified to improve the transition process is to introduce the topic of self-care skills and transition to adult care during the teen years. The self-management readiness assessment questionnaire and transition tools were used to assess patients' readiness to transition to more independent management of their illness (Walicka-Serzysko et al., 2019). These discussions should also include educational/vocational plans, behavioral risk counseling, screening for depression/anxiety, and reproductive health and family planning. Finally, conducting formal, transition-focused visits can help introduce patients to their new treatment team in a familiar clinic setting (Walicka-Serzysko et al., 2020).

6.8.12. Lung Transplantation

Lung diseases are still responsible for almost 60% of CF-related mortality. Lung transplantation is a surgical option that can prolong and improve the quality of life of people with CF. However, it requires a comprehensive pre-transplant evaluation and adherence to therapies and lifestyle recommendations to optimize the success of the transplanted lung (Walicka-Serzysko et al., 2017). Lung transplantation offers a survival benefit, where recent reports show that people with CF have a median survival time of 9.5 years after a lung transplant. CF providers are advised to discuss disease progression and treatment options, including the risks and benefits of lung transplantation, with patients with advanced lung disease (Waters et al., 2015). Referral to a lung transplant center should be discussed with patients whose FEV1<50% predicted or is rapidly declining (>decreases by 20% over 12 months). Overall, 6.3% of CF transplants performed in 2018 were in people under the age of 18, and the criteria for referral are similar to those for adults over the age of 18 (Waters et al., 2012). The discussion about a lung transplant can be seen by people with CF as another transition and should be facilitated through education, communication, and support for the individual and their family (Wojsyk-Banaszak et al., 2022).

A Closer Look

Nasal Polyposis

Nasal polyposis is a chronic inflammatory condition characterized by the growth of soft, painless, and non-cancerous polyps in the nasal passages and sinuses. These polyps are often associated with other conditions such as asthma, allergic rhinitis, and cystic fibrosis. They can lead to various symptoms, including nasal obstruction, loss of smell, sinus pressure, and chronic nasal discharge. The exact etiology of nasal polyposis is multifactorial, involving genetic predisposition, environmental factors, and immune system dysregulation. Research indicates that eosinophilic inflammation plays a significant role in the pathogenesis of nasal polyps, highlighting the importance of understanding the immune mechanisms involved in this condition.

Recent studies have explored the molecular pathways contributing to nasal polyposis. A study by Saito et al. (2021) identified elevated levels of interleukin-5 (IL-5) and eosinophils in the tissue of patients with nasal polyps, suggesting that these inflammatory mediators may drive polyp formation and persistence. Similarly, a systematic review by Fokkens et al. (2020) concluded that Th2-mediated inflammation, characterized by an imbalance of cytokines, significantly contributes to the development of nasal polyps. These findings support the hypothesis that targeting specific cytokines involved in the inflammatory process could offer therapeutic benefits.

In terms of treatment, the management of nasal polyposis has evolved significantly. Corticosteroids, both topical and systemic, remain the first-line therapy due to their anti-inflammatory properties. However, many patients experience recurrence after treatment. Recent research has investigated the efficacy of biologic therapies, particularly in patients with severe or refractory nasal polyposis. A randomized controlled trial by Bachert et al. (2019) demonstrated that the anti-IL-4 receptor monoclonal antibody dupilumab significantly reduced polyp size and improved symptoms compared to placebo. This study underscores the potential of biologics in managing nasal polyposis, offering hope for patients who do not respond adequately to conventional therapies.

Moreover, the relationship between nasal polyposis and comorbid conditions is an area of active investigation. A meta-analysis conducted by Li et al. (2023) found a significant association between nasal polyps and asthma, suggesting that these conditions share common pathophysiological mechanisms. The presence of nasal polyps in asthmatic patients was linked to increased severity of asthma symptoms and a higher rate of asthma exacerbations. These findings emphasize the need for comprehensive management strategies that address both nasal polyposis and associated respiratory conditions, ultimately improving patient outcomes and quality of life.

Summary

People affected by CF live longer and healthier lives, and their survival is expected to improve further with earlier diagnosis through routine newborn screening, the dissemination of evidence-based guidelines, interdisciplinary care centers, and the use of mutation-specific modulator therapies. The primary goals of treatment continue to be the optimization of lung function and nutritional status, and incremental advances in these therapies have had a profound impact on the health and quality of life of people with CF. Building partnerships with those affected and their families requires recognition of the emotional, social, and financial impact of this lifelong disease, as well as effective communication and coordination between primary care physicians and CF care center teams.

References

1. Aurora, P., Bush, A., Gustafsson, P., Oliver, C., Wallis, C., Price, J., Stroobant, J., Carr, S., & Stocks, J. (2005). Multiple-breath washout as a marker of lung disease in preschool children with cystic fibrosis. *American Journal of Respiratory and Critical Care Medicine, 171*(3), 249–256.
2. Aurora, P., Gustafsson, P., Bush, A., Lindblad, A., Oliver, C., Wallis, C. E., & Stocks, J. (2004). Multiple breath inert gas washout as a measure of ventilation distribution in children with cystic fibrosis. *Thorax, 59*(12), 1068–1073.
3. Bayfield, K. J., Douglas, T. A., Rosenow, T., Davies, J. C., Elborn, S. J., Mall, M., Paproki, A., Ratjen, F., Sly, P. D., Smyth, A. R., et al. (2021). Time to get serious about the detection and monitoring of early lung disease in cystic fibrosis. *Thorax, 76*(11), 1255–1265.
4. Bell, S. C., Mall, M. A., Gutierrez, H., Macek, M., Madge, S., Davies, J. C., Burgel, P. R., Tullis, E., Castaños, C., Castellani, C., et al. (2020). The future of cystic fibrosis care: A global perspective. *Lancet Respiratory Medicine, 8*(1), 65–124.
5. Beydon, N., Davis, S. D., Lombardi, E., Allen, J. L., Arets, H. G. M., Aurora, P., Bisgaard, H., Davis, G. M., Ducharme, F. M., Eigen, H., et al. (2007). An official American Thoracic Society/European Respiratory Society statement: Pulmonary function testing in preschool children. *American Journal of Respiratory and Critical Care Medicine, 175*(12), 1304–1345.
6. Breuer, O., Caudri, D., Stick, S., & Turkovic, L. (2018). Predicting disease progression in cystic fibrosis. *Expert Review of Respiratory Medicine, 12*(11), 905–917.
7. Bush, A., & Sly, P. D. (2015). Evolution of cystic fibrosis lung function in the early years. *Current Opinion in Pulmonary Medicine, 21*(6), 602–608.
8. Castellani, C., Duff, A. J., Bell, S. C., Heijerman, H. G., Munck, A., Ratjen, F., Sermet-Gaudelus, I., Southern, K. W., Barben, J., Flume, P. A., et al. (2018). ECFS best practice guidelines: The 2018 revision. *Journal of Cystic Fibrosis, 17*(2), 153–178.
9. Cheney, J., Vidmar, S., Gailer, N., Wainwright, C., Douglas, T. A., & the ACFBLAs Group. (2020). Health-related quality-of-life in children with cystic fibrosis aged 5-years and associations with health outcomes. *Journal of Cystic Fibrosis, 19*(5), 483–491.
10. De Boeck, K., Wilschanski, M., Castellani, C., Taylor, C., Cuppens, H., Dodge, J., & Sinaasappel, M. (2006). Cystic fibrosis: Terminology and diagnostic algorithms. *Thorax, 61*(8), 627–635.
11. De Boer, K., Vandemheen, K. L., Tullis, E., Doucette, S., Fergusson, D., Freitag, A., Paterson,

N., Jackson, M., Lougheed, M. D., Kumar, V., et al. (2011). Exacerbation frequency and clinical outcomes in adult patients with cystic fibrosis. *Thorax, 66*(8), 680–685.

12. Desiraju, K., & Agrawal, A. (2016). Impulse oscillometry: The state-of-art for lung function testing. *Lung India, 33*(5), 410–416.
13. Esther, C. R., Jr., Muhlebach, M. S., Ehre, C., Hill, D. B., Wolfgang, M. C., Kesimer, M., Ramsey, K. A., Markovetz, M. R., Garbarine, I. C., Forest, M. G., et al. (2019). Mucus accumulation in the lungs precedes structural changes and infection in children with cystic fibrosis. *Science Translational Medicine, 11*(504), eaav3488.
14. Evans, D. J., Schultz, A., Verheggen, M., Hall, G. L., & Simpson, S. J. (2019). Identifying pediatric lung disease: A comparison of forced oscillation technique outcomes. *Pediatric Pulmonology, 54*(6), 751–758.
15. Farrell, P. M., Rosenstein, B. J., White, T. B., Accurso, F. J., Castellani, C., Cutting, G. R., Durie, P. R., LeGrys, V. A., Massie, J., Parad, R. B., et al. (2008). Guidelines for diagnosis of cystic fibrosis in newborns through older adults: Cystic fibrosis foundation consensus report. *Journal of Pediatrics, 153*(5), S4–S14.
16. Gangell, C. L., Horak, F., Jr., Patterson, H. J., Sly, P. D., Stick, S. M., & Hall, G. L. (2007). Respiratory impedance in children with cystic fibrosis using forced oscillations in clinic. *European Respiratory Journal, 30*(5), 892–897.
17. Heltshe, S. L., Goss, C. H., Thompson, V., Sagel, S. D., Sanders, D. B., Marshall, B. C., & Quon, B. (2016). Short-term and long-term response to pulmonary exacerbation treatment in cystic fibrosis. *Thorax, 71*(3), 223–229.
18. Horsley, A. R., Belcher, J., Bayfield, K., Bianco, B., Cunningham, S., Fullwood, C., Jones, A., Shawcross, A., Smith, J. A., Maitra, A., et al. (2022). Longitudinal assessment of lung clearance index to monitor disease progression in children and adults with cystic fibrosis. *Thorax, 77*(5), 357–363.
19. Kent, L., Reix, P., Innes, J., Zielen, S., Le Bourgeois, M., Braggion, C., Lever, S., Arets, H., Brownlee, K., Bradley, J., et al. (2014). Lung clearance index: Evidence for use in clinical trials in cystic fibrosis. *Journal of Cystic Fibrosis, 13*(1), 123–138.
20. King, G. G., Bates, J., Berger, K. I., Calverley, P., De Melo, P. L., Dellacà, R. L., Farre, R., Hall, G., Ioan, I., Irvin, C. G., et al. (2020). Technical standards for respiratory oscillometry. *European Respiratory Journal, 55*(5), 1900753.
21. Kraemer, R., Baldwin, D. N., Ammann, R. A., Frey, U., & Gallati, S. (2006). Progression of pulmonary hyperinflation and trapped gas associated with genetic and environmental factors in children with cystic fibrosis. *Respiratory Research, 7*, 138.
22. Lucy, P., Sanja, S., Melinda, S., Hartmut, G., Neil, S., Valerie, W., Sanders, D. B., Davis, S. D., & Ratjen, F. (2023). Evaluation of clinically relevant changes in the lung clearance index in children with cystic fibrosis and healthy controls. *Thorax, 78*(5), 362.
23. Miller, M. R., Hankinson, J., Brusasco, V., Burgos, F., Casaburi, R., Coates, A., Crapo, R., Enright, P., Van Der Grinten, C. P. M., Gustafsson, P., et al. (2005). Standardization of spirometry. *European Respiratory Journal, 26*(2), 319–338.
24. Nguyen, T. T., Thia, L. P., Hoo, A. F., Bush, A., Aurora, P., Wade, A., Chudleigh, J., Lum, S., & Stocks, J. (2014). Evolution of lung function during the first year of life in newborn screened cystic fibrosis infants. *Thorax, 69*(10), 910–917.

25. O'Neill, K., Tunney, M. M., Johnston, E., Rowan, S., Downey, D. G., Rendall, J., Reid, A., Bradbury, I., Elborn, J. S., & Bradley, J. M. (2016). Lung clearance index in adults and children with cystic fibrosis. *Chest, 150*(6), 1323–1332.

26. Pattie, P., Ranganathan, S., Harrison, J., Vidmar, S., Hall, G. L., Foong, R. E., Harper, A., Ramsey, K., & Wurzel, D. (2022). Quality of life is poorly correlated to lung disease severity in school-aged children with cystic fibrosis. *Journal of Cystic Fibrosis, 21*(2), e188–e203.

27. Perrem, L., Stanojevic, S., Shaw, M., Davis, S., Retsch-Bogart, G., & Ratjen, F. (2020). Changes in the parent cystic fibrosis questionnaire-revised (CFQ-R) with respiratory symptoms in preschool children with cystic fibrosis. *Journal of Cystic Fibrosis, 19*(4), 492–498.

28. Perrem, L., Stanojevic, S., Shaw, M., Jensen, R., McDonald, N., Isaac, S. M., Davis, M., Clem, C., Guido, J., Jara, S., et al. (2020). Lung clearance index to track acute respiratory events in school-age children with cystic fibrosis. *American Journal of Respiratory and Critical Care Medicine, 203*(8), 977–986.

29. Quittner, A. L., Buu, A., Messer, M. A., Modi, A. C., & Watrous, M. (2005). Development and validation of the Cystic Fibrosis Questionnaire in the United States: A health-related quality-of-life measure for cystic fibrosis. *Chest, 128*(4), 2347–2354.

30. Quittner, A. L., Modi, A. C., Wainwright, C., Otto, K., Kirihara, J., & Montgomery, A. B. (2009). Determination of the minimal clinically important difference scores for the Cystic Fibrosis Questionnaire-Revised respiratory symptom scale in two populations of patients with cystic fibrosis and chronic Pseudomonas aeruginosa airway infection. *Chest, 135*(6), 1610–1618.

31. Quittner, A. L., Sawicki, G. S., McMullen, A., Rasouliyan, L., Pasta, D. J., Yegin, A., & Konstan, M. W. (2012). Psychometric evaluation of the Cystic Fibrosis Questionnaire-Revised in a national sample. *Quality of Life Research, 21*(7), 1267–1278.

32. Ramsey, K. A., Ranganathan, S. C., Gangell, C. L., Turkovic, L., Park, J., Skoric, B., Stick, S. M., Sly, P. D., & Hall, G. L. (2015). Impact of lung disease on respiratory impedance in young children with cystic fibrosis. *European Respiratory Journal, 46*(6), 1672–1679.

33. Ramsey, K. A., Rosenow, T., Turkovic, L., Skoric, B., Banton, G., Adams, A. M., Simpson, S. J., Murray, C., Ranganathan, S. C., Stick, S. M., et al. (2016). Lung clearance index and structural lung disease on computed tomography in early cystic fibrosis. *American Journal of Respiratory and Critical Care Medicine, 193*(1), 60–67.

34. Ranganathan, S. C., Hall, G. L., Sly, P. D., Stick, S. M., Douglas, T. A., & AREST-CF. (2017). Early lung disease in infants and preschool children with cystic fibrosis: What have we learned and what should we do about it? *American Journal of Respiratory and Critical Care Medicine, 195*(12), 1567–1575.

35. Rayment, J. H., Stanojevic, S., Davis, S. D., Retsch-Bogart, G., & Ratjen, F. (2018). Lung clearance index to monitor treatment response in pulmonary exacerbations in preschool children with cystic fibrosis. *Thorax, 73*(5), 451–458.

36. Robinson, P. D., Latzin, P., Verbanck, S., Hall, G. L., Horsley, A., Gappa, M., Thamrin, C., Arets, H. G. M., Aurora, P., Fuchs, S. I., et al. (2013). Consensus statement for inert gas washout measurement using multiple- and single-breath tests. *European Respiratory Journal, 41*(3), 507–522.

37. Sakarya, A., Uyan, Z. S., Baydemir, C., Anık, Y., Erdem, E., Gokdemir, Y., Karadag, B., Karakoc, F.,

& Ersu, R. (2016). Evaluation of children with cystic fibrosis by impulse oscillometry when stable and at exacerbation. *Pediatric Pulmonology, 51*(11), 1151–1158.

38. Sanders, D. B., Bittner, R. C. L., Rosenfeld, M., Hoffman, L. R., Redding, G. J., & Goss, C. H. (2010). Failure to recover to baseline pulmonary function after cystic fibrosis pulmonary exacerbation. *American Journal of Respiratory and Critical Care Medicine, 182*(5), 627–632.

39. Sanders, D. B., Bittner, R. C., Rosenfeld, M., Redding, G. J., & Goss, C. H. (2011). Pulmonary exacerbations are associated with subsequent FEV1 decline in both adults and children with cystic fibrosis. *Pediatric Pulmonology, 46*(4), 393–400.

40. Sanders, D. B., Hoffman, L. R., Emerson, J., Gibson, R. L., Rosenfeld, M., Redding, G. J., & Goss, C. H. (2010). Return of FEV1 after pulmonary exacerbation in children with cystic fibrosis. *Pediatric Pulmonology, 45*(2), 127–134.

41. Sands, D., & Borawska-Kowalczyk, U. (2009). Polska adaptacja Kwestionariusza Jakości Życia przeznaczonego dla dzieci i dorosłych chorych na mukowiscydozę oraz ich rodziców (CFQ-R). *Pediatria Polska, 84*(2), 165–172.

42. Sawicki, G. S., Rasouliyan, L., McMullen, A. H., Wagener, J. S., McColley, S. A., Pasta, D. J., & Quittner, A. L. (2010). Longitudinal assessment of health-related quality of life in an observational cohort of patients with cystic fibrosis. *Pediatric Pulmonology, 46*(1), 36–44.

43. Spano, J., & Milla, C. E. (2021). Defining the clinical utility of the lung clearance index. Are we there yet? *American Journal of Respiratory and Critical Care Medicine, 203*(8), 937–939.

44. Stanojevic, S., Davis, S. D., Perrem, L., Shaw, M., Retsch-Bogart, G., Davis, M., Jensen, R., Clem, C. C., Isaac, S. M., Guido, J., et al. (2021). Determinants of lung disease progression measured by lung clearance index in children with cystic fibrosis. *European Respiratory Journal, 58*(1), 2003380.

45. Stanojevic, S., Davis, S. D., Retsch-Bogart, G., Webster, H., Davis, M., Johnson, R. C., Jensen, R., Pizarro, M. E., Kane, M., Clem, C. C., et al. (2017). Progression of lung disease in preschool patients with cystic fibrosis. *American Journal of Respiratory and Critical Care Medicine, 195*(9), 1216–1225.

46. Tiddens, H. A., Donaldson, S. H., Rosenfeld, M., & Paré, P. D. (2010). Cystic fibrosis lung disease starts in the small airways: Can we treat it more effectively? *Pediatric Pulmonology, 45*(2), 107–117.

47. Van Horck, M., Winkens, B., Wesseling, G., de Winter-de Groot, K., de Vreede, I., Jöbsis, Q., & Dompeling, E. (2017). Factors associated with changes in health-related quality of life in children with cystic fibrosis during 1-year follow-up. *European Journal of Pediatrics, 176*(8), 1047–1054.

48. VanDevanter, E. J., Heltshe, S. L., Skalland, M., Lechtzin, N., Nichols, D., & Goss, C. H. (2021). The effect of oral and intravenous antimicrobials on pulmonary exacerbation recovery in cystic fibrosis. *Journal of Cystic Fibrosis, 20*(6), 932–936.

49. Vermeulen, F., Proesmans, M., Boon, M., Havermans, T., & De Boeck, K. (2014). Lung clearance index predicts pulmonary exacerbations in young patients with cystic fibrosis. *Thorax, 69*(1), 39–45.

50. Walicka-Serzysko, K., Postek, M., & Sands, D. (2017). Silent lung zone—Application of multi-breath nitrogen washout test (MBNW) in the diagnosis of small airways diseases in children—

Preliminary report based on literature and own experience. *Developmental Period Medicine, 21*(4), 369–379.

51. Walicka-Serzysko, K., Postek, M., Milczewska, J., & Sands, D. (2019). Change in lung clearance index with microbiological status in children with cystic fibrosis. *Pediatric Pulmonology, 54*(6), 729–736.

52. Walicka-Serzysko, K., Postek, M., Milczewska, J., & Sands, D. (2020). Lung function deterioration in school children with cystic fibrosis. *Pediatric Pulmonology, 55*(12), 3030–3038.

53. Waters, V., & Ratjen, F. (2015). Pulmonary exacerbations in children with cystic fibrosis. *Annals of the American Thoracic Society, 12*(Suppl. S2), S200–S2006.

54. Waters, V., Stanojevic, S., Atenafu, E. G., Lu, A., Yau, Y., Tullis, E., & Ratjen, F. (2012). Effect of pulmonary exacerbations on long-term lung function decline in cystic fibrosis. *European Respiratory Journal, 40*(1), 61–66.

55. Wojsyk-Banaszak, I., Więckowska, B., Stachowiak, Z., Kycler, M., & Szczepankiewicz, A. (2022). Predictive value of impulse oscillometry and multiple breath washout parameters in pediatric patients with cystic fibrosis pulmonary exacerbation. *Pediatric Pulmonology, 57*(10), 1466–1474.

Chapter 7

TUBERCULOSIS

Contents

Introduction

Tuberculosis (TB) is a bacterial infection caused by *Mycobacterium tuberculosis*, primarily affecting the lungs but also capable of affecting other parts of the body. While TB is one of the top 10 causes of death worldwide, it is considered rare in many developed countries. Despite being preventable and treatable, TB remains a significant global health issue, especially in low- and middle-income countries.

According to the World Health Organization (WHO), an estimated 10 million people fell ill with TB in 2019, with 1.4 million deaths reported, including among individuals with HIV. While the global incidence rate has been declining, with a 9% reduction from 2015 to 2019, overall progress to reduce transmission and infection is slow, and challenges such as drug-resistant TB and inadequate funding for TB programs persist.

In developed countries, TB is considered rare due to effective public health measures, such as widespread vaccination (For example, Bacillus Calmette-Guérin or BCG vaccine) and robust healthcare systems. For example, in the United States, the TB incidence rate is low, with approximately 2.7 cases per 100,000 people in 2019. However, certain populations, such as homeless individuals, those with compromised immune systems, and foreign-born individuals from TB-endemic countries, remain at higher risk (Acharya et al., 2020).

Despite its rarity in some regions, TB requires continued attention and resources to achieve global elimination. Efforts such as early detection, access to quality care, and addressing social determinants of health are crucial in the fight against TB and its associated stigma and impact on vulnerable populations. This chapter is organized as follows. Firstly, the global disease burden and clinical context are discussed in detail, followed by an overview of approaches to diagnosis, treatment, and prevention. The aim is to look at tuberculosis through the lens of the health system and, in the final part of the chapter, provide recommendations for improving implementation strategies and strengthening health systems, including care, the supply chain and information systems. As current tools to combat TB are woefully inadequate, we conclude with sections on critical research and development and economic analyzes of new interventions for diagnosis, treatment, and vaccines. The focus is on data or models on the economic costs and benefits of current or potential future interventions to combat this disease, where available (Aggarwal et al., 2017).

The chapter recommends actively seeking cases in countries with high disease burden, investing more in health systems, delivering care at the community level rather than in hospitals, and providing more support for research into new tools — that is, the development of better diagnostics, treatments, and vaccines. Most of these approaches were already included in previous WHO policies but were not emphasized. They are now part of the WHO Strategy to End Tuberculosis, with which this report is fully aligned.

Orientation and Directional Terms

Term	Definition	Illustration
Mycobacterium tuberculosis	A bacterial species that causes tuberculosis (TB), an infectious disease that primarily affects the lungs but can also impact other parts of the body.	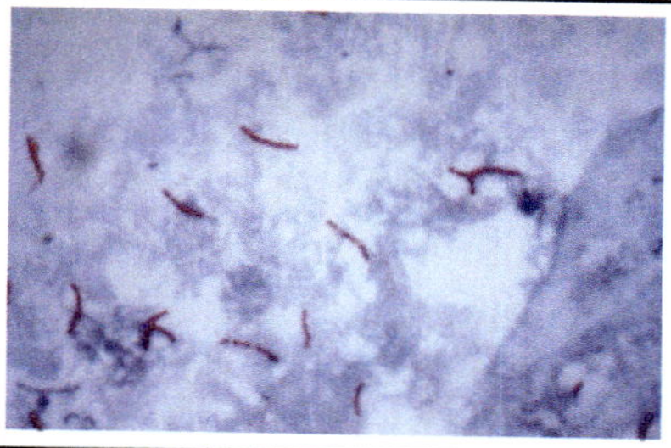
World Health Organization (WHO)	A specialized agency of the United Nations responsible for international public health, aiming to promote health, keep the world safe, and serve the vulnerable.	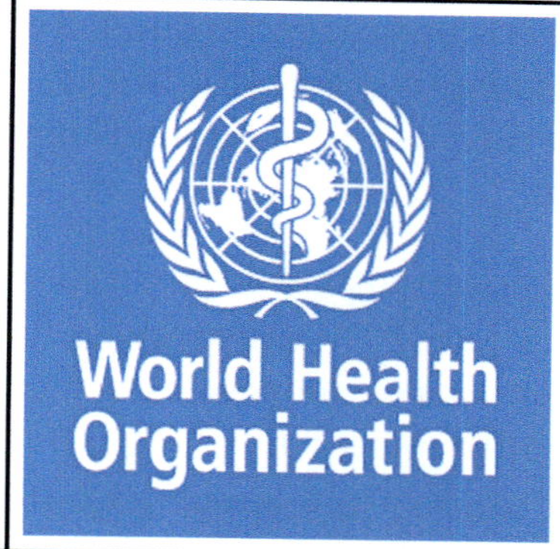
HIV (Human Immunodeficiency Virus)	A virus that attacks the body's immune system, weakening the ability to fight infections and diseases, potentially leading to AIDS (Acquired Immunodeficiency Syndrome).	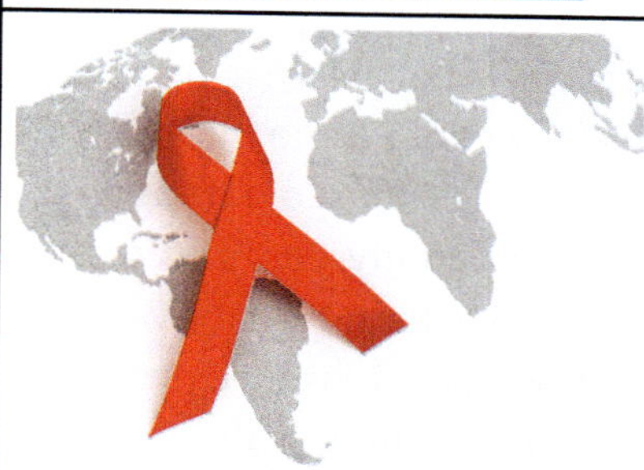
Bacille Calmette-Guérin (BCG)	A vaccine primarily used against tuberculosis (TB), made from a weakened strain of Mycobacterium bovis to provide immunity against TB.	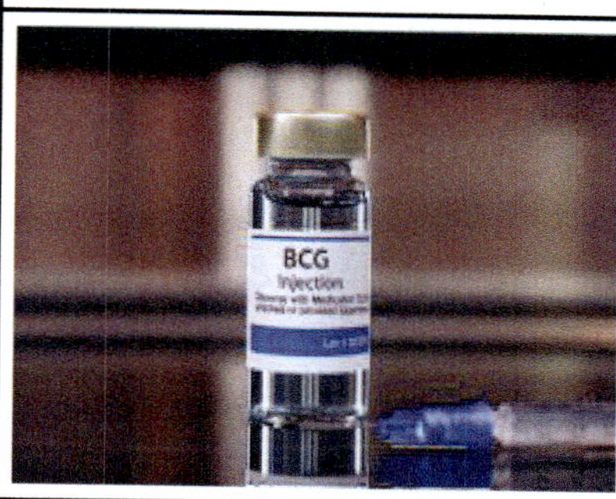
Chemotherapy	A treatment method that uses powerful drugs to kill or inhibit the growth of cancer cells or microorganisms causing diseases, including infections like tuberculosis.	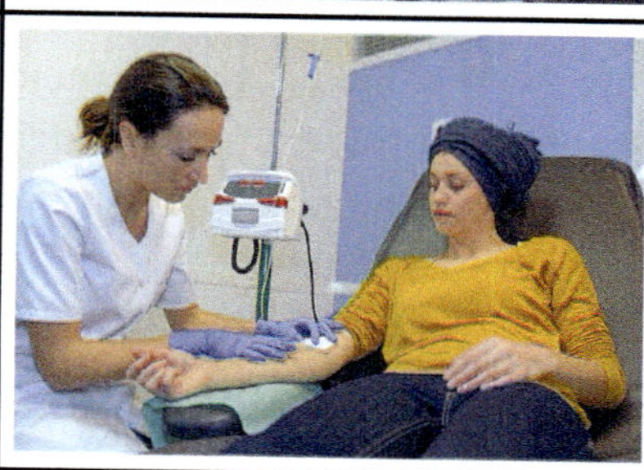

7.1. An Overview of Tuberculosis

Despite 90 years of vaccination and 60 years of chemotherapy, TB remains the leading cause of death from an infectious agent worldwide, overtaking human immunodeficiency virus/ acquired immunodeficiency syndrome (HIV/ AIDS) for the first time. The WHO estimates that there are around 10.4 million new cases and 1.8 million deaths from TB every year. A third of these new cases (around 3 million) remain unknown to the healthcare system and many do not receive adequate treatment (Bhatt et al., 2007).

TB is an infectious bacterial disease caused by *M. tuberculosis* (Mtb). It is transmitted from person to person via the respiratory tract and most commonly affects the lungs, but it can damage any tissue. Only about 10% of people infected with Mtb develop active TB disease in their lifetime, while the rest of those infected can successfully contain the infection. One of the challenges of TB is that the pathogen remains in a latent state for many years in many infected individuals and can be reactivated to cause disease. The risk of TB disease progression after infection is highest shortly after initial infection and increases dramatically in persons co-infected with HIV/AIDS or other immunocompromising diseases (Brecik et al., 2015).

Treatment of TB disease requires multiple medications over many months. These long courses of medication are a challenge for both patients and health systems, particularly in low- and middle-income countries (LMICs) where the disease burden often far exceeds local resources. In some areas, the incidence of drug-resistant TB is increasing, requiring even longer treatment regimens with more expensive and poorly tolerated drugs.

The diagnosis in LMICs is primarily conducted by microscopic examination of stained smears of sputum from suspected patients, however, smear microscopy can only detect 50–60% of all TB cases (smear-positive). While more sensitive methods for diagnosing TB and detecting drug resistance have recently become available, they are more expensive. The time between the onset of the disease and diagnosis and the start of treatment is often long, and such delays allow transmission of the disease. Although Bacille Calmette–Guérin (BCG) remains the most widely used vaccine worldwide, its efficacy is geographically highly variable and incomplete. Model calculations show that more effective vaccines are probably needed to eliminate TB in high-incidence areas.

The basic strategy to combat TB for the past 40 years has been to diagnose and treat sick people who visit a health facility.

The premise is that if patients with the active disease are cured, mortality will disappear, the prevalence and transmission of the disease will decrease, and therefore the incidence should also decrease. The reality in many countries is more complex, and the overall decline in incidence (only about 1.5% per year) is unacceptably slow (Brown et al., 2011).

Chemotherapy for the treatment of TB is one of the most cost-effective of all health interventions. These findings have been instrumental in the global promotion by the WHO and the Stop TB Partnership of the Directly Observed Treatment Short Course (DOTS) strategy, a package of interventions that combines the best practices in the diagnosis and treatment of TB patients. The DOTS strategy for TB control promotes standardized treatment with monitoring and patient support, including the strategies of Direct Observation of Therapy (DOT) and beyond, where a health care worker personally observes the patient taking the medication.

Between 1990 and 2010, the absolute number of TB deaths worldwide fell by 18.7%, from 1.47 million to 1.20 million, and by 22% between 2000 and 2015. By 2015, an estimated 49 million lives had been saved. The internationally agreed targets to combat TB, enshrined in the United Nations (UN) Millennium Development Goals, aimed to "halt and reverse the increase in tuberculosis by 2015," and this target was achieved in all six WHO regions and in most, but not all, of the 22 countries with a high burden of the disease (Campbell et al., 2001).

Despite progress, major gaps remain. Although the Sustainable Development Goals (SDGs) aim to end the TB epidemic altogether, the decline in incidence is disappointing. One in three patients remains "unknown" to the health system," where many are undiagnosed and untreated, and rates of case detection and treatment success remain too low in high-burden countries. Worryingly, rates of multidrug-resistant (MDR) TB — defined as resistance to the two main TB drugs isoniazid and rifampicin — are increasing worldwide, with extensively drug-resistant (XDR) TB against many second-line drugs and strains resistant to all commonly used drugs emerging. These resistant strains are now primarily the result of transmission rather than inadequate treatment (Carroll et al., 2011).

In addition, the problem of TB has been exacerbated by co-infection with HIV/AIDS. While co-infection with HIV/AIDS and TB accounts for only 11% of the total TB burden worldwide, in some areas of sub-Saharan Africa with a high TB burden, up to three-quarters of TB patients are co-infected with HIV/AIDS.

In these countries, TB control efforts are being overwhelmed by the rising number of TB cases occurring alongside the HIV/AIDS epidemic, and after decades of steady decline, tuberculosis incidence is also increasing in some high-income countries (HICs), mainly as a result of outbreaks in vulnerable groups.

If the ultimate goal of infectious disease control is to interrupt transmission, then controlling TB requires early and accurate detection of cases, rapid initiation and adherence to effective treatment that prevents transmission, and, where possible, preventive treatment of latent tTB. It is widely recognized that new strategies and more effective tools and interventions are needed to achieve the post-2015 targets. These interventions must not only be cost-effective but also affordable and able to deliver at scale (Chahine et al., 2014).

TB control will require three new advances — the development of new point-of-care (POC) diagnostics, more effective drug regimens to combat drug-susceptible and drug-resistant TB and more effective vaccines. As outlined in this chapter, this requires new strategies and tools. These include moving away from traditional passive DOTS case finding and towards more active case finding in high

TB burden regions, which includes the provision of services targeted at the most vulnerable populations and integrated with other services, particularly HIV/AIDS services, and care that is delivered at the primary health care and community levels. Especially in countries with a high burden of TB, many people with tuberculosis are asymptomatic, so waiting until patients are sick enough to seek treatment is not enough to significantly reduce transmission and incidence (Chai et al., 2018). A more proactive and aggressive approach is needed to address the barriers in the healthcare system for effective TB control.

The strategies recommended by the WHO to combat TB have evolved considerably over time. In early formulations, the central tenets of the global TB control strategy were clinical and programmatic in nature, and focused primarily on the provision of standardized drug regimens; the underlying assumption was that the problem could be largely solved with existing biomedical resources (Chatterji et al., 2014). However, in many LMICs, health system weaknesses in governance, financing, health workforce, procurement, and supply chain management, and information systems have hindered TB control and have not been adequately addressed in TB control efforts. The current global TB strategy, formulated as the End TB Strategy, is the most comprehensive approach to date and includes three key pillars:

- Integrated, patient-centered care and prevention;
- Social and political action to address determinants of disease;
- Recognition of the urgent need for research to provide new tools.

Health systems are important and need to be strengthened, as with other health interventions, the success of TB treatment and control in a country often depends on the strength of its health system. A health system can be defined in many ways, perhaps best defined as "all activities whose primary purpose is to promote, restore or maintain health" (Chiang et al., 2010).

In a sense, the greatest risk factor for contracting TB is breathing, therefore, people from all social and economic classes are at risk.

Although the low-socioeconomic populations are disproportionately affected by TB, the claim that TB is "only a disease of the poor" is misleading and counterproductive if it leads either to further stigmatization of the disease or to the view that middle- and high-income countries need not worry about the disease. In the case of HIV/AIDS co-infection, evidence suggests that in Africa, where there are high rates of TB, HIV/AIDS is more prevalent in the wealthier segments of the population (Chikhale et al., 2018).

The analytical framework on which this chapter is based defines the main functions of the health system, the end goals, and the contextual factors that influence the health system (Figure 7.1).

It draws on the WHO framework as well as the health systems and national accounts frameworks developed by Frenk (1994); Hsiao & Heller (2007); and Roberts and others (2004) (OECD, Eurostat & WHO, 2011).

The four key health system functions represented in the framework are as follows:

- **Governance and Organization:** The policy and regulatory environment; stewardship and regulatory functions of the Ministry of health and its relation to other levels of the health system; and structural arrangements for insurers and purchasers, health care providers, and market regulators.
- **Financing:** The way funds are collected, funds, and risks are pooled, finances are allocated, and health care providers are remunerated (Cole et al., 1998).
- **Resource Management:** The way resources—physical, human, and intellectual—are generated and allocated, including their geographic and needs-based allocation.
- **Service Delivery:** Both population- and individual-level public health interventions and health care services are provided in community, primary health care, hospitals, and other health institutions.

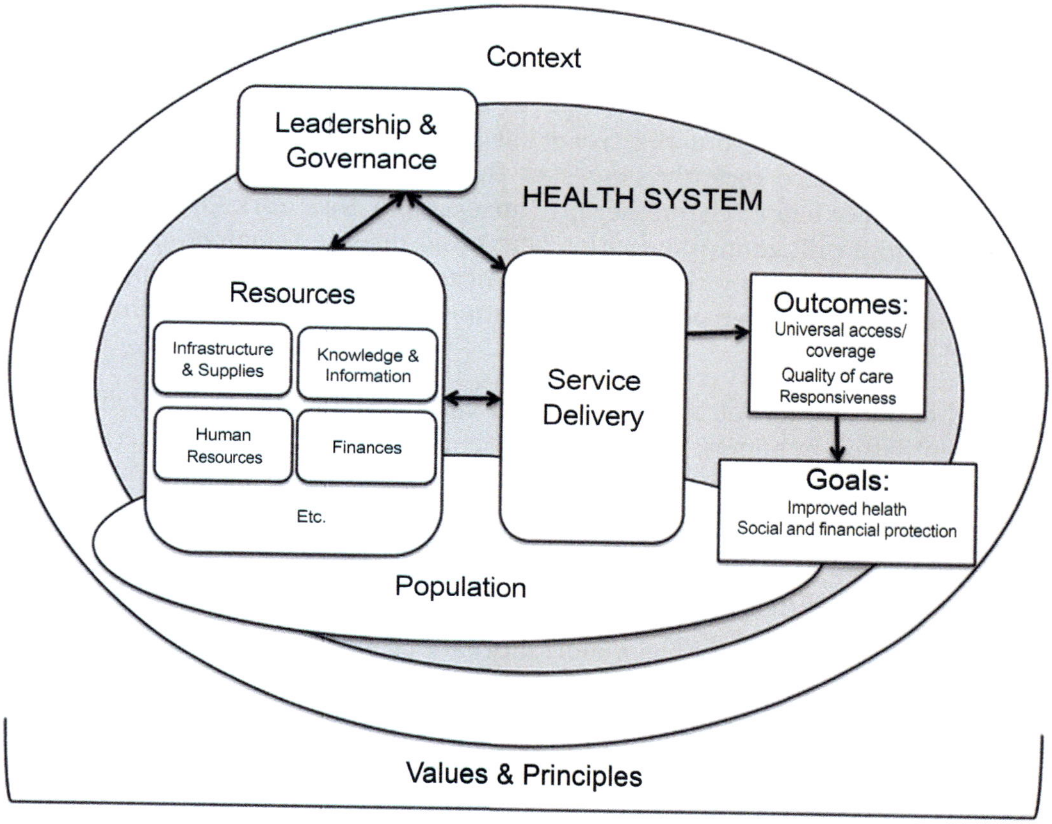

Figure 7.1. *Schematic health systems framework.*

Source: https://www.researchgate.net/publication/344610783/figure/fig3/AS:971444032909320@1608621714509/Health-systems-framework-by-Van-Olmen-et-al-43.ppm.

Each of these functions is influenced by the economic, demographic, legal, cultural, and political context.

As the framework indicates, the objectives of the health system include better health, financial protection, and user satisfaction (Degiacomi et al., 2017). Personal health services and public health interventions should be organized to achieve an appropriate balance between equity (including the reduction of out-of-pocket spending and impoverishment of individuals and families), efficiency, effectiveness (that is, the extent to which interventions are evidence-based and safe), responsiveness, justice, and customer satisfaction (as perceived by service users).

7.2. Historical Trends, Current Burden, and Global Response

TB has been one of the main causes of death worldwide for centuries and has now overtaken HIV/AIDS and malaria as the biggest cause of death from an infectious disease worldwide (Deidda et al., 1998).

7.2.1. Historical Trends

TB rates have been declining in North America and Western Europe since the early 19th century, before the introduction of chemotherapy in the 1950s. The decline may be due in part to the natural waning of the epidemic, but the trend has persisted too long for this to be the only explanation. Researchers have recently suggested that the dramatic differences between cities where TB declined sharply before chemotherapy (for example, New York City in the United States and London in the United Kingdom) and cities where the disease remained high (Cape Town in South Africa) may be explained by the quality and organization of the local health care system (Dorhoi & Kaufmann, 2015). Other possible explanations for the 150-year decline are subject to debate and include the following:

1. Reduced opportunities for transmission per case, possibly due to lower housing density, better ventilation in homes, isolation of patients in sanatoria, and a decrease in contacts among older patients (Flynn & Chan, 2001),
2. Reduced susceptibility of contacts, possibly due to improved nutrition and genetic pressure (Gande et al., 2004),
3. Lower virulence of the pathogen, even if there is little evidence for this.

While untreated TB traditionally has a mortality rate of 50%, there are differing opinions on the role of natural selection in resistance to pulmonary TB in humans before the availability of anti-TB drugs (Gavalda et al., 2014). It is not possible to decipher all the factors that contributed to the decline in TB before the widespread introduction of chemotherapy, or the reasons why progress has stalled since then. What is clear is that TB death rates in Western Europe declined by 5% per year in the pre-chemotherapy era, with the decline in the United States and Western Europe linked to active case finding, such as through X-ray screening.

By the 1990s, however, TB had emerged as a major global health problem, largely due to an increase in the number of cases in the former Soviet Union and sub-Saharan Africa. While the number of cases declined in other parts of the world, the per capita incidence of TB increased in these two regions.

In the Russian Federation and other countries of the former Soviet Union, TB cases and deaths rose dramatically between 1990 and 2000, however the exact reasons for this occurrence are almost as difficult to understand as the decline in Europe and North America. What is clear is that there was a marked deterioration in case-finding and cure rates in Russia, but this probably does not explain the entire increase (Gavalda et al., 2009). Other factors include increased transmission due to the mixing of prison and civilian populations, increased susceptibility to disease after infection likely related to alcoholism and stress, poor nutrition, emphasis on hospitalization and prolonged hospital stays, poor service delivery, the spread of drug resistance, and more recently, the rise in HIV/AIDS infections (Gengenbacher & Kaufmann, 2012).

7.2.2. Current Burden

7.2.2.1. Global Progress

Although the overall burden of the disease remains high, significant progress has been made in the fight against TB worldwide. Between 1995 and 2013, the rate of TB cases increased from 46% to 64%, and in the same period, between 41 million and 56 million people were successfully treated and as many as 49 million lives were saved by 2015 (Ginsberg et al., 2007). The prevalence of TB had also fallen by 47% worldwide in 2015, and the mortality rate attributable to TB had fallen by 45% compared to the baseline year of 1990.

Since the mid-2000s, the global incidence of TB has been declining, albeit slowly, as has the absolute number of new cases reported each year. However, the incidence rates in countries with a high TB burden in Southeast Asia and sub-Saharan Africa remain discouragingly high (Figure 7.2).

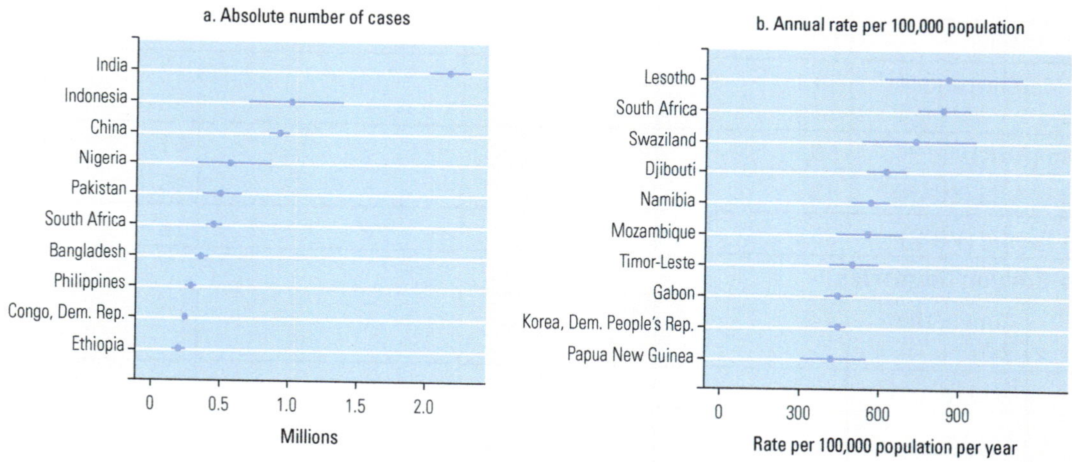

Figure 7.2. *Estimated TB incidence: Top-10 countries (2014).*

Note: TB: tuberculosis. The range shows the lower and upper bounds of the 95% uncertainty interval. The bullet indicates the best estimate.

Source: https://www.ncbi.nlm.nih.gov/books/NBK525174/figure/ch11.sec2.fig2/.

Despite global progress, uncertainties remain about the burden and trends in the disease, for example, while the WHO and Institute for Health Metrics and Evaluation (IHME) estimates of TB prevalence in 2012 were similar, the trends differed where the WHO estimated a decline in cases, while the IHME estimated an increase in cases over the same period.Country progress by key international TB goals and targets in 22 countries with a high burden of TB, i.e., the 22 countries defined by the WHO as accounting for approximately 80% of global TB cases in 2015—is shown in Table 7.1 (Goude et al., 2009).

Table 7.1. *2015 Target Assessment: Global, WHO Regions, and 22 High-Burden Countries*

TB/HIV: 2015. Global Plan Targets			**MDR-TB: 2015. Global Plan Targets**			
TB patients with known HIV status (%).	Notified HIV-positive TB patients started on ART (%).	People living with HIV newly enrolled in HIV care who were started on IPT.	Estimated MDR-TB cases that were detected and notified (%).	Treatment success rate: confirmed MDR-TB cases, 2011 cohort (%).		
Target	100%	100%	50%	100%	≥75%	
Global						
Global		48	70	–	45	48
WHO Region						
African (AFR)		76	69	–	74	47
Americas (AMR)		69	65	–	47	56
Eastern Mediterranean (EMR)		11	38	–	22	64
European (EUR)		59	54	–	61	46
South-East Asia (SEAR)		43	81	–	45	54
Western Pacific (WPR)		35	60	–	16	52
22 High-Burden Countries						
AFR	Congo, Dem. Rep	44	48	–	9	59
–	Ethiopia	71	68	–	40	72
–	Kenya	94	84	–	6	70
–	Mozambique	91	72	17	19	31
–	Nigeria	88	67	3.5	18	63
–	South Africa	90	66	>100	>100	45
–	Uganda	91	65	–	12	77
–	Tanzania	83	73	0.4	10	75
–	Zimbabwe	92	77	3.5	53	81
AMR	Brazil	65	–	–	39	56
EMR	Afghanistan	26		23	6	29
–	Pakistan	2.8	–	–	20	70
EUR	Russian Federation	–	–	–	33	37
SEAR	Bangladesh	1.1	100	0	22	68
–	India	63	88	–	57	50
–	Indonesia	2.3	21	–	13	60

–	Myanmar	12	74	19	22	71
–	Thailand	83	59	–	12	–
WPR	Cambodia	82	89	55	24	86
–	China	39	67	–	8	50
–	Philippines	2.1	–	–	47	41
–	Vietnam	70	61	–	24	72
Classification						
–	–	≥80% tested	≥80%	≥50%	≥80% detected and notified	≥75%
–	–	50–79% tested	50–79%	25–49%	50–79% detected and notified	50–74%
–	–	<50% tested	<50%	<25%	<50% detected and notified	<50%

7.2.2.2. Remaining Challenges

Despite significant progress, TB remains a formidable global health threat where the overall rate of decline in incidence is frustratingly slow by all accounts (1.5% per year), and some countries and regions are still reporting increases in TB incidence, particularly for drug-resistant TB. Based on notification reports and surveys, there were an estimated 10.4 million new cases in 2015, and assuming a lifelong latent infection, about one-third of humanity could still be infected with Mtb (Grosset, 2003).

Estimates of TB incidence and prevalence remain imprecise, especially in countries with high TB burdens, where precision is most needed. Over the past decade, national TB prevalence surveys have been conducted in more than 20 countries, including 15 of the 22 countries with the highest burden, providing important data for these countries regarding TB burden. There is a high need to invest in high-quality routine surveillance that builds on existing systems and provides robust data for assessment and future planning (Grzegorzewicz et al., 2012). With a quarter of TB patients living in India, the national survey planned for 2017–2018 will be very important.

There are many factors responsible for the persistence and mortality of the disease. First, case detection is inadequate: in 2014, only about 64% of people who contracted TB were reported as newly diagnosed cases, which leaves around 3 to 4 million cases either undiagnosed or diagnosed but not reported to national TB programs.

The emergence of highly drug-resistant TB, including MDR-TB (resistance to at least isoniazid and rifampicin) and XDR-TB (MDR and resistance to at least one fluoroquinolone and one injectable antituberculous antibiotic), has proven to be a serious obstacle to effective control of TB in many settings. The most recent estimates of the burden of MDR-TB indicate that approximately 480,000 new cases of MDR-TB occur each year, of which only 20% receive treatment. Sufficiently strong surveillance and laboratory testing for drug resistance are not yet sufficient to determine whether MDR-TB is increasing or decreasing in most countries where MDR is a problem (Hariguchi et al., 2020).

HIV/AIDS is another factor that makes effective control of TB difficult, especially in the countries of southern Africa. Of the 10.4 million new TB cases in 2014, 1.2 million occurred in HIV-positive people. Of the approximately 1.5 million deaths from TB in 2014, 400,000 people were co-infected with HIV/AIDS (Hunter, 2011). Globally, around half of patients diagnosed with TB have been tested for HIV/AIDS, with this figure rising to 79% in the African region. The treatment of TB patients co-infected with HIV/AIDS with antiretroviral therapy (ART) has increased to 77% globally, which is critical as the risk of clinical TB is reduced by 64% when HIV-positive patients are treated with ART.

Although dramatic improvements in TB control have been achieved over the past 25 years, the benefits have not been evenly distributed across geographic regions. The decline in mortality rates has often been driven by rapid economic development in Asian countries. Three WHO regions — the Americas, Southeast Asia and the Western Pacific — were able to reduce prevalence by 50% by 2013, but the other three regions have not yet reached this target (Huszar et al., 2020).

In 2014, the WHO region of Africa had the highest incidence rates (about 280 cases per 100,000 population) and 28% of the estimated number of cases worldwide. Asia accounted for 58% of the total cases, and China and India alone accounted for more than one in three (35%) of new TB cases worldwide in 2013. Approximately 78% of all TB deaths and 73% of TB deaths among HIV-negative people occurred in the Africa and Southeast Asia regions.

Spatial and temporal variations in TB incidence in Africa are strongly correlated with the prevalence of HIV/AIDS infection (Ioerger et al., 2013). Globally, an estimated 11% of all new adult TB cases in 2015 were infected with HIV/AIDS. In the WHO African region, the percentage of new TB cases with HIV/AIDS ranged from 8% in Eritrea to 77% in Swaziland.

Many of the global successes in the fight against TB have stalled: in some East Asian countries, particularly in the Hong Kong Special Administrative Region (China), Japan, the Republic of Korea and Singapore, the incidence of TB is no longer declining. Part of the explanation could be that more cases are occurring due to the reactivation of a previously infected, aging human population (Kaufmann & Schaible, 2005). In addition, immigration from high-incidence countries is one reason why the decline in TB in North America and Western Europe has plateaued. Immigrants who are infected in their country of origin contribute to varying degrees to further transmission and outbreaks in the country where they live or work.

7.2.3. Global Response

After the WHO declared in 1993 that TB was a global health emergency, it introduced the DOTS strategy in 1994 (Kawate et al., 2013). Prior to the introduction of DOTS, there were at least five recommended regimens for the treatment of TB with varying efficacy, serious adverse effects and costs (Kolly et al., 2014). DOTS aimed to create a single common best practice strategy that would be applicable to all countries and would include not only adherence to treatment but also securing political commitment and adequate and sustained funding:

- Ensure early case detection and diagnosis through quality-assured bacteriology;
- Provide standardized treatment with supervision and patient support;
- Ensure effective drug supply and management;
- Monitor and evaluate performance and impact.

Increasing drug resistance forced the WHO to introduce DOTS-plus in 1998 with two additional requirements: (1) the ability to conduct drug susceptibility testing (DST) and (2) the ability to ensure access to second-line drugs (Stop TB Working Group on DOTS-Plus for MDR-TB 2003).

DOTS was further expanded in 2014 to include six programmatic interventions that are critical to an effective global TB control strategy.

The history of TB control thus reflects an attempt to tackle its increasingly fundamental causes by addressing the root causes of the epidemic in the health system.

Important organizational initiatives have attempted to intensify the fight against TB: the TB Alliance in 2000; the Green Light Committee at WHO in 2000; the Stop TB Initiative in 2001; the Global Fund to Fight AIDS, TB, and Malaria (Global Fund), established in 2002 as a major funder of country programs; UNITAID in 2006; and the Stop TB Partnership in 2008, established to work with WHO to coordinate the many provider, advocacy, and donor groups working to fight TB. The Stop TB Partnership has 1,200 partners in 100 countries, while the Global Laboratory Initiative was established in 2007 to strengthen laboratory capacity in LMICs.

The increased attention and initiatives have been accompanied by a significant increase in international and national funding for TB. In 2016, funding for its prevention, diagnosis, and treatment amounted to 6.6 billion US dollars, almost double the amount spent in 2006 (Koul et al., 2011). Overall, about 84% (US$ 5.5 billion) of reported TB funding came from domestic sources.

Nevertheless, low-income countries (LICs) have benefited from Global Fund funding, which accounts for about 67% of total TB funding to these countries. In 2016, the largest share of TB funding (USD 4.9 billion) was spent on drug-susceptible TB, with about USD 1.7 billion going to MDR-TB. The WHO estimates that the funding gap to achieve the SDG for TB is in the order of USD 2 billion per year (Koul et al., 2007).

7.2.4. Evolving Targets

The original DOTS targets aimed to achieve a global TB detection rate of 70% and a treatment success rate of 85%. In 2000, the United Nations Millennium Declaration (UN General Assembly, 2000), which established the Millennium Development Goals (MDGs), launched a concerted global effort to alleviate poverty and improve global health. Surprisingly, the MDG targets did not specifically mention TB, which at the time was causing more than 9 million new cases and 1.5 million deaths annually.

However, MDG 6, which aimed to stop and gradually reduce HIV/AIDS, malaria, and "other infectious diseases,"" contained sufficient language to set international targets for TB control (Kuhn et al., 2016).

The Stop TB Partnership's Global Plan to Stop TB 2001–2015 set two targets in addition to the overall MDG 6 target, bringing the total number of targets frequently cited in TB literature to three:

- Halt and reverse the global growth in TB incidence;
- Decrease TB prevalence 50% from 1990 baseline levels by 2015;

- Decrease TB mortality 50% from 1990 baseline levels by 2015.

The current UN Sustainable Development Goals (SDG) aim to reduce the number of TB deaths by 95% and the incidence rate by 90% by 2035, effectively eliminating the disease. These are ambitious goals, and experts have set milestones in five-year increments to track progress and hold government agencies accountable. With evidence that transmission and treatment errors remain high in many countries, other metrics, such as case detection and treatment success rates, are important indicators of progress.

Dye and others (2013) have modeled the requirements to eliminate TB as a public health problem (less than 1 case per 100,000 population) by 2015. A projection of the decline in incidence at current rates (about 1% annually) shows that the MDG targets would not be met for more than 50 years. An updated model requires incidence to decline by 10% in 2020 and 17% per year thereafter (Figure 7.3). However, as La Rosa and colleagues state, such a "rate of decline has never been achieved at any geographic scale, over any time period, and is not possible with the current tools and systems for their implementation worldwide" (La Rosa et al., 2012).

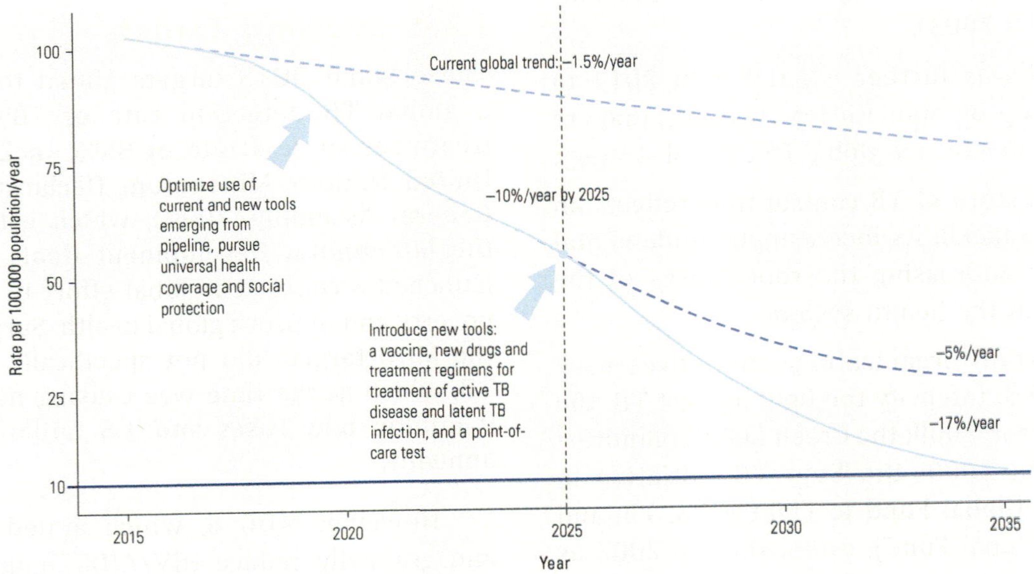

Figure 7.3. *Projected acceleration of the decline in global tuberculosis incidence rates to target levels, 2015–2035.*

Source: https://www.ncbi.nlm.nih.gov/books/NBK525174/figure/ch11.sec2.fig3/.

It is difficult to imagine that significant progress can be made by 2035 without the development and application of new tools and investment in TB health systems.

This includes reintroducing active case finding, developing more effective care strategies, investing in the supply chain and information management systems, researching, and developing new diagnostics, and introducing new and more effective treatments and vaccines (Leung, 1999).

The WHO's current strategic plan for TB control, the End TB Strategy (Li et al., 2015), is a multifaceted program that is far more comprehensive than the previous versions. By recognizing the success of previous programs in reducing mortality and prevalence, and the failure of current programs to reduce incidence to a level that will enable countries to achieve the SDG targets by 2035, a broader and more ambitious program is proposed. These are very ambitious and important goals, which will depend largely on investment in research and development of new instruments, and more effective use of existing instruments.

7.3. Infection and Disease in Individuals and Populations

TB is a bacterial infectious disease caused by Mtb, which is transmitted by aerosols and most commonly affects the lungs. Mtb is essentially unique to humans, although the related pathogenic mycobacterium, *Mycobacterium bovis*, causes disease in cattle, and was the cause of scrofula and TB of the lymph nodes prior to pasteurization of milk. Another related pathogen, *Mycobacterium leprae*, is the cause of leprosy in humans.

As there is no animal reservoir for Mtb, the pathogen has evolved to survive in humans for long periods of time, with only a proportion of people developing clinical disease with lung damage.

TB is transmitted from person to person via aerosol droplets from the throat and lungs of people with active respiratory disease. People with pulmonary or laryngeal TB produce droplets in the air when coughing, sneezing or simply speaking (Li et al., 2016), qne infectious droplets are inhaled and deposited in the alveoli and bacilli, where they are taken up by macrophages.

7.3.1. Stages of TB Disease and Intervention Points

TB is best understood, not as a single clinical entity, but as a spectrum that generally correlates with immune responses. A high but unknown percentage of people infected with Mtb develop latent or persistent infection, but only about 10% develop disease during their lifetime (Li et al., 2019). In immunocompromised individuals, the risk is about 8% per year (Locher et al., 2015). A proportion of highly exposed individuals who are likely to be infected with Mtb do not develop tuberculin skin tests (TSTs) but remain healthy, suggesting that they are protected by currently unknown immune mechanisms.

Another unknown proportion of individuals with tubercle bacilli in sputum remain asymptomatic but must be assumed to be able to transmit the infection (Louw et al., 2011).

Along the continuum of care, there are several potential entry points for interventions, including preventing infection, preventing the establishment of latency, preventing the transition from latent TB to active disease (chemoprophylaxis) and treating individuals with active disease to achieve cure and thereby reduce morbidity, mortality, and transmission intensity (Figure 7.4).

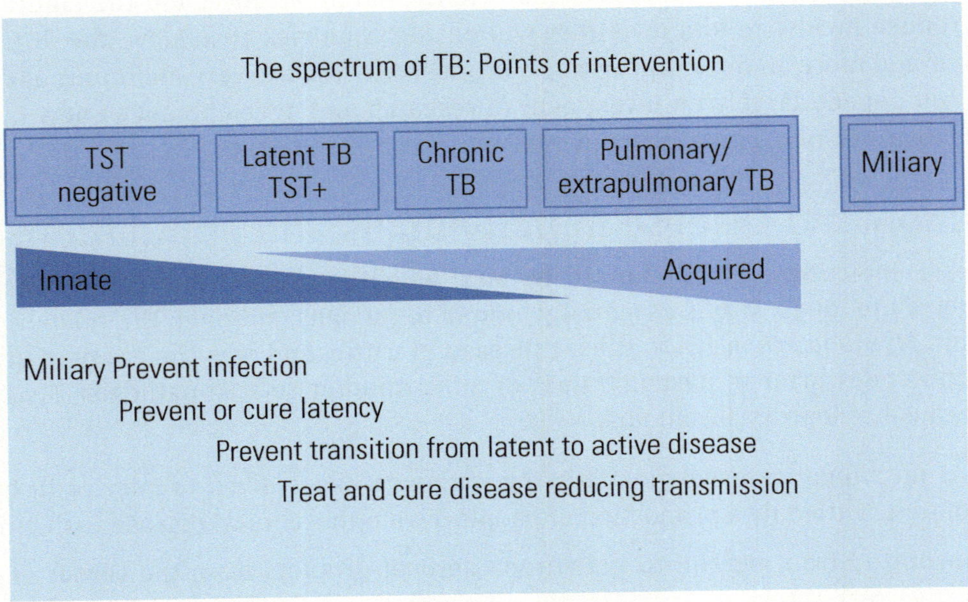

Figure 7.4. *The TB spectrum and possible points of intervention.*

Note: TB: tuberculosis; and TST: tuberculin skin test.

Source: Bloom, B. R., Atun, R., Cohen, T., et al., (2017). Tuberculosis. In: Holmes, K. K., Bertozzi, S., Bloom, B. R., et al., (eds.), Major Infectious Diseases (3rd edn.). Washington (DC): The International Bank for Reconstruction and Development / The World Bank; Figure 11.4, The TB Spectrum and Possible Points of Intervention. Available from: https://www.ncbi.nlm.nih.gov/books/NBK525174/figure/ch11.sec3.fig4/ doi: 10.1596/978-1-4648-0524-0_ch11.

Infection with Mtb can lead to subclinical infection, which is cured by innate or acquired immune responses, latent infection that persists, chronic or asymptomatic TB in which tubercle bacilli are found in sputum of otherwise apparently healthy individuals, and active TB disease. In a small proportion of individuals, infection can lead directly to rapidly progressing disease, known as primary progressive TB. Miliary TB is widely disseminated, occurring primarily in children and severely immunodeficient individuals.

In most healthy people, infection with Mtb often causes no symptoms as the person's immune system kills or fights off the bacteria through innate and acquired immunity. Acquired cell-mediated immunity develops two to eight weeks after infection, and granulomas—that is, infiltrating macrophages and lymphocytes—seal off the infection and limit further replication and spread of the organism (Lu et al., 2014), although this is only partially protective (Lu et al., 2019). There is a widespread belief that infection does not confer significant immunity (Luies & du Preez, 2020), which is used to explain why reinfection is not uncommon (Lun et al., 2013). However, a recent analysis of numerous studies shows that although latent TB infection protects against active disease, almost certainly through a protective innate or acquired immune response, this protection is only partial.

Molecular fingerprinting techniques can be used to distinguish bacteria that have emerged during a relapse of a previous infection from reinfection with new strains. The original strain of infection can reemerge after an apparent cure or ineffective treatment and cause the active disease to relapse (Lun et al., 2021). Reactivation rates vary between 1% and 30% per year in different populations. Whether latent bacilli remain viable throughout the lifespan of all infected individuals is unknown, but the risk of reactivation persists into old age (Makarov et al., 2014).

The phenomenon of reactivation, often long after infection or after treatment, reflects the limitations of the immune response in providing protection and highlights the challenge in developing effective vaccines that can provide long-term protection (Makarov et al., 2009). Bacille Calmette-Guérin (BCG) is the only licensed vaccine available today. It has been used for more than 90 years with a good safety record, except in immunocompromised children. However, the vaccine's effectiveness in preventing TB in adults varies in different parts of the world, while it consistently protects children against the most severe forms of the disease: disseminated miliary TB and tuberculous meningitis (Makarov et al., 2015). The BCG vaccination is explained in more detail in the section on prevention.

Primary infection leads to active TB (primary progressive TB) in some people if the host's immune response cannot effectively suppress replication of the bacilli. The symptoms of active pulmonary TB are cough, sometimes with blood in the sputum, chest pain, weakness, weight loss, fever, and night sweats. Clinical TB is the sum of complex interactions between the pathogen and a person's immune response that facilitate mycobacterial replication and cause disease, including emaciation and granulomatous inflammation with tissue damage, for example, caseation, vasculitis, and fibrosis. The most common clinical manifestation of TB is pulmonary disease, and in most infectious patients, the bacilli are visible microscopically on stained sputum smears (50–70% of lung cases). While extrapulmonary TB accounts for 10–30% of cases, it is more common in women and children (especially lymphatic TB) and in HIV/AIDS-infected individuals.

In the absence of other predisposing conditions, only 5–10% of infected individuals develop progressive primary disease within five years of infection (Manjunatha & Smith, 2015). After five years, the annual risk of developing TB due to reactivation of a latent infection is significantly lower. In HIV-positive individuals, however, the risk is in approximately 10% per year after infection. The risk of developing an active disease is relatively high in infancy, but lower in older children, while increasing rapidly in adolescence (earlier in girls) and slower increases in adulthood (Marrakchi et al., 2014). The lifetime risk of contracting TB after infection clearly depends on the prevailing transmission rate but is generally estimated to be around 10%.

Latent TB, which exists in an unknown percentage of people infected with Mtb, has a significant impact on the epidemiology and population dynamics of TB. It represents a huge reservoir of potential disease and further transmission. At the same time, long-term latent infection appears to provide partial protection against the development of disease.

Whether infection remains latent or develops into active disease following Mtb infection is thought to depend largely on the host's ability to develop protective innate and cell-mediated immunity. Currently, there is little evidence that serum antibodies provide protection, although recent studies using serum from TST-negative, highly exposed individuals suggest that they may possess antibodies that enable macrophages to kill some bacilli *in vitro* (Mdluli et al., 2015). Human

T cells are very heterogeneous. Animal studies indicate that both CD4 cells and cytotoxic CD8 T cells are important for protection against Mtb infections, and studies show CD4+ cells are functionally heterogeneous. At the simplest level, two antagonistic subclasses of CD4+ — Th1 and Th2 — have been described, each with its own set of cytokine mediators. Th1 responses, characterized by the production of interferon gamma (IFN-γ), are associated with protection, whereas Th2 responses, characterized predominantly by Th2 cytokines (For example, IL-4, IL-10), are associated with antibodies, inflammatory responses, and tissue damage. Recently, a unique subset of human Th1 cells has been described that appears to correlate strongly with protection against mycobacterial disease. These Th1* cells represent a unique subset of human CD4+ T cells that express the chemokine receptors—CCR6, CCR4 and the nuclear transcription factor RORγ, which appears to exclusively produce IFN-γ against mycobacteria (Mdluli & Ma, 2007).

The importance of TB among infectious diseases is due to the high mortality rate of untreated or improperly treated cases. About two-thirds of untreated smear-positive TB cases die within five to eight years, while most die within the first two years. As shown in Figure 7.4, the rest remain latent, chronically ill or asymptomatic, or recover over time. The mortality rate in untreated microscopic smear-negative cases is lower, but still in the order of 10–15% (Migliori et al., 2020). Even in smear-positive patients receiving anti-TB drugs, the mortality rate can exceed 10% if adherence to treatment is low or if HIV/AIDS infection rates and drug resistance are high.

7.3.1.1. *M. tuberculosis* Strains

There is remarkable evidence that the major strains of Mtb evolved together with the great migrations of humans from Africa to Asia, Europe, and the Americas (Mudde et al., 2022). Many Mtb strains can be uncovered by molecular analysis and this diversity is thought to exacerbate drug resistance and compromise the effectiveness of disease control measures. While early targeted genetic analyzes suggested only minimal diversity of Mtb within species (Nahid et al., 2019), genomic studies have revealed much greater variation. Subsequent studies have led to a better understanding of Mtb strains and their global distribution. Other studies aim to determine whether differences between or within (Pawlowski et al., 2012) strains alter the pathogen's ability to infect hosts or are associated with differences in the natural history of disease. The number and scope of such studies is still limited, but a recent study has linked differences in Mtb strains to the likelihood of disease transmission among exposed households in Brazil (Pethe et al., 2013).

There is increasing evidence that strain lineages differ in the strength and mechanism of stimulation of the host immune system after infection (Peyron et al., 2008), the ability to compete within the host, the rate of acquisition of mutations and drug resistance as well as specific acquired mutations, each of which can influence the course of the infection, the disease and the response to therapy within the host. In general, the fitness of pathogens decreases with the accumulation of mutations. A large body of evidence suggests that MDR-TB strains are heterogeneous in their transmissibility in animal models and human populations. It is likely that limited transmissibility may change if compensatory mutations occur that restore fitness. Of particular concern is the increased transmissibility of the Beijing strain with antibiotic resistance. Mathematical modeling also suggests that strain diversity may influence the occurrence of drug resistance and interventions (Philips & Ernst, 2012), however, additional data are needed for better predictions, especially from whole genome sequencing and long-term monitoring of strain types in human populations.

7.3.1.2. TB and HIV/AIDS Co-Infection

The extent to which HIV/AIDS fuels the transmission of TB (in addition to reactivation) remains poorly understood. One analysis suggests that in 2000, 1–2% of all transmissions were from HIV-positive, smear-positive TB cases. Co-infection with TB and HIV/AIDS is geographically heterogeneous, for example, in countries such as Eastern Europe and Southern Africa, up to 75% of all TB patients are HIV-positive, while in other countries such as China and India, only a small proportion of TB cases are HIV-positive (Portevin et al., 2004).

The proportion of TB infections attributable to people co-infected with HIV/AIDS depends on the prevalence of HIV/AIDS and the infectivity of HIV/AIDS-associated Mtb compared to TB cases not affected by HIV/AIDS. This proportion is influenced by biological factors (For example, the likelihood of smear-positive lung disease) and how quickly those affected are diagnosed and receive effective treatment. The duration of HIV/AIDS-associated TB appears to be shorter than the duration of HIV-negative TB or about the same, depending on the setting.

It is clear that HIV/AIDS infection causes a multifaceted suppression of innate and acquired T cell responses. In a sense, TB is often a sentinel for HIV/AIDS infection in areas with high HIV/AIDS epidemics. Even before there is a significant decrease in CD4+ T cells, active disease can occur in individuals with latent TB. HIV/AIDS infection not only suppresses the immune response to Mtb, but stimulation of T cells by Mtb antigens may contribute to T cell activation, leading to increased production of HIV/AIDS and acceleration of the disease process.

Clinically, both the prevalence of extrapulmonary TB and disseminated TB are increased in HIV-positive patients. Low CD4 cell counts are associated with an increased frequency of extrapulmonary TB, positive mycobacterial blood cultures, and atypical chest X-ray findings, reflecting the inability of the impaired immune response to contain the infection. The increase in TB incidence attributable to HIV/AIDS appears to have peaked in most countries as HIV/AIDS incidence has declined (Portevin et al., 2005).

7.3.1.3. Effect of TB on the Distribution of Other Diseases

TB influences the presence and nature of other diseases, as well as having a protective effect. Microbial infections have the potential to influence the balance between functional subsets of CD4+ T cells by stimulating innate immune responses and altering cytokine profiles, which may have a positive or negative impact on health. Mtb infection may also protect against asthma, possibly by shifting the innate and acquired Th2 response towards a Th1 subset that reduces the inflammatory response. A study of Japanese children found that strong tuberculin responses following BCG vaccination were associated with less asthma, rhinoconjunctivitis, and eczema in later childhood. In a study of South African children, an inverse association was found between Mtb infection and atopic rhinitis. Comparisons between different countries have shown that asthma tends to be more common where TB is less prevalent (Rao et al., 2013).

Interactions between other infections have also been studied. Strong Th2 responses are observed in protective immune responses to helminth infections, and helminths can shift the balance of immune responses to enhance allergic reactions and thus impair Th1 immune responses to BCG and Mtb. Conversely, a vaccine based on mycobacteria could potentially prevent allergic reactions and reduce asthma. Mtb infection, like BCG, may protect against leprosy, and natural TB transmission may have contributed to the decline of leprosy in Europe (Rawat et al., 2003).

There is currently no information on whether the human microbiome influences responses to mycobacteria, but this is an area of research that should be investigated. The synergistic and antagonistic interactions between bacterial, viral, and parasitic infections are complex and unresolved, but these examples raise the general likelihood that mycobacteria are influenced by the presence of other infections.

7.3.2. Risk Factors for TB

Risk factors influence the likelihood of infection, disease or outcome and operate at many levels, including physiological, genetic, environmental, and behavioral. Once a person has been exposed to another with infectious pulmonary TB, their risk of developing subclinical TB infection depends on factors that influence either the infected person's ability to transmit the disease or the exposed person's susceptibility to infection and disease. Infected persons who have acid-fast bacilli in smear or culture (Reece & Kaufmann, 2012), who have cavitary disease (destructive lesions in the lungs in which bacilli proliferate vigorously), frequent coughs or who have delayed treatment are important vectors of TB infection.

Risk factors relevant to the exposed host mostly reflect the social and environmental determinants of high exposure and include living in densely populated areas, incarceration, and working in occupations such as healthcare that involve frequent social or direct contact with TB patients. Most studies suggest that the risk of TB infection among similarly exposed contacts does not vary greatly depending on host characteristics. However, some recent studies report that genetic loci are associated with differential risk of infection among household contacts exposed to an infectious case, while there is evidence that smoking increases the risk of TB (Remuiñán et al., 2013).

In contrast to infection, the course of the disease is known to be highly dependent on host risk factors. The most important of these include HIV/AIDS co-infection, low body mass index, exposure to tobacco and biomass fuels, diabetes mellitus and heavy alcohol consumption. Host-specific risk factors also affect TB outcomes, including the risk of treatment failure, relapse after treatment and TB-related death. In addition to HIV/AIDS, smoking, and diabetes are recognized biological risk factors for poor treatment outcomes, and some studies have considered other comorbidities such as iron overload, renal dysfunction, and hematologic malignancies (Russell et al., 2019).

There is much evidence to suggest that malnutrition is associated with TB in LMICs. In national surveys in India, the population-attributable risk of TB was twofold or more increased in malnourished adults and adolescents and was highest in rural areas.

Table 7.2 lists the risk factors for TB progression and summarizes the relative risks for selected factors for which meta-analyzes have been conducted. Although HIV/AIDS is a much stronger risk factor for disease progression than other exposures, the relatively common occurrence of other determinants means that they explain a higher proportion of global TB cases than HIV/AIDS. Table 7.3 estimates the most common attributable risk factors in different economic strata in India using data from the Indian National Family Health Survey. This data shows that people living in poverty often have a combination of risk factors, which further increases their risk of disease.

Table 7.2. *Key Risk Factors for TB from Meta-Analyses of Randomized Controlled Trials*

Key Risk Factor	Odds Ratio
Cigarette smoking	2.01–2.66
Indoor air pollution	1.4
Low body mass index	2.45[a]
Alcohol use (daily or alcohol use disorder)	2.94
Diabetes mellitus	3.11

Table 7.3. *Attributable Fraction of Key Risk Factors for TB Disease Progression in India, by Socioeconomic Strata*

Population-Attributable Fraction (%)			
Lowest Socioeconomic Stratum	**Middle Socioeconomic Stratum**	**Highest Socioeconomic Stratum**	
Cigarette smoking	16	10	6
Indoor air pollution	29	25	6
Low body mass index	34	27	20
Alcohol use, daily	4	2	1
HIV/AIDS seroprevalence	9	10	6

HIV/AIDS is found in only about 11% of TB patients worldwide, whereas other risk factors, such as diabetes mellitus and smoking, are more widespread. The population attributable fraction is the proportional reduction in disease or mortality in the population that would occur if exposure to a risk factor were reduced to an alternative ideal exposure scenario, for example no smoking. A global estimate of the population attributable factors for TB is given in Table 7.4. It is not possible to estimate precisely the number of people with each of the risk factors because of the uncertainty of the background risk data and the overlap of risks. Nevertheless, the larger number of smokers and the rapidly growing number of people with diabetes mellitus suggest that the proportion of all cases attributable to malnutrition and diabetes, and smoking is respectively five times higher and eight times higher than the proportion attributable to HIV/AIDS (Sacksteder et al., 2012).

The risk factors also vary according to socio-economic status, as shown with the example of India. While infection with Mtb is a risk for people of any economic class, data from India suggest that some known risk factors for TB are most pronounced in the lowest socioeconomic group, a finding that is likely true for most populations.

Other, less common comorbidities also modify the risk of disease. Individuals who have silicosis, renal disease, solid, and hematologic malignancies are more likely to develop active TB, have undergone gastrectomy or ileojejunal bypass surgery or have received the tumor necrosis factor-alpha (TNF-α) inhibitor infliximab for the treatment of rheumatoid arthritis. Although these exposures are rare, some dramatically increase the risk of TB. Older forms of weight loss surgery, for example, can significantly increase the risk. To date, although there have been several case reports of TB in patients who have undergone gastric bypass, no systematic epidemiologic studies have been conducted on this risk factor (Schluger, 2005).

Table 7.4. *Global Prevalence, Relative Risk, and Attribution Rate for TB Cases*

Key Risk Factor	Global Prevalence	Relative Risk	Attributable Fraction (%)	References
HIV/AIDS	0.008	8.3	5.5	WHO (2009a)
Undernourishment	0.11	2.1	10.7	Lönnroth et al. (2010)
Diabetes mellitus	0.085	3.0	14.5	Jeon & Murray (2008)
Heavy alcohol use	0.075	2.9	12.5	Lönnroth et al. (2008)
Cigarette smoking	0.21	2.6	25.1	Lin, Ezzati, & Murray (2007); Slama et al. (2007)
Indoor air pollution	0.41	1.5	17.0	Lin, Ezzati, & Murray (2007)

In addition to low body mass index, several micronutrient deficiencies have been associated with the progression of TB. *In vitro* studies suggest a role for vitamin D in host susceptibility to disease, as shown from a clinical trial in Pakistan, a 25-hydroxyvitamin D—25(OH)D— level of less than 9 nanograms per milliliter increased the risk of progression to active disease fivefold. In the United States, vitamin A deficiency has been associated with a 2.8-fold increased risk of TB, although this finding was not statistically significant. Seasonal variations in vitamin D levels in South Africa further correlate with TB reports.

Dietary factors may also interact with genetic polymorphisms to increase TB risk. Polymorphisms in the 25(OH)D receptor have been associated with TB risk, and several studies have demonstrated a gene-environment interaction between 25(OH)D levels and 25(OH)D receptor mutations; there is ample evidence that 25(OH)D3 is essential for human macrophages to kill Mtb *in vitro*. Vitamin D is produced in the skin by exposure to ultraviolet light, and seasonal variations in vitamin D levels have been linked to the number of TB cases. This finding and the role of the skin pigment melanin in the absorption of ultraviolet light could explain the increased susceptibility of dark-skinned people to TB infection and more severe disease. But correlation does not equal causation, and there is an urgent need for well-designed clinical studies to determine the importance of these factors.

Recently, much work has focused on identifying the genetic determinants of TB progression. Twin studies support the hypothesis that genetic factors play a role in susceptibility to TB, and several loci have been identified through candidate gene studies (Sensi, 1983). Some of these are rare variants that lead to alterations in the interferon-γ signaling pathway, which is required for the development of acquired immunity against mycobacteria. Several defects in this signaling pathway result in a Mendelian susceptibility to mycobacterial disease that predisposes people not only to disseminated infections with nontuberculous mycobacteria but also to TB (Shirude et al., 2013). Other studies have identified candidate genes that influence the innate immune response. Several genome-wide association studies have also been conducted and summarized: some have identified alleles that occur in "gene-free" regions of the human genome, but these have not been consistently validated in separate populations. A locus on chromosome 11 has been associated with susceptibility in several populations. Of particular interest is a locus on chromosome 5 that encodes a component of interleukin 12 (IL-12), which is required for T cell differentiation. This locus appears to confer resistance in highly susceptible HIV-positive populations in East Africa and there is evidence of positive selection (Shirude et al., 2014).

7.4. TB Diagnosis and Screening

In simple terms, the DOTS strategy for TB control is to test individuals attending a health facility for clinical symptoms of TB and provide appropriate drug treatment over a period of 6–24 months. With timely diagnosis and correct treatment, almost all people with drug-sensitive TB can be cured, and even a short course of treatment reduces the bacterial burden and the likelihood of transmission. Nevertheless, the rate of TB cases worldwide remains low: in 2012, about 66% (5.7 million) of the estimated 10.4 million people who contracted TB were newly diagnosed cases, with an estimated 3 to 4 million cases undiagnosed or unknown to health systems. The detection of cases in children is of particular concern: in 2010, an estimated 1 million children contracted TB, with approximately 32,000 children contracting MDR-TB (Sotgiu et al., 2015).

In most countries, the most common diagnostic test is microscopic examination of acid-fast bacilli in a sputum smear — a technique dating back to the 1880s. It is convenient but insensitive, and only diagnoses around half of all TB cases in adults and even fewer in children and HIV-positive people. Diagnostic certainty is established when the organism is detected in a laboratory following clinical evaluation of symptoms (usually cough) consistent with TB. In the absence of diagnostic laboratory tests, clinicians must review the clinical information and decide whether to initiate TB treatment, weighing the risks of untreated TB against the adverse drug reactions and the social and financial costs of months of therapy (Stanley et al., 2013). Treatment is often initiated - whether appropriate or not - before it is clear whether the patient has TB and whether the infection is drug-sensitive or drug-resistant.

7.4.1. Diagnosis of MDR and XDR TB

The diagnosis and treatment of MDR-TB has largely stalled worldwide. Only 30 out of 107 countries treat 75% or more of patients with MDR-TB, and in many countries, there is a high level of follow-up. Of the estimated 450,000 people who developed MDR-TB in 2012, only 94,000 (20.9%) were detected, and only 77,000 were started on second-line treatment. MDR- and XDR-TB also pose a threat to healthcare workers and healthcare infrastructure. An unknown number of nurses and doctors have contracted MDR- and XDR-TB, and there were an estimated 210,000 deaths from MDR-TB in 2014.

The diagnosis of drug-resistant TB and its treatment are complex, requiring laboratory capacity for drug susceptibility testing and 9 to 20 months of daily administration of drugs that are both more toxic and less effective than the drugs typically used to treat drug-resistant TB (Stec et al., 2016). Inadequate human resources, poor access to laboratory services, and low capacity to perform drug susceptibility testing and analysis are partly responsible for the low case rate of MDR-TB. Health system approaches that favor hospital-based management of MDR-TB often have limited access to service delivery, and the diffusion of new diagnostic tools and treatment regimens is often weak in health systems where MDR-TB is prevalent (Stout et al., 2016). Several economies—including Estonia, Hong Kong SAR, China, Latvia, and Singapore—that have strengthened their health systems by improving access to diagnosis and treatment in primary care have been able to halt the rise in MDR-TB incidence. Strong laboratory capacity that has enabled rapid and definitive drug susceptibility testing, strong supply chain management systems, and the successful implementation of effective treatment regimens have contributed to this success (Su et al., 2019). In this context, it is technically difficult for countries to diagnose the patterns of drug resistance. For this reason, the WHO has established the Supranational Reference Laboratory Network for TB, which consists of 24 quality control laboratories located on all continents and capable of performing sophisticated drug resistance testing.

7.4.2. Recent Advances in TB Diagnostics

The diagnosis of TB has developed steadily over the last 10 years. As a result, the WHO issued 10 new policy statements on TB diagnosis between 2007 and 2012, covering a range of approaches (Sutherland et al., 2019).

Among the new diagnostic options that have emerged in recent years, the Xpert MTB/RIF test has received the most attention. Xpert MTB/RIF is an automated deoxyribonucleic acid (DNA) amplification test that provides rapid and sensitive detection of TB and rifampicin resistance. It uses a cartridge-based system that integrates real-time sample processing and polymerase chain reaction, can be operated by relatively untrained healthcare personnel and provides results in less than two hours. The system is expensive, costing about $17,000 per unit, and the tests, which are currently subsidized, cost about $10. The ability to diagnose TB and identify MDR-TB from sputum in less than two hours is a major advance in linking diagnosis and rapid initiation of treatment. However, Xpert MTB/RIF is not currently a technology for POC diagnosis. In December 2010, the WHO recommended that the device be used for the initial diagnosis of patients with suspected MDR-TB or HIV/AIDS-associated TB disease. Subsequently, several countries, including China, India, and South Africa, have purchased Xpert devices at reduced prices and taken advantage of volume pricing for the purchase of test cassettes.

The Xpert system is a significant advance in accelerating the diagnosis of TB, particularly MDR-TB, and is likely to be a valuable novel tool for large hospital and TB diagnostic laboratories. It is, however, dependent on a sophisticated and expensive device and therefore each sample tested is a relatively high cost. However, a multicenter study in four African countries failed to demonstrate reduced TB-related morbidity. A new device model under development, the GeneXpert Omni, which is portable and battery-powered, has the potential to become a POC diagnostic test in many more locations and is due to be launched in 2017.

As shortening the time between diagnosis and initiation of appropriate treatment is an important factor in reducing transmission, technologies that enable POC diagnosis and drug sensitivity testing are ideal. Some innovative research is underway to achieve this goal, but POC testing remains a formidable challenge. Given the sheer number of patients waiting in line at crowded outpatient clinics, it is unlikely that cough screening and sputum testing can be done effectively in many of the highest-risk outpatient settings — or in all resource-limited settings. Even DNA amplification methods are not sensitive enough to detect many patients in the early stages of the disease, and therefore potentially infectious TB cases are overlooked, diagnosis is delayed, and patients with XDR-TB are unlikely to respond immediately to current therapy. Ultimately, traditional control methods will still be necessary for the foreseeable future (Tahlan et al., 2012).

A recently developed molecular approach that examines gene expression from peripheral blood cells rather than sputum has the potential to identify the subset of healthy individuals with latent TB who are likely to progress to active disease. Rather than detecting components of the pathogen, this novel method measures gene expression signatures in peripheral white blood cells that are elevated in healthy individuals with latent infection prior to progression to active TB. In a panel of 16 gene probes in three separate cohorts in different countries, it was possible to predict individuals who developed active disease six months to one year before the clinical onset of symptoms. One year before diagnosis, the specificity of the test was around 61%, and in HIV-positive individuals it was significantly higher at around 80%. Molecular research into host responses offers new opportunities to diagnose infection and define the gene signatures of individuals who do not develop active disease, potentially leading to a better understanding of the genes required for disease resistance. In a similar approach, gene expression in whole blood from patients with latent TB or other disease was compared to that of patients with active TB using a validated multi-cohort analytical framework. The diagnostic capacity of a set of three genes was found to be 88–90% in active and latent TB in samples from children and adults in 10 countries (Tima et al., 2016). Such molecular host signatures could potentially serve as biomarkers for determining determinants of protection from infection or disease in future studies and vaccine trials.

7.5. TB Treatment

Treatment is aimed at curing the disease process, rapidly stopping transmission and preventing relapse. Current treatment requires a variety of antibiotics taken over many months and depends on predicted or proven antibiotic susceptibility. Context-specific treatment guidelines are usually developed by local health authorities under the guidance and supervision of the WHO. Clinical trials in the 20th century developed today's first-line drugs. Treatment success rates of 85% or more for new drug-susceptible cases are regularly reported to the WHO from a variety of clinical settings.

However, the effectiveness of treatment has been undermined by the development and transmission of MDR-TB. Therefore, the treatment of MDR-TB, defined as resistance to isoniazid and rifampicin (the two most effective TB drugs), takes longer and requires more expensive and toxic drugs. For most patients with MDR-TB, the current WHO-recommended regimens take 18–24 months, and treatment success rates are much lower, approximately 60%. The WHO now conditionally recommends the use of seven drugs to reduce the duration of treatment for uncomplicated lung disease to nine months. New drug combinations, for example bedaquiline or delaminid, which are thought to act on new molecular targets, are currently being introduced, but an ideal combination is probably still several years away (Trefzer et al., 2012).

Patients who are effectively treated for TB usually show a clinical response within 8–12 weeks, both subjectively (reduced cough, fatigue, fever, and sweating; increased appetite) and objectively (conversion of sputum smear or culture from positive to negative; weight gain). Non-response to treatment is usually due to poor drug quality, underdosing or malabsorption, lack of adherence to treatment, drug resistance (which may escalate during treatment), paradoxical reactions or inflammatory immune reconstitution syndrome (IRIS), adverse drug reactions, or another disease process (bronchiectasis, malignancy, pneumoconiosis, autoimmune disease or organ failure).

One of the embarrassing shortcomings in the field of TB control is the ambiguous definition of "cure." In the 21st century, it should be shocking that there are essentially no accurate biomarkers of treatment response or even a cure, nor the ability to predict relapse after treatment. In clinical trials, a cure for TB is defined as no relapse after one year of treatment. In LMICs, the general criterion for a cure in individual patients is two negative sputum smears with one month apart. However, sputum smears are not sensitive or accurate enough to ensure that the infection is truly cured. Although bacterial culture is more sensitive, it is also more time-consuming and is used less frequently in resource-poor countries. There are no microbiological or molecular biomarkers to determine whether a person's infection has been sterilized by treatment. Relapse can be due to either reactivation of a previously treated strain or reinfection with a new strain. Reinfection in previously treated patients can be as common as relapse and can further be distinguished from relapse by comparing the mycobacterial DNA sequences of the original isolate and the relapse (Varela et al., 2012).

7.5.1. Treatment Regimens

Effective TB treatment must overcome the organism's ability to survive in various microenvironments under extreme conditions, including immunologic attack, prolonged antibiotic exposure, and nutrient and oxygen deprivation. Standardized treatment regimens and fixed-dose combination preparations facilitate good clinical care in resource-limited settings. Table 7.5 shows the current treatment regimens with an intensive phase followed by a continuation phase.

Table 7.5. *TB Treatment Regimens Currently Recommended by the WHO*

Type of Case and Phase	Length of Regimen (Months)	Drug Used
New TB Case		
Intensive phase	2	Rifampicin, isoniazid, pyrazinamide, ethambutol.
Continuation phase	4	Rifampicin, isoniazid (low risk of isoniazid resistance) or rifampicin, isoniazid, ethambutol (high risk[a] of isoniazid resistance).
Previously Treated TB Case (Relapse or Default)[b]		
Intensive phase	2	Rifampicin, isoniazid, pyrazinamide, ethambutol, streptomycin

Continuation phase	1	Rifampicin, isoniazid, pyrazinamide, ethambutol
–	5	Rifampicin, isoniazid, ethambutol.
Previously Treated TB Case (Treatment Failure)c		
Intensive phase	8	MDR-TB regimen (see below)
Continuation phase	12	MDR-TB regimen (see below)
MDR-TB Cases		
2010 guideline	20	Kanamycin (or amikacin), moxifloxacin[d] (ethionamide, cycloserine (or terizidone), pyrazinamide
Intensive phase	8	Bedaquiline or delamanid, where sensitivity following the initial regimen cannot be assured (up to six months)
Continuation phase	12	Moxifloxacin,[d] ethionamide, cycloserine, pyrazinamide
2016 short regimen (conditional recommendation)	–	–
Intensive phase	4–6	Kanamycin, moxifloxacin,[d] prothionamide, clofazimine, pyrazinamide, high-dose isoniazid, ethambutol
Continuation phase	5	Moxifloxacin,[d] clofazimine, ethambutol, and pyrazinamide

Note: MDR TB = multidrug-resistant tuberculosis defined as resistance to isoniazid and rifampicin; WHO = World Health Organization.

a = Using local epidemiological data.

b = Low risk of MDR TB using local epidemiological data. The WHO recommends treatment guided by drug-susceptibility testing, especially rapid molecular tests, and suggests that standard first-line treatment be used if there is no evidence of drug resistance to isoniazid and rifampicin.

c = Defined as smear positive after five months of first-line treatment, relapse or default after second or subsequent course of treatment, or active tuberculosis after contact with an MDR TB case.

d = Or high-dose levofloxacin or gatifloxacin.

7.5.2. First-Line Treatment of Drug-Susceptible TB

Rifampicin and isoniazid are the most effective drugs against susceptible TB and are taken for the entire duration of initial treatment (Xu et al., 2017). Pyrazinamide synergistically enhances the sterilizing effect of rifampicin and shortens the duration of treatment to six months when combined with the first two months of treatment. Ethambutol is added to the regimen for two months to reduce the development of drug resistance during treatment and is continued for the full duration of therapy in situations with a high background prevalence of isoniazid resistance.

As effective as standard treatment has been, the resistance to isoniazid, rifampicin, and pyrazinamine is increasing in many countries, suggesting that new regimens increasingly need to be incorporated into TB treatment.

7.5.3. Second-Line Treatment of MDR TB

The treatment of drug-resistant TB continues to evolve, and recommendations are changing rapidly, however four factors renders it difficult to arrive at clear, generalizable recommendations. First, individual strains differ in their susceptibility and, where possible, tailored therapies are more appropriate. Second, susceptibility testing for pyrazinamide and second- and third-line agents are neither widely available nor consistently reliable. Third, many agents have limited availability due to their high cost or limited production. Finally, there are few comparative studies that provide data on which to base optimal treatment decisions.

Drug-resistant disease is curable, but the cure rate is lower than for drug-susceptible disease in several studies. In some studies of MDR-TB, only 54–70% of patients achieve treatment completion or cure. The treatment requires new drugs, with treatment regimens containing between three and seven drugs that have not been used before. In general, these second- and third-line drugs are less effective and must be administered over a longer period, ranging from 9 to 24 months. They are also more difficult to administer as most therapies contain agents such as kanamycin and amikacin, which must be administered by injection. These drugs are far more toxic than first-line drugs and cause several drug-specific side effects. Nevertheless, MDR-TB cure rates of 60–80% have been achieved in situations with severe resource constraints and in patients with advanced disease, regardless of HIV/AIDS status (Yee et al., 2003).

Key strategies that have contributed to successful treatment include intensive management of side effects, nutritional supplementation, treatment adherence measures and collaboration between the public health service, and non-governmental organizations (NGOs). These approaches should be routinely incorporated into programs wherever possible.

In general, MDR-TB has significant human, economic, and social consequences (Zhang et al., 2019). For example, the cost of treating MDR-TB with conventional therapies ranges from US$2,500 to US$10,000, compared with US$100 to US$1,000 for drug-susceptible TB cases, implying significant costs for high-burden countries. In South Africa, for example, although MDR-TB and XDR-TB account for less than 3% of all TB cases detected, they consume an estimated 35% of the national health budget allocated to TB control. In some countries, the cost of treating MDR-TB is estimated to exceed the total budget for TB control.

In May 2016, the WHO issued a conditional recommendation for the use of the shorter MDR-TB regimen, which shortens treatment duration (to 9–12 months), increases adherence and retention in treatment, and reduces costs (approximately USD 1,000 in drug costs per patient). Routine analysis of mutations conferring resistance to isoniazid can further influence the choice of MDR-TB treatment: isolates with mutations in the promoter region of the inhA gene are susceptible to high-dose isoniazid but resistant to ethionamide, while isolates with katG mutations are resistant to high-dose isoniazid but sensitive to ethionamide.

Ongoing clinical trials are beginning to form the basis for the WHO guidelines listed in Table 7.5 and are discussed in more detail in the 'Research and development' section. In this rapidly changing field, encouraging data suggest that higher cure rates are possible, perhaps with shorter treatment durations using newer agents. Bedaquiline and delamanid, two newly approved drugs, both lead to faster killing of organisms and higher cure rates in MDR-TB when administered with an optimized regimen. The oxazolidinone antibiotic linezolid, which is mainly used to treat Gram-positive infections, also accelerates killing and increases cure. Clofazimine, a riminophenazine dye used to treat leprosy, is now recommended for the abbreviated MDR-TB cure. These new treatments can cause significant side effects, for example Clofazamine can cause skin discoloration. Bedaquiline therapy has been associated with a higher mortality rate, although the reasons are unclear, while linezolid causes a range of dose-limiting toxicities, including neuropathy and myelosuppression (Zhang et al., 2019).

7.5.4. Treatment in Specific Situations

The therapies for the treatment of TB in children are identical to those for adults. Correct dosing by weight is crucial, and the most appropriate formulation of combination drugs is constantly being promoted.

TB in pregnancy can be treated with isoniazid, rifampicin, pyrazinamide, and ethambutol. In contrast, streptomycin, amikacin, and kanamycin can cause fetal ototoxicity and should not be used if possible. The safety of other drugs used to treat MDR-TB has not been well studied in pregnancy. Treatment should be individualized and reviewed by experts, and contraceptive counseling during MDR-TB treatment is essential.

Glucocorticoids can limit the inflammatory damage associated with TB, and there is evidence to support the use of glucocorticoids in tuberculous meningitis. In addition, surgery may be necessary to improve the chances of recovery by removing localized disease and to decompress vital structures affected by the tuberculous cavities.

A particularly devastating form of TB, tuberculous meningitis, occurs rapidly and is often fatal. Current treatments are less effective for tuberculous meningitis, and higher doses of drugs may be required to achieve therapeutic levels in the central nervous system (Zhang et al., 2019).

7.5.5. Drug Toxicities and Interactions

Timely detection and effective treatment of adverse drug reactions is critical to the integrity of a treatment program. TB antibiotics, like other drugs, can interfere with the metabolism and excretion of drugs. Rifampicin induces the expression of hepatic cytochrome P450 enzymes, significantly lowering the levels of several clinically important drugs such as HIV/AIDS protease inhibitors, warfarin, phenytoin, carbamazepine, and estrogen-containing contraceptives. The antiretroviral drugs nevirapine and efavirenz interact with rifampicin. However, only the interaction with nevirapine is clinically significant and the current recommendations are to use efavirenz with rifampicin. The newer drugs bedaquiline and delamanid, which appear to be effective against MDR- or XDR-TB in small studies, prolong the QT interval with the risk of cardiac arrhythmias, and linezolid has serious effects on bone marrow and neurological function. Clinically significant interactions should be regularly reviewed online.

7.5.6. Antiretroviral Therapy

In 2014, there were 10.4 million new cases of TB, of which 1.2 million (11%) were among people living with HIV/AIDS. Over the past 30 years, antiretroviral therapy for HIV/AIDS infection has improved to the point where effective therapy is widely available in LMICs, with significant improvements in mortality among patients co-infected with HIV/AIDS and TB (Zhang et al., 2019).

Early initiation of ART reduces the risk of mortality in HIV-positive patients co-infected with TB and is therefore recommended regardless of CD4 count. To reduce the risk of death, ART should be started within two weeks of TB treatment. The aim of ART is long-term viral load suppression, which is determined by regular viral load measurements. Cotrimoxazole prophylaxis against Pneumocystis pneumonia, toxoplasmosis, bacterial sepsis and malaria reduces mortality in patients co-infected with TB and HIV/AIDS, and should be administered until the CD4 count is back above 200 cells/μL after at least six months of ART.

A significant adverse effect of combination treatment is the development of IRIS, which is characterized by persistent or recurrent fever and an exacerbation of the focal tuberculous process (in severely immunosuppressed patients with a CD4 count below 50 cells per microliter) who start combination ART shortly after starting TB treatment. IRIS can usually be controlled with steroids and non-steroidal anti-inflammatory drugs.

7.5.7. Antidiabetic Treatment

Diabetes is a major risk factor for TB but has received less attention in LMICs than HIV/AIDS. This is likely to change given increasing life expectancy and the global prevalence of obesity and type 2 diabetes. All patients with TB should be screened for diabetes (Zhang et al., 2019). In diabetic patients, glycaemic control should be regularly monitored during TB treatment as part of integrated clinical care, and treatment should be optimized with oral antidiabetics and insulins.

7.5.8. Surgery

Given the fact that treatment outcomes in MDR-TB patients are only about 50%, surgery, which was an important tool in the era before the introduction of antibiotics, has re-established itself as an adjuvant therapeutic strategy. A systematic review and meta-analysis evaluating the evidence for the effect of surgery as an adjunct to chemotherapy found that there are few strong data on which to base recommendations, but there appears to be some improvement in successful outcomes with surgery performed in adults treated for MDR-TB.

7.5.9. Palliative Care

TB remains one of the main causes of death in LMICs. Suffering and the dying process are important clinical consequences of advanced TB that should be recognized and communicated by an experienced physician who can initiate effective palliative treatment. Terminally ill patients may choose to improve their quality of life by discontinuing TB treatment. Physical ailments, mental health problems and unresolved social issues at the end of life can be addressed by trained community health workers (CHWs) once the need has been identified. These structures require ongoing local support and advocacy (Zhang et al., 2018).

7.5.10. The Cascade of Care and Completion of Treatment

The DOTS strategy for TB control promotes standardized treatment with patient monitoring and support, which may include direct observation of therapy in which a health care worker personally observes the patient taking the medication. The scientific evidence for the effectiveness of DOT therapy compared to self-medication is mixed. Despite the positive effect of the DOTS strategy in mobilizing support and treatment activities, a systematic comparison of the effectiveness of DOT versus self-medication in 11 randomized control trials did not find unique effectiveness in ensuring compliance or cure.

DOTS has been associated with a lower prevalence of drug resistance in the United States, in other HICs, and in many LMICs such as Cambodia, China, and Ethiopia. However, in high-endemic countries, particularly those with a high HIV/AIDS burden, the strategy has not reduced incidence and transmission to the extent required, even when adequate diagnosis and effective treatment are provided. As discussed in the section on research and development, additional strategies are needed when the forces of infection, environment, and HIV/AIDS drive the rate of infection despite effective treatment of cases (Zhang et al., 2018).

Some countries have experimented with involving community members to make treatment monitoring more acceptable to individual patients, but the operational problems are considerable, and a meta-analysis after the introduction of DOTS that included community members in China found that 52% of patients were still self-administering therapy. Patients who do not adhere to treatment need to be identified early and offered practical interventions to help them return to treatment, including hospitalization for supervised treatment and physical rehabilitation. Clinicians who know the patient and the community are in the best position to decide which patients need the intensive treatment adherence support that DOTS provides.

It is important to emphasize that early case detection, whether through passive or active case finding, is a necessary but not sufficient condition for effective TB control. A recent analysis of the cascade of TB care in India highlights the challenges in ensuring treatment completion. In this important study of approximately 2 million cases of conventional TB evaluated under the Revised National TB Control Program, the authors established a framework and traced the cascade of care from the number of prevalent cases to those who reached TB diagnostic centers, those who were diagnosed with TB, those who enrolled for treatment, those who completed treatment, and finally those who survived relapse-free after one year. The results showed that for conventional TB, 45% completed treatment and 39% were disease-free after one year. Of the patients diagnosed with MDR-TB, only 14% completed treatment and 11% were disease-free after one year. These striking results clearly show the importance of supporting treatment to enable better treatment completion in India and most LMICs.

7.6. TB Prevention

There are three obvious strategies to prevent TB: Vaccination, infection control, and chemoprophylaxis or isoniazid preventive therapy (IPT). Probably the most useful, but perhaps least recognized, preventive measure is simply the early diagnosis and prompt initiation of effective treatment of TB cases to reduce the burden of infection and transmission. TB is unusual among infectious diseases as the appropriate (and effective) treatment of the individual patient may be the most effective public health measure to protect the population (Zhang et al., 2018).

7.6.1. Vaccination: Natural and Acquired Immunity

7.6.1.1. BCG Vaccine

The most commonly used vaccine worldwide is BCG, which is administered to around 100 million children every year. BCG was isolated in 1908 after attenuation by 431 passages of virulent *M. bovis* isolated from a human TB case and was found to be protective to some degree in several animal models of TB. In the first human study in 1921, it was found to protect a highly exposed child in a high-risk household.

BCG has several advantages: it can be administered at birth or at any time after birth; a single vaccination results in long-lasting positivity of the skin test for tuberculin; it is relatively stable; it leaves a scar, which is useful for epidemiological surveillance of access to immunization; and it is inexpensive.

There is much evidence to suggest that BCG immunization of young children is an effective preventive measure against tuberculous meningitis and disseminated (miliary) TB (Zhang & Mitchison, 2003). Randomized control trials and case-control studies have shown a consistently high protective effect of BCG against severe forms of disease in children (73%), meningitis, and miliary TB (77%). The most comprehensive analysis of the effect of BCG vaccination indicates that the administration of BCG to children born in 2002 prevented approximately 29,000 cases of childhood meningitis and 11,500 cases of miliary TB in the first five years of life. This corresponds to one case of meningitis for every 3,400 children vaccinated and one case of miliary TB for every 9,300 children vaccinated. A recent report shows that delaying BCG vaccination until six weeks after birth produces a stronger and longer-lasting specific cellular Th1 immune response. In some countries, children have been repeatedly vaccinated over time, and there is some evidence from Taiwan, China, that multiple vaccinations can increase protection. However, a worrying drawback is the occurrence of widespread BCG infections in HIV-positive children (Zhang & Mitchison, 2003).

Successful vaccines ideally prevent both infection and disease in individuals exposed to the pathogen. While it is generally believed that BCG protects against disease rather than infection, recent evidence using interferon-gamma release assays (IGRAs), which can distinguish Mtb infection from BCG vaccination, suggests that BCG may also protect against infection to varying degrees.

The cost-effectiveness of BCG was estimated in 2006 to be US$40 to US$170 per disability-adjusted life year (DALY), US$8,000 to US$11,000 per life saved, or US$5,000 to US$8,000 per case of disease prevented (Dye, 2006), making it a very cost-effective intervention.

Despite positive evidence for the effects of BCG on children, BCG remains the most controversial of all vaccines currently in use, as its protective efficacy varies widely in different parts of the world, from 77% protection in adolescents in the UK to 0% protection in all age groups in southern India. Since young children account for only a small proportion of TB transmission, BCG vaccination of infants has only a relatively small impact on transmission within populations. This finding is confirmed by the results in parts of Europe and North America where BCG vaccination was not carried out. There, TB declined at rates that were not measurably different from those in regions that used the vaccine (Zhang & Mitchison, 2003). In a more recent analysis using South African data, some found that BCG vaccination would reduce TB in HIV-negative individuals by about 17%, to which would be added the value of preventing transmission to HIV-positive individuals. He estimated that BCG booster vaccination would be highly cost-effective for all combinations of cost (US$1 to US$10 per child) and efficacy (10–80%).

BCG vaccination has also shown a highly variable protective effect against TB in adults in randomized trials and observational studies. The explanations for these variations remain unclear. Suggestions include the fact that BCG lacks more than 100 genes from Mtb, including some putative protective antigens, the genetic composition of different human populations, differential persistence of different BCG strains or preparations, and interference from atypical mycobacteria in the environment. Many years ago, it was shown that guinea pigs immunized with different types of environmental atypical mycobacteria were differentially protected against Mtb, for example *Mycobacterium kansasii*, were as effective as BCG in animals (Zumla et al., 2015). It is often forgotten that *Mycobacteriaum microti*, a murine mycobacterium, was as effective as BCG in humans in the British Medical Research Council vaccine trials. This suggests that if environmental exposure to mycobacteria provides some protection in a population, the effects of BCG observed in that population will be comparatively less than in a naïve population. This could explain the large differences in the efficacy of BCG in populations living in different geographical locations, with children in tropical latitudes showing less protection. For example, in the South Indian trial area, two-thirds of individuals were positive to a skin test with purified protein derivative of *Mycobacterium avium* at age 9 years and 97% were positive at age 15–19 years (Tuberculosis Prevention Trial, 1979). Knowledge of the extent of exposure to non-tuberculous mycobacteria in the environment is important for the planning and evaluation of new vaccines against TB.

7.6.1.2. A Rationale for Vaccines: Latent Infection Can Prevent Reinfection

It is widely believed that it is unlikely to develop a protective vaccine against TB, as natural infection with Mtb cannot prevent reinfection. However, there is remarkable epidemiologic evidence that latent infection with Mtb actually provides substantial protection against reinfection by eliciting protective immune responses that are likely to persist. An early experiment by Heimbeck (1938) employing Norwegian nurses, as well as a study by Sutherland, Svandova, & Radhakrishna (1982) demonstrated that in healthy young people, a positive TST provided up to 80% protection against reinfection compared to a negative TST (ranging from 45–81% in several studies). In a recent study from South Africa, where it was possible to measure infections in the apparently uninfected group and directly observe TB cases, the estimated immunologic protection from latent TB infection was 79% (Zumla et al., 2015). These results encourage the view that new vaccines with better efficacy than BCG could provide a relatively high level of protection if the protective immune responses generated are maintained over time, as is the case with latent TB.

7.6.1.3. Innate Immune Responses

The body's immune response is crucial for protection against infection and disease, through both innate and acquired immunity. This is perhaps best illustrated by the fact that while only 10% of individuals infected with TB will contract the disease in their lifetime, immunocompromised individuals have a contraction risk of nearly 10% per year. Immunocompromised individuals, such as those infected with HIV/AIDS or those receiving anti-TNF immunotherapy for autoimmune diseases, have a significantly higher incidence of TB. In immunocompromised HIV-positive patients in KwaZulu-Natal, the average time from diagnosis to death from XDR or drug-resistant TB was an astonishing 16 days (Zumla et al., 2015). And the increased prevalence of drug-resistant TB in immunocompromised individuals is consistent with the notion that the efficacy of antibiotics depends to some degree on the antimicrobial immune response. It is intriguing that in countries with a high burden of TB, there is a population of healthy contacts who have almost certainly been repeatedly exposed to infection and yet are TST negative, IGRA negative and apparently healthy. This suggests that mechanisms of innate immunity may be able to kill the relatively small number of infectious tubercle bacilli early after respiratory infection, even before they can grow to numbers capable of sensitizing and expanding T cells that can respond to TB antigens. These mechanisms are not yet understood, and further research is needed.

7.6.1.4. Preventive Therapy

There are two approaches to preventive therapy. Cotrimoxazole is routinely recommended for HIV-positive people who are at high risk of many opportunistic infections, and in countries with high disease burden, between 50 and 87% of HIV-positive patients receive this preventive therapy.

The main approach to preventing the development of TB in high-risk individuals, particularly household contacts and HIV-positive individuals, is to screen them with a TST and ideally offer individuals who are HIV-positive chemoprophylaxis, IPT against latent infection (Xu et al., 2017). In perhaps the most dramatic studies, a community-based trial of IPT among BCG-vaccinated Alaskan Eskimos, a community at high risk of infection, resulted in a 60% reduction in TB incidence that persisted for more than two decades in treated households. Overall, an analysis of randomized controlled trials has shown that preventive therapy offers clear benefits. Since 2011, the WHO has recommended that HIV-positive individuals who do not have symptoms suggestive of TB be treated with IPT for at least six months. The risk of clinically active TB disease is reduced by 60% in immunocompetent, HIV-negative individuals and by 32–62% in HIV-positive adults treated with 3 to 12 months of preventive therapy (Xu et al., 2017). Since these guidelines came into force, the number of HIV-positive people receiving IPT has risen sharply and stood at around 933,000 in 2014. The high risk of TB in people co-infected with Mtb and HIV/AIDS motivates those advocating for wider use of preventive therapy, particularly in Africa. However, questions have been raised about screening methods to ensure that those most likely to benefit receive this treatment and that those with subclinical TB are not inadvertently treated with isoniazid monotherapy, which could lead to resistance. Studies of contact children of active cases have shown that daily administration of isoniazid for 12 months provides 30–60% protection against active TB. More recent work suggests that isoniazid can be continued in HIV-positive adults for longer than six months with minimal side effects and prolonged protection.

At the population level, a randomized trial conducted in high-incidence urban communities in Brazil found that the incidence of TB after five years was 15% lower in communities that received an intervention compared to those that did not. Despite this, the widespread implementation of isoniazid preventive therapy (IPT) remains limited. Of the countries with the highest TB burden, only Brazil and South Africa have policies in place to expand the use of IPT. Even in the United States, where resources are more readily available, the implementation of contact investigation and IPT has fallen short of recommended guidelines (Xu et al., 2017).

In countries with high rates of TB infection, studies on IPT in HIV/AIDS-infected, tuberculin skin test (TST)-positive adults showed an average protection of around 60%. However, the protective effect diminished shortly after IPT treatment concluded, and little to no impact on mortality was observed. In contrast, IPT has been shown to reduce both TB incidence and mortality in HIV-positive children.

A key randomized controlled trial, the Temprano study, compared early versus delayed initiation of antiretroviral therapy (ART) and IPT in 2,050 HIV-positive individuals with high CD4+ counts in Côte d'Ivoire. Results revealed that six months of IPT reduced the risk of severe HIV/AIDS-related illness by 44% and the risk of death from any cause by 35% compared to delayed ART initiation and no IPT. Furthermore, the combination of early ART and IPT reduced TB incidence by 73% (Xu et al., 2017). In Brazil, a six-month IPT regimen not only reduced TB incidence during treatment but also showed sustained protection over a seven-year follow-up period. This evidence suggests that combining early ART with IPT, as now recommended by the WHO, should be a standard approach in HIV/AIDS and TB control.

The use of IPT is associated with real challenges: before taking isoniazid alone, active disease must be ruled out, if possible by radiography, as well as the poor adherence to six or more months of daily treatment in healthy people. Even in the United States, less than 50% of people who started IPT completed the six months of treatment. Adverse effects include the risk of hepatitis, particularly in individuals concurrently infected with HIV/AIDS, when IPT is administered over a long period of time. In the United States, adverse effects are on the order of 1%, but increase to 4% when IPT is administered with rifapentine. Recently, a cluster randomized trial of mass screening and IPT for TB control was conducted among gold miners in several mines in Thibela, South Africa, a community known to be at high risk of TB. The miners received IPT for 9 months and the effect on disease prevention was followed for 12 months. Despite the positive effect of isoniazid in preventing TB during the treatment period, IPT had no significant sustained effect on TB control in the South African gold mines. Most discouragingly, the results of a systematic review and meta-analysis of the treatment cascade for latent TB indicate that preventive treatment is completed only 19% of the time (Xu et al., 2017).

Apart from HIV-positive individuals and children with household contacts, it remains unclear how feasible and cost-effective it would be to scale up IPT in countries with high TB burdens. It is a challenge for health systems in LMICs that struggle to treat diagnosed TB patients and maintain IPT for healthy contacts. A more recent approach to shortening preventive therapy stems from studies of a combination of long-acting rifapentine plus isoniazid, which shortened treatment duration from nine to three months and was better tolerated, albeit more expensive.

The crucial question of the best preventive therapy to combat MDR-TB remains unanswered. The significant adverse effects of MDR-TB therapies are a serious disadvantage compared to preventing the 10% of cases expected from preventive treatment, and no optimal therapy with newer drugs has yet been found (Tima et al., 2016). The alternative is to register all these contacts, monitor them carefully and initiate treatment at the first sign of disease.

It is perhaps not so far-fetched to imagine that with advances in research, more effective drug therapies for latent infections could have a profound impact on reducing the global burden of TB. It is not known what proportion, of the one-third of people globally who have a positive TST, retain viable tubercle bacilli that can reactivate and transmit the disease. However, if a viable drug treatment could kill the infection in all these people, this enormous reservoir of the pathogen could be eliminated in a short time. Rather than passively tracking down patients with disease, screening the population for people infected due to tuberculin positivity, and applying the hoped-for effective mycobacterial-killing treatment, the enormous burden of latent TB could potentially be reduced or eliminated. This approach should be considered in future research.

7.6.1.5. Impact of Effective Treatment on Transmission

Of the measures available to control transmission, it has long been taught that effective treatment is paramount. Treatment can only be administered to known or suspected cases and, to be effective, requires knowledge of drug resistance. Traditionally, it was thought that drug-resistant TB required at least two weeks of effective treatment to significantly reduce the risk of transmission regardless of sputum smear status (Tima et al., 2016). However, for drug-resistant TB, the two-week rule appears to have failed during the outbreaks in New York City and Miami in the 1980s and 1990s, when patients with unsuspected drug resistance on conventional four-drug therapy transmitted their infection after isolation ended. Therefore, current guidelines generally recommend isolation of MDR-TB patients until conversion to smear or culture.

The rate at which TB cases become non-infectious through treatment has recently been re-examined using the classical model of transmission from humans to guinea pigs. This model demonstrated that TB transmission was detected by transiting hospital exhaust air past a group of guinea pigs that were highly susceptible to TB. The study suggests that MDR-TB transmission, like drug-susceptible TB, responds rapidly to effective treatment, well before sputum smear or culture conversion. In a series of five exposure studies, with predominantly smear-positive, coughing patients with confirmed MDR-TB were enrolled and immediately started on treatment, while the disease's transmission to guinea pigs appears to have originated predominantly from patients with unsuspected XDR-TB who did not respond to effective treatment.

7.6.2. Infection Control of TB Transmission in Congregate Settings

Transmission and reinfection, particularly of drug-resistant strains, is a major cause of the global TB epidemic (Sutherland et al., 2019). The benefits of isoniazid prophylaxis in high-risk HIV-positive populations, for example, were quickly negated by ongoing transmission and reinfection soon after isoniazid was discontinued. Similarly, the challenge in high-transmission settings is to provide greater protection against reinfection than is currently possible through BCG vaccination at birth and subsequent natural exposure to Mtb and mycobacteria in the environment.

Control of transmission was not explicitly mentioned in the original Global Plan for TB Control 2006–2015, but the 2006 outbreak of XDR-TB, which occurred mainly in hospitals, dramatically focused attention on the problem. Since then, control measures have focused on healthcare facilities, although it is well known that transmission also occurs in homes, schools, churches, shelters, refugee camps and correctional facilities, as well as other community settings. Nevertheless, healthcare facilities dominate the list of environments that increase transmission at the population level because they bring together infectious and vulnerable people.

7.6.2.1. Hospitals as Epicenters of Transmission

An important epicenter of transmission includes hospitals where TB patients are present. Since exposure in hospitals is better documented than in many other settings, it is likely that transmission in hospitals is underestimated, for example, infecting strains for which DNA fingerprints are not available are not counted.

The significant decline in the TB epidemic in New York City from 3,800 cases in the 1980s to 577 in 2015 shows that multi-faceted efforts are needed in large urban, multicultural settings with large numbers of visitors, migrants, and homeless people and rising rates of HIV/AIDS. The DOT approach was undoubtedly helpful in ensuring adherence among a proportion of TB patients, but perhaps more significant were the major efforts to implement infection control in hospitals, prisons, shelters, and community housing (Su et al., 2019).

Using a network analysis, many concluded that most strain-specific XDR-TB transmissions in KwaZulu-Natal occurred in hospitals, due to prolonged stays, community accommodation, and delayed detection of drug resistance. Similar transmission patterns also exist in Tomsk Oblast in Siberia, where a retrospective study of the causes of drug resistance in the Tomsk region showed a more than six-fold higher risk among treatment-resistant patients hospitalized for drug-susceptible TB than among patients who were not hospitalized (Stout et al., 2016). Anyone familiar with common treatment practices in Eastern Europe will understand why this might be the case.

Although new cases of TB in Tomsk are mainly treated on an outpatient basis, hospitalized patients are housed in poorly ventilated multi-bed rooms that are tightly sealed against the cold. Drug sensitivity is usually only tested if patients do not respond to first-line treatment, usually after months of ineffective treatment, and the use of conventional methods require additional months. During this long period of ineffective treatment, there is ample opportunity for transmission and reinfection. This scenario is not unique to Tomsk, as delays in drug susceptibility testing occur in most TB programs where laboratory services are inadequate. Treatment failure is the usual indication for drug susceptibility testing, and molecular methods are slow to reduce the time needed for first-line and much less frequently second-line drug results. However, despite hospital transmission, outpatient treatment is very effective, and Tomsk is one of the few high-burden places in the world where MDR-TB rates may be declining.

7.6.2.2. Principles of TB Transmission Control

Since the resurgence of TB in 1985–1992 in the United States and several European countries, where institutional transmission has played an important role, a three-tiered hierarchical approach has been adopted based on a paradigm used in industry: administrative controls, engineering (or environmental) controls, and personal protection (respiratory protection). Administrative controls include the rapid diagnosis of symptomatic, potentially infectious cases and drug resistance and the prompt initiation of effective therapy. This has recently been promoted under the acronym FAST (Find cases Actively by cough surveillance, Separate temporarily, and Treat effectively) to communicate the key components and facilitate implementation. Environmental controls focus on natural and mechanical ventilation and the evolving technology of ultraviolet germicidal sustainable air disinfection (UVGI). Personal respiratory protection is the final level of protection, assuming incomplete protection from administrative and engineering controls. Ironically, despite being the last level of protection, respirators are often the only protection available to healthcare workers. They cannot always be worn and are unlikely to be worn when treating a patient with unsuspected TB.

7.6.2.3. Efficacy Measures of TB Transmission Control

Measuring the effectiveness of transmission control measures has been difficult course, and process indicators include questions about whether windows are open, or the availability of respirators, although these factors may have too little to do with exposure to be useful. However, to the extent that undiagnosed TB patients and undiagnosed drug resistance are important exposure factors, process indicators tied to unprotected exposure time can be measured and reported. For example, facilities can document the percentage of patients screened for cough and whose sputum was sent to a laboratory, the turnaround time from submission to receipt of results, and the time from admission to initiation of effective treatment based on drug susceptibility testing. Such measures should become routine in hospitals with access to rapid diagnostic tests.

There are a few studies that address not only the effectiveness of TB control methods but also their cost. Aside from the great difficulty in measuring the effectiveness of measures to prevent transmission, isolating the costs of infection control measures can be challenging, as many infection control measures are integral to hospital functions in general. Assuming that unsuspected, untreated patients are in the hospital, ventilation is one of the most important measures, with natural ventilation in appropriate climates at the top of the list of recommendations. The additional cost of designing and building a naturally ventilated patient waiting area is however difficult to separate from routine hospital capital costs. Some insights can be gleaned from unpublished data from a high-risk hospital in Vladimir, Russia, a TB control training center.

7.6.2.4. Cost-Effective Air Disinfection

Natural ventilation alone does not provide sufficient ventilation for airborne infection control in many areas. However, mechanical ventilation systems are often prohibitively expensive and often fail due to lack of maintenance. Room air cleaners (with filters, UVGI or both) are often sold to hospital administrators as a simple, low-cost solution, but they rarely move enough air to achieve the 12 or more equivalent air changes per hour recommended to control airborne infections. Re-trapping and recirculating the same air through the unit (short-circuiting) also results in a low rate of effective clean air delivery.

As found in the Vladimir study, UVGI germicidal irradiation in upper rooms (with fans for air mixing) is one of the most effective and cost-effective methods for high-volume air disinfection. While hospital studies have shown an effectiveness of 70–80%, similarly with mechanical ventilation and room air purifiers, caution is required. Although they are under development, international standards and guidelines for safe and effective use and maintenance are not widely available. There is currently no authority regulating this small industry and few experts are qualified to design installations. Nevertheless, they is a logical choice as a backup technology for natural ventilation, such as the recommendation of low speed ceiling fans to ensure the necessary mixing of indoor air. With the development of LED UVGI (light emitting diodes) and the prospect of solar-powered systems with battery backup, germicidal UVGI in upper rooms could become more sustainable in the near future (Stout et al., 2016).

7.6.2.5. Masks and Respirators

Assuming that both the control of the source of infection as well as the technical or environmental control strategies are insufficiently effective, the final measure is respiratory protection, that is the use of a device that excludes infectious droplet nuclei from the inhaled air.

Masks and respirators are easily confused, for example surgical masks are intended to protect the environment by blocking aerosolization of some of the exhaled droplets and droplet nuclei, but they do not adequately protect the wearer and play only a limited role in controlling TB transmission when worn by patients for short periods. MDR-TB patients who wore masks were 53% less likely to infect guinea pigs that inhaled the ward's exhaust air (Su et al., 2019). More recently, Mphaphlele and others (2015) used the same transmission model in South Africa to test the effectiveness of various control measures to prevent transmission from patients in hospital rooms to guinea pigs. The study confirmed the earlier report and showed 70–80% efficacy of UVGI air disinfection in the upper rooms.

In contrast, respirators are designed to protect the wearer, where properly fitted, certified N-95 (or equivalent) respirators can provide 85–90% protection. However, as an intervention, respiratory protection often fails, either because the face seal is leaking due to improper fit or wrong adjustment or, more importantly, because the masks are not worn consistently. The cost of respiratory protection programs is easy to estimate, but their effectiveness is not.

7.6.2.6. Lessons for Household Transmission

As TB is largely transmitted by aerosol droplets, transmission is influenced by the built environment of the household. A study from South Africa found evidence that transmission of the infection, as determined by DNA fingerprinting of the strains, was greater in modern brick houses with windows than in older huts (Su et al., 2019). The reason for this could be that residents in modern homes kept windows closed to maintain cleanliness, while the cottages were simply better ventilated. Another study measured the effects of increased natural ventilation in traditional dwellings. This showed that natural ventilation was facilitated by opening doors and windows, and it was extrapolated that such a change could reduce the risk of household transmission by 80%.

7.7. Turning the Tide Against TB

Despite the progress made in TB control over the last two decades, there are still serious gaps. Although TB can be treated and cured, it is still one of the deadliest infectious diseases in the world today.

Three key elements are needed to achieve effective TB control and achieve the SDG: (1) early and accurate diagnosis and drug susceptibility testing, (2) patient access to and completion of effective treatment, and (3) prevention of the transition from latent infection to disease. Of course, these categories are inseparable; each influences and interrelates with the others, and all face both technical and systemic challenges. Without greater effectiveness of these key elements, it will not be possible to bend the curve and dramatically reduce transmission and incidence rates in all countries. To win the fight against TB, we must therefore invest in new technologies — diagnostics, treatments and vaccines — and address the systemic and strategic challenges that influence the extent to which technological advances reach the people who need them and translate into better health.

7.7.1. Earlier Diagnosis: Toward Active Case Finding

7.7.1.1. Limitations of Passive Case Finding

Even with modern technology, it has been difficult to implement effective case detection in low-resource communities with weak health systems (Stec et al., 2016). The main paradigm for diagnosing TB cases is passive case finding, which depends on people infected with the disease to seek medical care. However, passive case finding faces many challenges. TB is most common in marginalized communities that are less visible to traditional health systems. Patients tend to be poor, are often migrants, belong to disadvantaged groups, and suffer from other diseases, such as HIV/AIDS and diabetes, that increase their susceptibility to TB. Even when symptoms are present, up to a third of TB patients in many countries either do not seek treatment or are treated by traditional healers before seeing a doctor, leading to more severe disease, delayed treatment and increased transmission. TB control assumes that transmission of the disease will be reduced and eventually interrupted if active cases are detected and treated. However, the issue of unsuspected cases is a serious problem that has received little attention. Traditional guidelines focus on known or suspected cases with classic symptoms and active disease, whereas some forms of TB, such as asymptomatic and chronic TB, do not show clinical symptoms for months or years and can transmit the infection over long periods of time.

There is strong evidence that the problem of unsuspected or asymptomatic cases of TB, as well as unsuspected cases of drug resistance, is significant and contributes to the fact that one-third of TB patients are "unknown to the health care system" These patients are capable of transmitting the disease but are not sick enough to seek treatment or to be detected through passive case finding. For example, at a teaching hospital in Lusaka, Zambia, 900 newly admitted patients (70.6% HIV-positive) who were able to produce sputum without induction were screened. Examination by fluorescence microscopy and automated liquid culture detected TB in 22% of patients, of whom 13.4% were unsuspected (Stec et al., 2016). This included 18 MDR-TB cases, of which 5 were unsuspected. At the same hospital, 94 patients with coughing were admitted primarily for obstetric or gynecologic indications (73.4% HIV-positive) and had their sputum processed in the same manner. Additionally, Xpert MTB/RIF was used for rapid diagnosis for these patients, and TB was diagnosed in 28% of the 94 sputum samples, of which the Xpert device detected 80.8%, compared to 50% with standard smear microscopy. Results of this nature are not new: similar findings were reported more than a decade ago in a low HIV/AIDS setting in Lima, Peru, where 250 of 349 consecutive new admissions to a female general medical ward were screened for TB by sputum smear, culture, and X-ray. Of these, 16% had culture-proven TB, of which one-third were unsuspected, including 6 unsuspected MDR cases.

The DOTS strategy in countries with high disease burden, even if implemented more effectively, will simply not be enough to meet the challenge of unsuspected cases or drug resistance. In a landmark population-based active case-finding study of HIV/AIDS and TB in sub-Saharan Africa, where the prevalence of HIV/AIDS infection is 23%, Wood and others (2007) found that despite a highly effective DOTS TB control program with high adherence rates, 63% of adult cases of pulmonary TB were not known to the health system. Among HIV-negative individuals, 67% of prevalent smear-positive cases were identified through passive case finding, the recognized target for adequate DOTS implementation. However, in persons with HIV/AIDS infection, only 33% of cases with smear-positive TB were identified through passive case finding.

Similar results were found in a large survey of 47,000 individuals in Cambodia, where 12% of individuals were clinically examined and sputa tested by smear and culture. Only a third of TB cases were detected by sputum smears. Importantly, 44% of sputum-positive cases and 23% of smear-negative culture-positive cases showed none of the signs of clinical TB (Stanley et al., 2013). A surprising demographic finding was that more than half of all infections detected were in people over the age of 50, a trend also seen in other Asian countries.

Clearly, in many parts of the world where the TB burden is low and control programs have been effective, the need for active case finding is not great and cost-effectiveness would argue against a recommendation. However, in high-burden communities, passive case finding fails to detect early and asymptomatic cases, leaving a third of TB patients unknown to the health system.

7.7.1.2. Active Case Finding: What Does the Evidence Show?

Active case finding — mass screening and surveillance — almost certainly contributed to the rapid decline in TB in European countries and the Americas (5–8% per year) after World War II — that is, before the introduction of antibiotics. In 1974, the WHO recommended that active case finding with radiographs be discontinued, as it was no longer necessary or cost-effective in populations with low TB prevalence and good access to quality health care, particularly in highly developed countries. The WHO reaffirmed this policy in 2014, again stating that it was not cost-effective and recommended that indiscriminate mass screening should be avoided. It did, however, advise the systematic screening for active TB in geographically defined subpopulations with extremely high rates of unreported cases (1% prevalence or more). Unfortunately, this WHO recommendation was not sufficiently emphasized to encourage countries and donors to initiate and support active case finding in countries with a high TB burden, or to influence transmission in these countries.

One strategy for active case finding is the use of radiography, particularly mobile X-ray machines, to detect lung lesions with computer-aided detection in people who are relatively asymptomatic (Shirude et al., 2014). This strategy can detect many more patients with infection than is possible through passive case finding, cough screening or self-reporting. In South Africa, for example, the only period in which the incidence of TB cases declined was between 1950 and 1975, when X-ray surveillance covered about 10% of the population annually. While TB control programs in Europe and North America dramatically reduced the annual risk of infection in successive cohorts, no such decline has occurred in countries with high TB and HIV/AIDS prevalence.

In recent studies in Kenya, chest radiography showed high sensitivity (94%) and reasonable specificity (73%) for the detection of TB (Shirude et al., 2013). X-ray examination represents a potentially valuable population-based screening tool to determine in which individuals' sputum should be examined with a culture or Xpert device for definitive diagnosis. With rapid technological development, computerized evaluation of X-ray images could allow cost-effective screening of larger numbers of individuals in a high-throughput manner. This is particularly true when combined with clinical symptoms, where it was found that a sensitivity of 95% and a negative predictive value of 98% can be achieved.

7.7.1.3. Active Case Finding in Targeted Regions

In many LMICs, patients with TB often visit one or more traditional providers before seeking appropriate medical care (Rao et al., 2013). Even with symptomatic surveillance for classic signs of TB — cough, fever, and weight loss— a significant number of cases are not detected, particularly in HIV-positive individuals.

In randomized cluster trials in Brazil, increased case detection had a significant impact on the reduction of TB. The WHO commissioned several studies on the effectiveness and acceptability of active case finding or systematic screening for active TB. The studies reported that active case finding is very well accepted by the population in sub-Saharan Africa.

In a recent review of undiagnosed TB that would not be found with passive case finding, Yuen and others (2015) found that, particularly in high-risk populations and those infected with HIV/AIDS, intensive case finding, and early initiation of treatment or preventive therapy would likely have the greatest impact with the least use of resources.

In another study in South Africa, a group of 2,800 individuals in households with a detected TB index case were enrolled to determine the prevalence of undetected TB and HIV/AIDS in the community. Field teams screened participants for TB symptoms, collected sputum samples for smear microscopy and culture, and provided HIV/AIDS counseling and testing. They found that 6,075 per 100,000 of the household contacts were sputum-positive, compared to 477 residents of randomly selected households without an index case. This result demonstrates the value of screening contacts of index cases in a high-burden area and cautions against random screening of the general population. Of the 169 previously unidentified cases with TB detected by culture, only 6% were found to be sputum-positive, and only 11% were symptomatic; the remaining 89% would not have been diagnosed with passive case finding.

However, the evidence is inconsistent. In a large, complex randomized community trial called the Zamstar study (Pethe et al., 2013), 64,000 individuals in Zambia and the Western Cape in South Africa were screened for TB symptoms, sputum was collected to identify ill individuals, and enhanced active case finding in the household with counseling was conducted in one arm. The study of households with index cases clearly identified a larger number of TB cases. The adjusted ratio for prevalence and the adjusted ratio for incidence did not differ significantly between enhanced case finding and usual practice or between the groups with and without households. The study found no evidence that enhanced case finding had an impact on the TB burden at the community level. Although the results did not reach statistical significance, they indicated that the household intervention reduced the burden of TB in these communities. A meta-analysis of controlled trials found that screening increased the number of cases found in the short term and that cases tended to be found earlier and with a less severe disease (Zumla et al., 2013). Treatment outcomes for individuals identified through screening were similar to outcomes for individuals identified through passive case finding. This analysis once again confirms that in many areas more than half of prevalent TB cases are undiagnosed.

A recent study on TB transmission modeling in South Africa found that the country is unlikely to meet the WHO 2050 targets with the current DOTS approach of passive case finding. The model predicts that interventions such as active case finding with early initiation of treatment and reduction of losses to follow-up could have a major impact instead. It is therefore important to define the high-burden target groups where active case finding is likely to be most effective.

Although most official data on TB incidence and prevalence are estimated for entire countries, an innovative epidemiologic approach has recently been developed that raises the question of whether regions of high TB burden within a country — so-called hot spots — might be suitable for targeted control measures. Such hot spots have been identified in some countries, such as Moldova, and it will be of interest to learn whether targeted control measures can improve their effectiveness at a lower cost than the usual nationwide programs (Zumla et al., 2015). These population experiments on TB control need to be supported and evaluated.

We therefore recommend identifying countries and high-risk populations that do not respond effectively to the standard DOTS strategy and developing targeted active case-finding interventions that could have a greater impact on earlier case detection and successful treatment.

Initiating active case finding interventions in countries with high disease burden will clearly require external financial support. However, given the limitations of current tools and the increasing threat of MDR-TB, active case finding may be the best strategy to reduce incidence and prevalence in high-burden areas in the long term. And although active case finding is more expensive than passive case finding, the additional costs are more than offset by the avoided diagnosis and treatment costs — that is hospital and community transmission of TB from unsuspected cases, especially MDR-TB cases. The questions of how much screening, in what locations and at what cost need to be answered if we are to prevent every additional case of drug-susceptible or MDR-TB. If the goal is to interrupt transmission and reduce incidence faster, actively searching for cases in high TB burden areas can make a demonstrable difference.

7.7.2. Community-Based, Integrated Delivery of TB Care

Service delivery—from screening and diagnosing patients to administering treatment and monitoring progress—is a key challenge in TB control, as in other health services (Acharya et al., 2020).

7.7.2.1. Dominance (and Cost) of Hospital

The cost of providing healthcare services is the biggest cost of TB control. While the average cost of diagnostics and testing does not vary significantly between income groups, the cost of medication and hospitalization does, particularly that of treatment. For example, the cost per patient for TB drug treatment was USD 14,659 in high-income countries, USD 840 in upper-middle-income countries, USD 273 in lower-middle-income countries and USD 258 in low-income countries, with a strong positive correlation with income. However, the average cost of treating drug-susceptible TB varied widely across countries with the same income levels.

Hospitalization accounted for an average of 74% of all costs for drug-susceptible TB (although this figure varied widely across studies) and 64% of all costs for MDR-TB. Conversely, the average cost of outpatient treatment was 12 times lower than the cost of hospitalization and accounted for 6% of total costs. In one study, India consistently had the lowest hospitalization costs in the LMIC group and Ukraine had the highest costs for hospitalization and outpatient treatment. In Ukraine, high hospitalization costs, where patients also incurred costs, led to treatment failures. In 2013, in countries with a high burden of TB and MDR TB (excluding China and Russia), almost 38% of funding (US$919 million) was spent on inpatient and outpatient treatment for drug-susceptible TB. In addition, Russia spent 1.6 billion US dollars on TB control in 2013, most of which went to hospital-based TB treatment. However, funding for neglected areas with high TB prevalence, such as prisons, remains woefully low (Pethe et al., 2013).

The efficient and effective delivery of TB health services is critical to improving TB outcomes globally. However, the provision of TB services is inefficient and ineffective, relying heavily on hospital services and vertical delivery of DOTS. For example, the average cost of treating a patient with drug TB between 2008 and 2010, and in most of the 22 countries with a high disease burden, was between 100 and 500 US dollars. However, the average cost ranged from US$100 to US$10,000 when Russia (a hospital-based service delivery model) was included.

In 2014, the WHO estimated that in most of the 22 countries with a high burden of drug-susceptible TB, the proportion of inpatient and outpatient hospital costs was between 30 and 60%, with length of stay ranging from 5 to 56 days. In the 22 high TB burden countries, the cost of inpatient and outpatient treatment for drug-susceptible TB relative to the national TB program budget was 1–10% in the Democratic Republic of Congo, Ethiopia, Tanzania, Thailand, and Uganda; 11–20% in Bangladesh, Kenya, Myanmar, and Pakistan; and over 40% in India (46%), Mozambique (51.8%), and Vietnam (74.2%). While the WHO report did not include data for China and Russia, previous studies suggest that in Russia, where drug-susceptible TB is predominantly treated in hospitals, patients remain under observation long after treatment is completed. As a result, inpatient hospital costs account for around 60% of total treatment costs. It is difficult to understand why China has shifted the majority of TB treatment from outpatient to inpatient care.

In South Africa, which has the second highest number of confirmed MDR-TB cases and the highest number of confirmed XDR-TB cases, MDR-TB accounts for only 3.5% of the TB disease burden but consumes almost half of the national TB program budget of 218 million US dollars. Patients with MDR-TB are hospitalized from the start of treatment until culture conversion. The cost per patient of treating MDR-TB was US$17,164, more than 40 times the cost of treating drug-susceptible TB, which was estimated to be between US$314 and US$392 for community-based treatment. About 95% of these costs were hospitalization costs. More recent studies in South Africa put the cost of inpatient treatment for MDR-TB at USD 6,772 (compared to USD 256 for the treatment of drug-susceptible TB), with hospitalization estimated to account for 45% of total costs (Nahid et al., 2019).

The cost situation in South Africa is similar to countries where drug-susceptible and MDR-TB are treated as inpatients, for example Estonia (USD 10,880) and Russia (Tomsk region, USD 14,657). These high costs contrast with the lower costs in countries where MDR-TB is treated in outpatient clinics and at home, such as Peru (USD 2,423) and the Philippines (USD 3,613). In Estonia and Russia, hospital costs accounted for 43% and 52% of the total cost of treating an MDR-TB patient, respectively. It is estimated that the global average cost per patient for MDR-TB treatment is US$13,259 (5th to 95th percentile US$2,797 to US$42,040) for an outpatient model and US$34,599 (5th to 95th percentile US$6,959 to US$109,154) for an inpatient model.

High hospital costs crowd out funding for cost-effective interventions, such as those targeting the social determinants of health, as well as new diagnostics and medicines that could be provided in the community or in primary care.

Globally, there are significant differences in the cost of treating patients with DOTS. In the 22 countries with high disease burden, the cost per successfully treated patient varies from less than US$100 to more than US$10,000 for standardized treatment. Even in countries with similar per capita incomes, the cost per successfully treated patient varies by a factor of 50. According to recent cost-effectiveness studies, the cost of treating an MDR-TB case ranges from nearly US$15,000 in a hospital-based program in Tomsk, Siberia, to US$2,400 in a community-based program in Lima, Peru (Manjunatha & Smith, 2015).

The failure to adequately prioritize MDR-TB or achieve adequate cure rates is a major problem, illustrated by the situation in two major countries. In India, the cure rate for MDR-TB is around 11%, and in China, only about 5% of MDR patients are treated, and the policy is entirely focused on hospital-based treatment, with high rates of relapse observed after discharge.

7.7.2.2. Efficiency and Effectiveness of Community-Based TB Treatment

There is ample evidence of the effectiveness of shifting hospital-based TB treatment to primary health care and community-based models, even for the treatment of MDR-TB. In addition to clinical effectiveness and improved outcomes, community-based models also appear to be better accepted by patients.

A more recent community-based model for TB treatment was developed in Bangladesh by BRAC, the world's largest NGO. People diagnosed with TB receive free treatment but are asked to pay a small deposit of around US$3.25 to ensure that they complete treatment. Once the treatment is successfully completed, the money is refunded. The cost of treatment per patient in 2010 amounted to 312 US dollars. For patients who cannot afford the deposit, the community provides the guarantee, creating a social incentive to complete treatment. The program's cure rates are up to 92%, which is comparable to a government program, while the cost of the community-based program is only half that of a government program (Migliori et al., 2020).

Several countries that have transitioned from hospital-based services to primary health care or community-based settings have improved the quality and outcomes of TB treatment—for example, Haiti, Latvia, Moldova, Romania, and Zambia. Ethiopia has introduced the use of health extension workers to improve access to primary health care services, including TB services, to increase treatment adherence and outcomes. Outreach village programs have also been used in rural areas. Similarly, India has used volunteers from the urban population to monitor DOTS. South Africa and Tanzania have used CHWs to expand access to TB services, and Rwanda has achieved effective community-based treatment. In addition to community-based care, a public-private mix with NGOs has been used in India, South Africa, and beyond, to expand access to TB services and improve outcomes.

For drug-susceptible TB, there is preliminary evidence that outpatient treatment in the community is no worse than inpatient care. Although current guidelines recommend isolating MDR-TB patients until smear or culture conversion, community-based treatment of drug-resistant TB is gaining acceptance due to its cost-effectiveness and the shortage of long-term hospital beds, as seen in South Africa.

The benefits of moving from facility-based services to community-based care are significant. In six studies, in which the outcomes of community-based and facility-based TB care were similar, the costs of community-based care were 33–70% lower (Figure 7.5). In the four countries where the outcomes of community-based and facility-based TB care were better, costs were 32–77% lower.

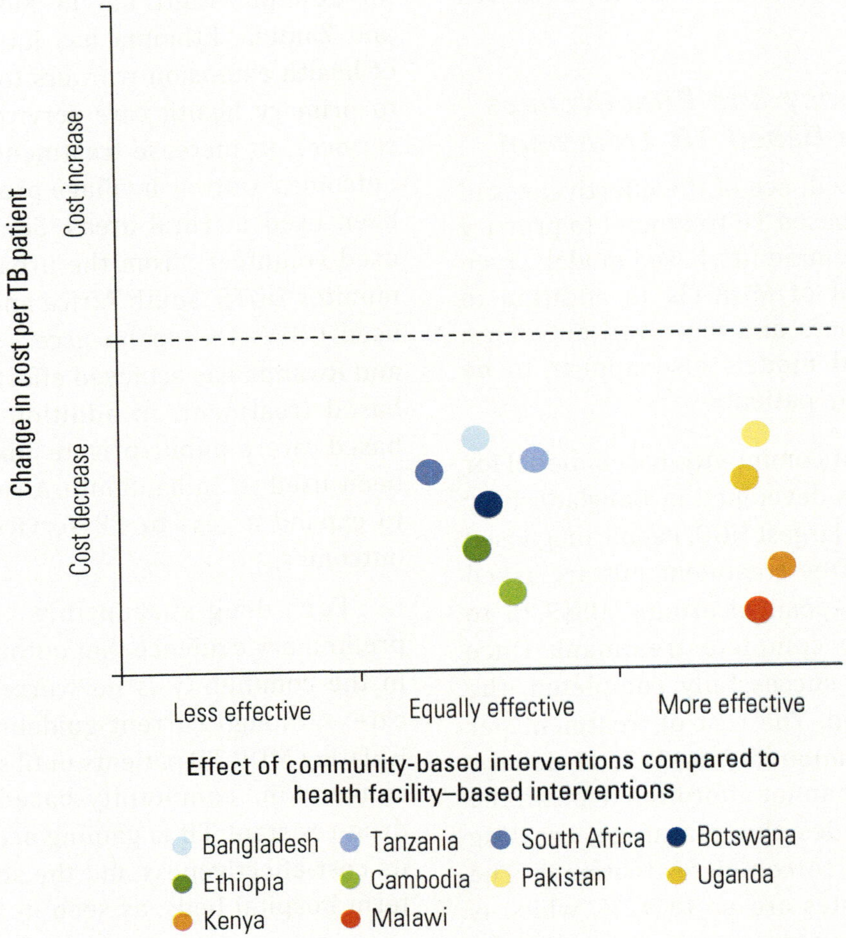

Figure 7.5. *Cost-effectiveness of community-based interventions compared to health facilities for TB treatment in selected countries.*

Source: http://www.ncbi.nlm.nih.gov/books/NBK525174/figure/ch11.sec7.fig5/.

Community-based DOTS treatment in Tanzania reduced costs by 35%: from US$203 per patient treated in a health center to US$128 per patient treated in the community, with nearly identical treatment outcomes. This program lowered costs by reducing the number of clinic visits (Makarov et al., 2014). In Malawi and Kenya, switching to a community-based model reduced costs even more: 67% and 77%, respectively (Table 7.6).

Table 7.6. *Costs and Effectiveness Comparing Community-based TB Care to Health Facility-based TB Care*

Study	Study Country	Community Cost (2012. US$)	Health Facility Cost (2012 US$)	Percent Difference in Cost per Patient	Effectiveness of Community-based Care vs. Health Facility-Based Care
Islam et al. (2002)	Bangladesh	172.80	259.20	33	Similar
Wandwalo, Robberstad, & Morkve (2005)	Tanzania	216.10	331.90	35	Similar
Dick & Henchie (1998)	South Africa	1,296.10	2,073.10	37	Similar
Moalosi et al. (2003)	Botswana	5,135.90	8,543.40	40	Similar
Datiko & Lindtjørn (2010)	Ethiopia	138.00	332.70	59	Similar
Pichenda et al. (2012)	Cambodia	639.30	2,131.10	70	Similar
Khan & Khowaja (2012)	Pakistan	320.83	471.16	32	Higher
Okello et al. (2003)	Uganda	796.52	1,405.63	43	Higher
Nganda et al. (2003)	Kenya	752.65	2,250.51	67	Higher
Floyd et al. (2003)	Malawi	1,040.94	4,477.99	77	Higher

7.7.2.3. Human Resource Challenges to Community-Based Care

Despite these findings, many countries have not yet moved to community-based models of TB care. Barriers to the adoption of innovative models of care are often related to health system governance, organization, and financing, funding streams (external and domestic) that reinforce vertical programming, provider payment systems that spend a large proportion of the budget on structures and inputs (hospitals and hospital activities) rather than health outcomes, and health workers who lack appropriate skills (particularly trained CHWs, who form the basis of community-based service delivery). A general reluctance to adopt innovations may also hinder the transition to community-based models, including public-private partnerships, which have helped improve outcomes while reducing costs in several countries (Lu et al., 2019).

Both active case finding and community-based TB treatment models require competent and motivated health workers, both in health facilities and in communities. The factors influencing patient adherence to treatment are complex and are related both to patients' willingness and ability to seek medical care and to their experiences within the health system. Clinical staff, who have limited resources, must provide accurate information to their patients and facilitate their access to quality treatment and consistently take it until they are cured.

Inadequate staff capacity remains a major barrier to TB control in the health system, particularly for MDR-TB, which requires longer and more complex interventions than drug-susceptible TB. Several factors such as weak planning, absolute shortage of health workers, limited training, inadequate skills, lack of incentives to motivate and retain staff, and inappropriate distribution of available health workers have contributed to the human resource crisis facing global TB control efforts.

While community-based TB treatment requires initial investments, including training, supervision, and management of CHWs, these initial investments are usually offset in the long term by the savings resulting from community-based treatment instead of hospital-based treatment (Lun et al., 2013).

7.7.2.4. Private Sector Challenges

In some countries with a high burden of disease, such as India, care provided by the private sector outweighs that provided by the public sector. In India, about 75% of health care is provided by the private sector, mostly on the basis of OOP payments. In many countries, a high proportion of healthcare providers are not medically trained, and adequate care is therefore often not provided. Patients with TB often seek out private providers first and may consult three to five providers before receiving a correct diagnosis of TB, extending the average time in starting treatment to 60–66 days.

In studies of surrogate patients who go to the doctor with cardinal symptoms of TB, correct diagnosis by doctors is only about one-third, and a survey of doctors on how they would treat a patient newly diagnosed with TB found that no more than one-third recommend the standard WHO treatment protocol. In this context, private doctors often do not register TB patients with the health system. Without notification, it is difficult for state and national TB programs to plan and improve TB control. These countries need to improve communication between private providers and the health system. Innovative approaches in India and Pakistan include creating public-private hybrids using interface organizations and information technology to improve TB treatment (Li et al., 2019).

7.7.2.5. From Vertical to Targeted, Integrated Delivery

Another challenge for the provision of TB services is the dominance of vertically organized and funded TB programs supported by external institutions and which bypass, rather than strengthen, weak health systems in LMICs in an effort to provide accessible and quality TB services.

The integrated provision of services has proven to be advantageous. By 2008, TB services were provided at the primary health care level in 20 of the 22 countries with high TB burden, and 83% of the 173 countries reported progress in TB control. However, these services were not effectively integrated with other disease control programs as part of comprehensive primary health care. In Cambodia, hospital-based DOTS care was the norm until stronger primary health care enabled the introduction of integrated community-based TB services. Similarly, the National Rural Health Mission in India has expanded integrated service delivery, including the rapid expansion of child health, TB and combined TB and HIV/AIDS services. Thailand expanded access to TB services in primary health care, as part of universal health coverage. In Vietnam, TB control services, previously operated through a vertical network, are now embedded in general health services. Integration between different health care sectors — for example, between civilian health care and prison health care — has been shown to improve patient outcomes.

Vertical delivery of TB services is particularly inefficient when TB and HIV/AIDS epidemics occur simultaneously. As noted above, the burden of TB and HIV/AIDS co-infection is substantial, particularly in sub-Saharan Africa, and there is a demonstrated need to integrate TB and HIV/AIDS services. New findings point to the advantages of integrating TB control with HIV/AIDS control and other targeted programs in primary health care. Integration improves outcomes — for example, through concurrent screening or by providing cotrimoxazole in routine TB care or isoniazid in routine HIV/AIDS care and in voluntary counseling and testing centers (Louw et al., 2011).

Treatment for both TB and HIV/AIDS should be integrated in the clinic as a standardized treatment package, with support for treatment adherence and HIV/AIDS resistance testing. It is important that all HIV-positive people are tested for TB. In 2004, WHO introduced integrated activities to improve the prevention, diagnosis, and treatment of TB in people living with HIV/AIDS, but success has been mixed. Creating positive synergies through effective integration of TB control with HIV/AIDS and other targeted programs is arduous. Integration must be location- and service-specific.

While the integration of diagnostic and laboratory services makes a lot of sense, the integration of patients with undiagnosed TB into health clinics and hospitals without adequate infection control measures poses a serious risk to people living with HIV/AIDS. An expected consequence of integrating HIV/AIDS and TB treatment is also that immunocompromised HIV-positive patients will be exposed to undiagnosed TB.

For effective TB control, health systems need to work with sectors that address the social determinants of health. However, it has been argued that the programmatic and biomedical focus promoted by DOTS may have hindered intersectoral collaboration and effective coverage of vulnerable populations in some cases, geographically concentrated groups, high-risk groups such as women, children, and young people, and disenfranchised population groups, for example people incarcerated in prisons.

7.7.3. Stronger Supply Chains

A robust and well-functioning supply chain is a complex but essential part of any country's healthcare system. An uninterrupted supply of high-quality medicines is essential to effectively treat TB and prevent transmission of the disease or the development of drug-resistant strains. Weak supply chain management systems with inadequate demand forecasting, ineffective drug procurement, long procurement cycles, substandard drugs and delays in the supply of diagnostics and drugs have led to treatment interruptions and exacerbated the epidemics of drug-resistant and MDR-TB. The lack of availability or poor quality of TB drugs in public clinics run by national TB programs or in private facilities causes patients to skip doses, increasing the risk of relapse and the emergence of drug-resistant forms of the disease.

Missing TB drugs have many causes — while some supply shortages are due to poor planning, distribution bottlenecks and lack of transparency in demand, some drugs have global shortages. The problem of global shortages affects many antimicrobials, particularly generic injectable agents. If a manufacturer has problems with the quality or production, global shortages can very often occur due to the small number of manufacturers.

7.7.3.1. Global Supply Chain

The global supply chain of TB drugs, from manufacturer to patient, can be divided into two distinct segments: the upstream supply chain (global supply chain) and the in-country supply chain (Figure 7.6). The global or upstream segment consists of the processes related to global demand forecasting, procurement, and financing. The in-country segment includes the quantification of demand by national TB programs, procurement by ministries of health, stockpiling, distribution, and collection of information on patients in relation to treatment and future demand.

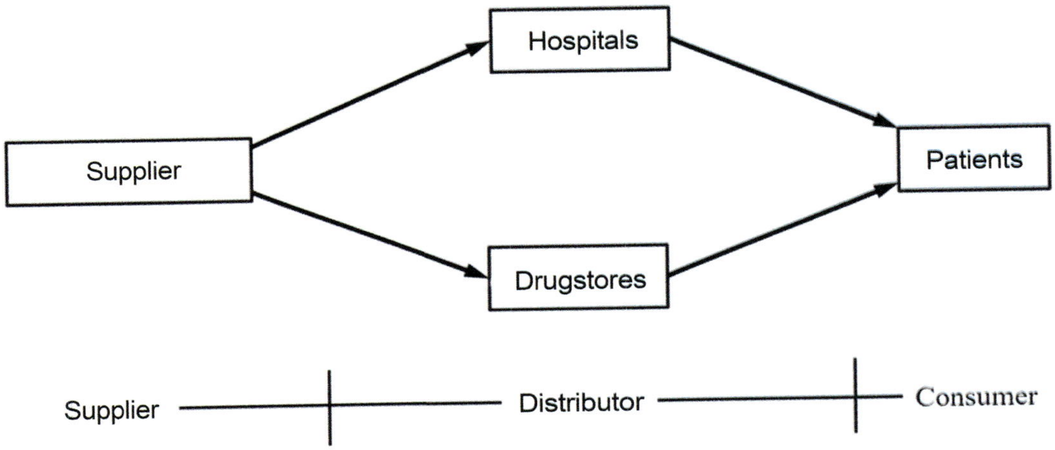

Figure 7.6. *A simplified supply chain from manufacturer to patient.*

Source: https://www.researchgate.net/publication/363005042/figure/fig2/AS:11431281099271755@1669234739269/Simplified-pharmaceutical-supply-chains-in-China.ppm.

The upstream supply chain for TB drugs is riddled with market failures. All current TB drugs are no longer patent-protected, which is of little interest to large pharmaceutical companies, and as a result, there are only a few manufacturers for most drugs. In particular, the timely provision of lifesaving second-line drugs for MDR-TB has been woefully inadequate. It is estimated that less than 0.5% of MDR-TB cases in 2002–2009 were treated with drugs of known quality (Kuhn et al., 2016). TB drug shortages are common in LICs, and there are shortages even in HICs, where standard isoniazid has been unavailable for more than a year.

Apart from the lack of interest from manufacturers in these low demand drugs with limited profit potential, the small market is further fragmented by the lack of coordination of procurement between low and high demand countries. The lack of adequate quantification at country level means that there are no solid global forecasts for TB drugs. The upstream supply chain for the donor-funded portion of the TB market currently operates through a pooled procurement mechanism run by the Global Drug Facility. The Global Drug Facility attempts to coordinate orders from multiple countries, particularly from countries with lower demand. For MDR-TB medicines, it also maintains a strategic rotational stockpile to reduce supply shortages and fluctuations in orders from the manufacturer. However, the global supply chain is far from optimal and requires significant strengthening of its technical capacity to manage a small market with highly uncertain demand and a fragile supply base. It is important to examine how the global supply chain for TB drugs has evolved over time. The Green Light Committee was developed in the 2000s to approve programs that deliver MDR-TB treatments and provide access to low-cost second-line drugs. However, the Green Light Committee approved only a small number of MDR-TB treatments, resulting in long delays in obtaining approvals and drugs, limited demand for second-line drugs, and limited supply as few manufacturers offer drugs that meet the stringent approval requirements.

In a typical healthy pharmaceutical supply chain, some upstream steps such as active pharmaceutical ingredient (API) manufacturing, formulation, and packaging are performed before the buyer places an order. These forecast-driven steps result in the finished product or API manufacturer having some inventory, which shortens the time to fulfill a confirmed order.

However, in the TB drug supply chain, many of these processes are order-driven and not forecast-driven. Manufacturers hold little and if any of the finished product inventory, as well as a small inventory of active ingredients only. All the steps in the upstream supply chain only begin after a confirmed order has been received, and the order flow from the pool buyer is irregular, that is, it comes in large quantities at certain times of the year. These problems lead to sub-optimal inventory management, poor batch size planning, sub-par manufacturing of the final product, higher costs, and excessively long lead times. These issues constrain national TB programs, which cannot plan much in advance due to uncertain funding and delayed disbursement, and therefore face further delays in receiving supplies once ordered. Taken together, these factors contribute to TB drug supply shortages at the national level.

Possible mechanisms to address these issues include the creation of an accurate global demand forecasting system, the development of supply contract structures that provide limited volume guarantees to manufacturers, and a buffer stock or stockpile to smooth demand. Their applicability and cost-effectiveness depend on a careful analysis of the nature of demand uncertainty, delivery lead times and the ability of global program staff to operate these mechanisms.

Some of these mechanisms are now being used by the Global Drug Facility (Koul et al., 2007), but they require adequate technical resources. Although procurement through the Global Drug Facility can lead to better coordination and pooling of orders from many LICs, a significant portion of the TB burden is in middle-income countries that are not procured through the Global Drug Facility. Overcoming the excessive fragmentation of the global TB drug market, especially for drugs with low demand for MDR-TB, requires not only robust technical solutions but also strong political will.

7.7.3.2. In-Country Supply Chains

In HICs, although the type of health care and financing varies considerably, medicines are primarily distributed by private sector organizations. In LICs, and particularly in many of the TB-endemic countries, drugs are primarily distributed to health facilities through a central medical warehouse, regional or district warehouses, or a transport fleet owned by the government or a central medical warehouse. TB drugs funded by global donors or national governments also flow primarily through this government-operated distribution system (Figure 7.7).

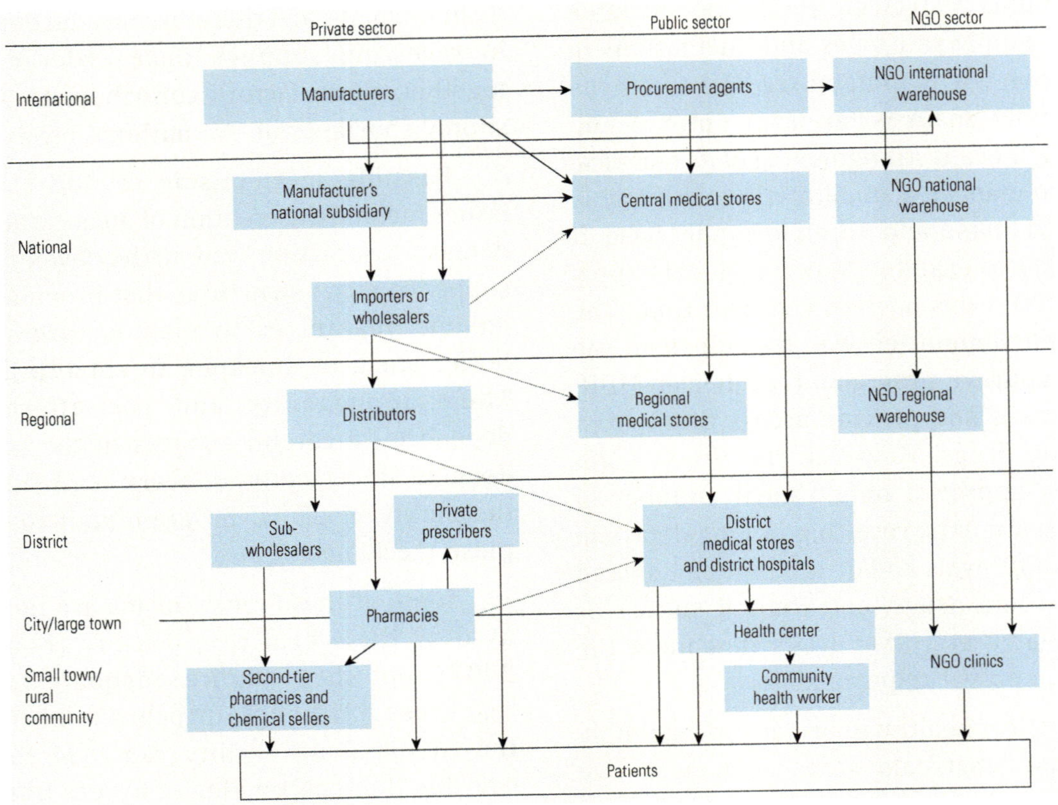

Figure 7.7. *Flow of medicines through the public, private, and NGO sector in low- and middle-income countries.*

Source: https://www.ncbi.nlm.nih.gov/books/NBK525174/figure/ch11.sec7.fig7/.

In most countries, there is a multi-level distribution structure where TB drugs are stockpiled at several levels (national, regional, district) before reaching TB clinics. The distribution system is directly aligned with the administrative structure of the health system for ease of management and control, as opposed to technical or operational requirements (Koul et al., 2011).

Successfully managing a multi-level distribution system for TB drugs is an information-intensive process. Data on stock levels at each tier, past consumption, and future orders must flow through the different levels of the system. This data is recorded in stock books, stock control cards and requisition forms at the district and health facility level but is rarely shared with the higher levels of the distribution system. The lack of consumption data prevents better planning of the overall supply. There is an urgent need for a simple and robust logistics management information system to systematically collect and report this data.

Staff must be well trained to forecast demand and place orders. However, staff in healthcare facilities are often unable to estimate the quantity of medicines needed, leading to under- or over-ordering. One solution is to deploy trained staff from district or regional delivery teams to visit the health facilities, check the stocks used, help them estimate the requirements for the next period and replenish this quantity from the stocks they carry. Zimbabwe has introduced such a system called Delivery Team Top Up, where a large-scale randomized pilot study in Zambia demonstrated that relatively simple changes to the information and commodity flow system significantly improved the availability of essential medicines. HIV/AIDS drug programs in several countries have also experimented with different variations of the distribution, request, and information flow model. TB drug distribution, unfortunately, lacks such innovation.

With the recent explosion of low-cost information technologies such as cell phones, new opportunities are available to collect and utilize information on consumption at the clinic level. However, technology will not solve all the problems related to the distribution system.

In addition to the lack of information, another key cause of poor supply chain performance is the lack of incentives: Public sector supply chains often lack the ability to reward good performance or dismiss incompetent employees, and therefore better mechanisms are needed to incentivize and motivate supply chain employees (Kawate et al., 2013). However, greater accountability in the TB drug distribution system requires more comprehensive information on stock levels and consumption data. These models have not yet been fully utilized, but they have the potential to be the backbone of planning in the supply system.

A healthy and robust supply chain for TB drugs in the private sector is as important as improving the publicly operated supply chain. A significant proportion of TB patients in countries with high disease burden, such as China and India, receive treatment in private clinics or obtain drugs from private pharmacies. In some countries, public-private models rely on the availability and quality of medicines in the private sector. While countries such as Brazil and China have created social insurance programs to help patients cover the cost of private sector services, in most countries patients pay out-of-pocket for TB treatment in the private sector.

TB drugs in the private sector are distributed through a network of importers, wholesalers, sub-wholesalers, pharmacies, and drugstores. Compared to private sector pharmaceutical supply chains in highly developed countries, private sector supply chains in most TB endemic areas are overly fragmented, with countless small wholesalers and distributors, middlemen between the manufacturer and the patient, and inadequate information and communication systems, resulting in poor coordination of the entire distribution channel. The fragmentation of the supply chain makes it difficult to achieve economies of scale and to improve or verify quality, especially given the severe resource constraints of regulatory authorities.

In some countries where pharmaceutical wholesale is highly fragmented, consolidation of wholesale and distribution in the supply chain is being driven by policies such as better enforcement of distribution practices and stricter reporting requirements. For example, when a nationwide campaign to enforce good supply practices was launched in China in 2004, the number of pharmaceutical wholesalers fell from 16,000 to 7,445.

7.7.4. Better Information Management and New Technologies

The lack of reliable and timely information hinders the organization of TB control and the effective performance of the control function by the ministries of health. In 2009, only 4 of the 22 countries with a high TB burden had well-functioning systems for recording causes of death (Hunter, 2011).

7.7.4.1. Challenges

As both a contagious and chronic disease, TB presents several challenges for the collection and management of information. First, there is the challenge of case finding and surveillance: once patients are identified, diagnosis requires a sputum smear and ideally a culture and drug sensitivity test, which is a challenge in low-income areas where good laboratory facilities are rare. Sputum smears can be taken in small clinics, but culture and DST are a specialized procedure. New diagnostic techniques, particularly GeneXpert, have greatly improved the situation and eliminate the need for a sputum smear or culture at initial diagnosis in facilities that have this equipment. However, many clinics need to send samples to other sites with equipment, and any patient found to be positive for Mtb will need further investigation to assess their response to treatment. Patients found to be rifampicin resistant must be followed up with susceptibility testing to allow for individualized therapy. It is therefore critical to collect laboratory data from all sites and sources, including GeneXpert. Newer, portable models in development (GeneXpert Omni) with potential for POC diagnostics have the ability to transmit results in real time via short message service or over the internet. Even in countries with highly developed healthcare systems such as South Africa, there are enormous problems in transmitting the data from a sputum sample to the appropriate clinic, doctor, and patient (Zumla et al., 2015).

Once a successful diagnosis has been made, patients need to be tracked in a longitudinal dataset that captures data on demographics, clinical condition, current, and previous medication, laboratory results, complications, response to treatment and treatment outcomes. In first-line TB treatment with DOTS, the recording is usually a paper register in the clinic. This usually complements other registries, including primary care visits and maternal health. While well-designed paper registers can be effective, it is usually difficult for busy staff to keep them up to date and accurate, and can result in a lot of duplicate data. This problem is exacerbated with large numbers of patients and mobile populations. Drug-resistant TB, therefore, poses a particular challenge due to the complexity of recording treatment and clinical data and long treatment times.

E-health systems are playing an increasingly important role in the treatment of TB and are particularly important for drug-resistant TB in LMICs. Labrique and others (2013) describe 12 key functions of m-health (and e-health tools in general). All of these are relevant to TB care:

- Customer education and communication to change behavior (short message service to remind customers to take medication or keep appointments).
- Sensors and point-of-care diagnostics (attachments for microscopy).
- Register and tracking of vital events (case finding and community registration).
- Data collection and reporting (collection of research data).
- Electronic (medical) health records.
- Electronic decision support (information, protocols, algorithms, checklists).
- Communication from provider to provider (telemedical consultations).
- Work and time planning of service providers (to support healthcare staff in the municipalities in caring for their patients).
- Provider education and training (web-based resources and videos on cell phone memory cards).
- Staff management (tracking of activities, patient contacts and health

worker locations).

- Supply chain management.
- Financial transactions and incentives.

7.7.4.2. New Technologies to Improve TB Information Management

Several recent e-health applications have addressed case findings. An m-health application was developed to assist non-clinical CHWs in screening patients in general medical clinics in Karachi, Pakistan. Staff used the built-in interactive questionnaire to identify symptoms and signs of TB in patients who had been coughing for two weeks or longer. In the intervention area, the number of TB cases reported to the national TB program increased from 1,569 to 3,140 cases between 2010 and 2011. CHWs in rural communities in LMICs are increasingly using m-health applications to find unknown patients with TB and other diseases.

Some groups have developed web-based electronic medical records (EMRs) for the management of drug-resistant TB, which were one of the first e-health applications for the management of TB. Partners In Health developed and launched a web-based medical record for the management of MDR-TB in Peru in 2001, which allowed physicians to view trends in laboratory data and medication changes and to generate reports for the national TB program and funders. The system was also used to collect core data for subsequent research studies after additional data collection and cleaning. For most patients, imaging data from chest X-rays taken with a digital camera were included, and psychiatric records were added later. The system was extensively evaluated to determine its performance and potential impact on the quality of data and care (Zhang, 2003).

Beginning in 2000, Peru expanded individualized treatment for drug-resistant TB, including improving laboratory facilities at the local, district, and national levels. Two e-health systems were introduced as part of the Peruvian system. The first was an early m-health application that assisted staff in collecting swab and culture data from 98 small clinics in northern Lima. The system reduced the average processing time for cultures from 23 to 8 days and for smears from 25 to 12 days and significantly reduced the number of errors. The intervention reduced the number of man-hours required to process results by 70% and was favored by all users.

Many researchers evaluated a web-based laboratory management and reporting system, eChasqui, also in Lima, in a large, randomized control trial of 1,671 patients in 44 clinics, 12 of whom were randomly assigned initial access to the system. The error rate (mainly missing results) decreased by 87% for cultures and 82% for DSTs. Wait times for cultures were reduced from a median of 8 days to 5 days and for DSTs from a median of 17 days to 11 days. In addition, the time to culture conversion was reduced by 20%. Similar results to those seen here for TB patients have been obtained for other diseases, particularly for HIV/AIDS.

Several EMR systems have been developed to support the management of MDR-TB, including the eTB Manager, which was originally developed in Brazil and is now used in many countries.

In 2008, a new EMR system was developed for the treatment of MDR-TB, based on the open-source EMR platform OpenMRS. The OpenMRS-TB system offered similar functionality to the Peruvian EMR system but was embedded in a universal EMR platform that was also used to support a range of clinical treatments, including HIV/AIDS, primary care, maternal health and oncology. It has been deployed in Haiti, Indonesia, Pakistan, and several

African countries. A version of OpenMRS-TB was developed and used in Peru for a large epidemiologic study of MDR-TB. A new version of OpenMRS-TB is currently being developed for clinical and research purposes as part of a collaboration between Partners In Health, Médecins Sans Frontières and ThoughtWorks. OpenMRS was developed as an open source software and supports open standards for coding medical data. It is also now used to support patient care in more than 40 LMICs, with versions to support the management of HIV/AIDS, maternal, and child health and, more recently, cardiac disease and primary care.

The design of OpenMRS offers several advantages for the development of research data management tools. As it focuses on the secure capture, storage, and management of clinical data, it includes auditing of data changes in the main database tables. This feature allows tracking the history of changes to data elements associated with the user's login. OpenMRS is based on a flexible data dictionary, the so-called concept dictionary, which allows new data elements to be added without changing the underlying structure of the database. The dictionary simplifies the translation and maintenance of elements in additional languages such as Spanish and has led to the development of a core dictionary that is aligned with coding standards such as ICD-10 and SNOMED-CT and is used by most users of the system. A major advantage of OpenMRS from a developer's perspective is the modular software architecture, which allows software modules from the OpenMRS module library or newly developed modules to be incorporated into the main system, adding functionality without changing the core system.

7.7.4.3. Telemedicine to Support Health Workers

While clinics can generally manage DOTS protocols for the treatment of drug-sensitive TB, the management of drug-resistant TB can be complex, particularly in patients with second-line resistance, including XDR-TB. Expertise in managing such patients is limited, which is one of the reasons why only a minority of patients receive fully effective treatment. Telemedicine is a potential strategy to support clinicians with limited knowledge of these complex treatment protocols. This can be as simple as an e-mail query to a specialist asking for advice on a particular patient's drug regimen and resistance, or a video conference with clinicians and patients. Many projects use "store-and-forward telemedicine," where text and attached images are usually sent by email. Studies have shown that even digital cameras with modest equipment can capture images of chest x-rays sufficient for the diagnosis and treatment of TB (Zhang, 2003).

Telemedicine approaches often work well in small projects but are difficult to scale up. Individual emails are not suitable for large numbers of referrals as it is difficult to ensure that all the correct information is recorded in the referral and the resulting assessment in the patient's records. A more effective approach is to share data in a secure, web-based EMR system such as Perus EMR, OpenMRS-TB or eTB Manager, which gives the remote specialist access to the individual patient's record. The remote specialist can view all clinical data, and lab results, as well as imaging and note an assessment directly in the medical record. Another challenge to scaling is that clinical expertise is limited and cannot be "spread too thinly." A more effective and scalable strategy may be to use telemedicine as part of training initiatives, along with better clinical guidelines and decision support for staff in the field.

7.7.4.4. SMS Reminders to Improve Adherence

Given the importance of good adherence in the treatment of TB and the prevention of drug resistance, there is great interest in tools and strategies to improve adherence. DOT is the best established approach, but questions have been raised about its scalability and cost. As cell phones are widely used in LMICs, m-health could provide tools to support adherence. Most work has focused on improving adherence through text messaging or interactive voice prompts. Some randomized control trials (Zhang et al., 2019) have shown improvements in adherence, but there have also been negative results.

The analysis of these studies suggests that messages tailored to the individual patient and the opportunity for patients to communicate with staff (rather than just automated prompts) improve adherence. To date, these tools have not achieved the adherence rates of effective DOT, and there is evidence of message fatigue among patients. Work continues to develop interventions based on established psychological models of behavior change and accompanied by rigorous assessment.

7.7.4.5. Information Technology to Manage Supply Chains

Another challenge in dealing with drug-resistant TB is establishing effective supply chains for medicines. Information systems are becoming increasingly important to forecast demand, track drug supplies and manage inventory in clinics.

The lack of supply of second-generation TB drugs is a key factor in the inadequate scale-up of treatment. While first-line drugs are inexpensive and usually widely available, second-line drugs are mostly used for drug-resistant TB and are often made to order. Orders must be placed months in advance to ensure continuity of treatment, and accurate forecasting is essential. Information systems can help with several steps in this process, such as forecasting, ordering, tracking supplies and managing inventory.

In Peru, the EMR was used to predict the need for drugs to treat drug-resistant TB. Combining data on the number of patients enrolled, duration of treatment, enrollment rates, and current therapies resulted in error rates of 3% or less for more than 1,000 patients in 2003 and 2004. A related study looked at medication prediction for 68 patients in the same cohort and compared it to standard manual methods. In one study, the Peruvian EMR predicted 99% of medication needs for one year, while the manual methods predicted 149% (Yee et al., 2003).

New tools are becoming available to manage supplies and inventory in LMICs. An information system for drug-resistant TB, such as eTB Manager, includes inventory management for each clinic linked to demand forecasting. These tools are now available for general use in drug forecasting. M-Health tools are also being used to track stock levels in local clinics in East Africa using text messaging (SMS for Life). They have been shown to drastically reduce stocks of malaria drugs, and are also used for TB drugs. Other systems have been developed to detect counterfeit drugs in countries such as Nigeria by allowing patients to text a unique code printed on the drug package to a toll-free number.

As mentioned above, the OpenMRS-TB EMR platform supports the management of a wide range of diseases and primary care. The use of open standards for the storage and exchange of data supports interoperability with other e-health systems, allowing systems with a variety of functions to be linked together, for example EMR systems, laboratory information systems, pharmacy systems, m-health applications, and national reporting systems such as the District Health Information System (DHIS 2).

Such approaches to e-health architecture are being used in several LMICs, including Bangladesh, India, Kenya, the Philippines and Rwanda. Many countries have now implemented DHIS 2 to collect, manage, and report on health data at district and national levels. The system can feed data directly from systems such as OpenMRS and some m-health applications, improving the accuracy and timeliness of data. Embedding the specialized data collection and analysis tools for TB care into broader e-health systems has great benefits, such as facilitating case finding through primary care visits and laboratory data, identifying potential risk factors such as diabetes, maintaining a complete and accurate medication list, and providing effective decision support based on the sharing of all relevant data.

The performance of e-health systems in LMICs and the clinical impact on TB management need to be further investigated. In addition, there is currently limited data on the cost of implementing such systems and maintaining good performance and utilization over the long term. However, there is some evidence that effective EMR and laboratory information systems in LMICs can save money by reducing errors and waste and speeding up patient management. Furthermore, it is most likely more cost-effective to embed TB management tools into existing e-health systems than to run parallel systems.

7.8. Research and Development

Winning the fight against TB requires not only new health care and health system strategies, but also technological advances that could accelerate cure, reduce transmission and incidence, and prevent disease. Despite the effectiveness of standard drugs to treat drug-sensitive TB, resistance is increasing, adherence to long treatment regimens is problematic and new drugs and therapies are needed.

Current TB therapy has many advantages: the standard drugs are remarkably safe, with low toxicity even in vulnerable populations such as pregnant women and children, full treatment is highly effective against drug-susceptible diseases, and the drugs themselves are affordable in the poorest parts of the world. Despite these advantages, first-line drugs are ineffective against MDR strains. And rifampin, perhaps the most effective agent in current first-line therapy, has pharmacologic interactions with many other drugs, particularly HIV/AIDS protease inhibitors, which are taken by many co-infected individuals.

The main limitation of the current regimen is the long time required for effective therapy, even a "short course" of chemotherapy is anything but short. Failure to complete six months of treatment results in a significant relapse rate, and as patients feel better within a few weeks, they often have little motivation to continue taking their medication. In addition, the long duration of treatment means that significant investment is required to ensure a continuous supply of medication. These requirements significantly increase the cost of an otherwise cost-effective endeavor. Combined with the training and logistics required to adequately deliver DOTS, this has led to remarkably poor outcomes and persistent treatment failures that result in millions of deaths every year. The challenge, then, is to develop not only new drugs, but ideally new regimens that are effective in treating drug-susceptible and drug-resistant TB and shorten treatment duration.

Better drugs and therapies could have a significant impact, and to increase their usefulness, they would require the following properties:

- Fast acting, thus shortening the therapy required for cure;
- Safety, so that they can be used in a wide range of patients without the need for extensive pre-testing;
- Easy to administer, preferably orally, so that no healthcare professional is required;
- Low interaction with other medications, especially antiretrovirals;
- Limited cost, making them affordable even in the poorest parts of the world.

There are two general ways to achieve these goals: optimizing the use of currently available drugs and developing completely new drugs.

Phase III clinical trials are often expensive and rare, and it will probably be impossible to test every new drug in series. There is therefore an enormous cost of developing new drugs (the average cost of developing a new drug to approval is in the order of $1 billion or more), which results in the former route, optimising the use of currently available drugs, to be the most attractive approach in making rapid changes to recommended therapy.

7.8.1. Optimizing the Use of Current Medications

Is it possible to redesign the current drug regimen to be more effective against a wider range of organisms? The evidence to date is mixed. Animal studies and pharmacokinetic observations in humans have suggested some modifications to TB therapy that could lead to better outcomes. For example, many patients receiving rifampin at the recommended dosage have low serum levels, and increasing the rifampin dose or using a different rifamycin could improve clearance of the infection. Several studies are looking at altered dosing regimens for rifampin or substitution of the long-acting drug rifapentine. When it is measured against a surrogate endpoint — conversion to culture after two months — rifapentine is no better than rifampin. In several short-term controlled trials, in which fluoroquinolones were used to shorten therapy, the failure rate to cure after two to four months was unacceptably high. None of these shortened therapies were effective enough to provide significant treatment benefits (Varela et al., 2012).

The fluoroquinolone trials included Phase III trials aiming to enable the approval of these therapies by the US Food and Drug Administration (FDA) if successful. However, conducting such a trial is an enormous undertaking. The current treatment regimen has been very successful in some patients, with a relapse rate of less than 5% in most cases. An enormous number of patients are required to demonstrate improved efficacy. Therefore, the fluoroquinolone trial was designed to demonstrate non-inferiority, a criterion that does not require the same level of evidence. Nevertheless, these trials require thousands of patients to build confidence in the results and investment in infrastructure in the low-income areas where the trials are conducted, making them extremely expensive and logistically difficult.

To reduce the costs associated with such trials, some studies are experimenting with alternative trial designs. For example, one study investigated the efficacy of the oxazolidinone linezolid. Instead of recruiting patients with drug-susceptible disease, these researchers studied patients with MDR-TB, a group in which success rates have historically been lower (Trefzer et al., 2012). They compared regimens, developed individually for each patient, with the same regimen plus linezolid. This study showed faster bacterial eradication and a lower relapse rate in patients treated with linezolid, suggesting that this drug has properties that may allow for shorter treatment, at least in this situation. However, treatment with linezolid was associated with very high toxicity, well above what patients with drug-sensitive disease could tolerate. Nevertheless, this class of agents is promising. In another study, delamanid (OPC-67683), a nitro-dihydro-imidazooxazole derivative, was found to accelerate sputum clearance of Mtb by 45% within two months, slightly better than standard treatment (30%). These studies suggest that the priority given to shortening treatment time to sputum conversion may compromise the need to ensure cure and prevent treatment failure and relapse.

7.8.2. Finding New Treatments

The development of novel active substances is in some respect better than optimizing the use of current drugs, however the duration of therapy cannot be shortened with current drugs. Additionally, since antibiotic resistance arises from mutations rather than the acquisition of broad resistance determinants, virtually all bacteria, including MDR-TB strains, should be sensitive to entirely new classes of antibiotics. However, these benefits must be weighed against the significant costs associated with the development of new drugs. Preclinical development costs tens of millions of dollars, while completing all the clinical trials required to get a drug approved can run into the hundreds of millions. It is also necessary to consider the risks, where only a small minority of compounds that enter clinical trials are approved, and many more do not make it to the clinics.

Nevertheless, the development of new drugs against TB has already achieved some notable successes (Hoagland et al., 2016). Two new drugs have recently received approval for use in humans against MDR-TB under certain conditions. Both bedaquiline and delamanid have been approved in Europe, and bedaquiline has also received FDA approval. These agents have interesting and novel mechanisms of action. Bedaquiline, a diarylquinoline, inhibits bacterial adenosine triphosphate synthesis by directly blocking the adenosine triphosphate synthase complex. Delamanid, a nitroimidazole, is converted to its active form by bacterial enzymes, which can release toxic nitric oxide. As expected for drugs with new molecular mechanisms, there is little cross-resistance to existing antibiotics (although altered activity of an efflux pump could reduce the efficacy of clofazimine and bedaquiline), however it is not clear how these agents should be used. In rather small clinical trials, bedaquiline was effective, but patients receiving the drug had a higher mortality rate for unknown reasons, largely after treatment was completed (Tima et al., 2016). Until more is known, the use of bedaquiline is likely to be restricted to people with drug-resistant TB. Less information is currently known about delamanid and its optimal use.

The path to approval of bedaquiline and delamanid is both interesting and illustrative. Both drugs have been tested in patients with MDR disease in a similar way to linezolid, by adding them to optimized therapies. Patients treated with the new drugs cleared the infection significantly faster and had lower relapse rates after stopping treatment. The small number of cases in these studies formed the basis for the "conditional" approval of both drugs for use in MDR infections. However, larger Phase III trials are required for final approval and an expanded indication for drug-susceptible diseases.

Several new therapies are currently being tested in clinical trials, such as the fluoroquinolone trials where many of these are targeting drug-susceptible TB to shorten the duration of therapy without compromising cure rates. At the time of writing, trials are planned, enrolling or ongoing to test whether treatment can be shortened to as little as two months with a variety of regimens. Of these trials, a phase III trial of pretomanid/moxifloxacin/pyrazinamide (PaMZ) was the most advanced, however, it was discontinued due to unexpected toxicity and its uncertain future.

In addition to the drugs that are either already approved or in late-stage clinical trials, several preclinical compounds are in development, including new members of existing classes, such as oxazolidinones, which may be less toxic than linezolid, as well as completely new classes of agents. Agents with novel mechanisms of action are particularly attractive, as not only are they generally effective against drug-resistant diseases, but they may also utilize pathways that allow for more rapid elimination of the disease.

However, two problems have arisen with these new compounds. First, many antibacterial active compounds appear to target a very limited number of bacterial processes, including inducing cross-resistant mutations. Therefore, there is far less diversity than desired. Secondly, and perhaps more worryingly, much is still unknown about the basic biology of infection. A major goal of new drug development is to shorten the course of therapy, however, there are no *in vitro* correlates that predict with certainty that an early-stage drug will lead to a more effective therapy. This represents a significant obstacle to drug development, and the differences in drug efficacy between laboratory studies and patients raise the question of whether *in vitro* and animal models adequately predict the most effective agents.

Do the standard markers of rapid elimination in clinical trials correlate with final treatment success? It is likely that some drugs used in TB are slower acting and are not considered effective in trials for early clearance of bacteria and, conversely, that some drugs are fast acting but do not maintain their effect and control the infection in the longer term. The lack of biomarkers for the state of viability and the extent of the TB bacillus in the host result in the necessity for larger studies (Sotgiu et al., 2015).

Even under the best of circumstances, it is unlikely that serial testing of single drugs in large trials will ever be affordable. Moreover, these drugs will never be used alone, but always in combination with other drugs, and these combinations could be more effective (or possibly less effective) than would be predicted for individual drugs. In fact, experiments in animal models suggest that some drugs may work synergistically to bring about a much faster recovery, which has led to the model of testing treatment regimens rather than individual drugs. In this model, which has been promoted by the TB Alliance, new drugs would be tested and approved in combinations. Although the properties of individual drugs may never be determined (and would not necessarily be approved as single agents in this model), this strategy would provide a much faster and more practical route to drug approval, albeit with the risk of missing information on individual agents.

Given the cost of developing new drugs and therapies and the fact that the most vulnerable populations live in the least developed countries, a huge challenge remains: how can countries afford new, more effective therapies and how can the international community help ensure they are available to populations in need? There are currently few incentives from the private sector for pharmaceutical companies to invest in TB drug development, or antibiotic development more generally, and some kind of public-private mechanism needs to be developed.

7.8.3. Developing New Vaccines

In the last two decades, renewed efforts have been made to develop vaccines against TB that would provide stronger protection than BCG. There are at least three strategies by which vaccines are being tested in clinical trials to contribute to TB control. One strategy, such as using IGRAs to detect infection with Mtb, allows the determination of vaccines that can prevent infection with TB (infection prevention trial). A second strategy is to test whether vaccines can prevent the recurrence of TB or MDR-TB after treatment (recurrence prevention trial) or possibly be used therapeutically together with chemotherapy to accelerate cure. Finally, the ultimate goal is large-scale immunization for disease prevention (POD). Approximately 40 vaccine candidates are in various stages of preclinical testing, and 15 vaccine candidates are currently in clinical trials (Sacksteder et al., 2012).

Candidates in the pipeline include (1) recombinant vaccine candidates that express Mtb antigens in BCG, adenovirus, cytomegalovirus (CMV) or other vectors; (2) genetically attenuated whole-cell Mtb strains that lack either virulence determinants or the ability to replicate; and (3) a variety of subunit protein antigen candidates with adjuvants that could be used as boosters in children or adolescents primed with BCG. All these vaccines are being tested in preclinical studies in experimental animals, and some are being tested in non-human primates.

The scientific basis for developing an effective vaccine includes (1) a comprehensive understanding of the immunologic mechanisms of protection against infection or disease; (2) molecular correlates of the mechanisms that would reduce the need for large, multi-year efficacy studies; (3) definition of the Mtb antigens that elicit these protective mechanisms; (4) means of delivery of these antigens that elicit or trigger protective rather than pathogenic responses; and (5) animal models that are more predictive of protection in humans than current models appear to be. However, none of these criteria have yet been met by a TB vaccine candidate.

Some special considerations are needed when testing vaccines. Since vaccines, unlike most drugs, are administered to healthy children or adults, their safety must be paramount. In addition, they must be tested in high TB burden sites that have laboratories capable of analyzing the immunological correlates of protection. They must not interfere with the ability to test for Mtb infection in IGRAs, and pre-exposure to environmental mycobacteria at the sites where they are tested must not interfere with the detection of protection.

Animal studies and human Mendelian genetic studies indicate that both CD4+ and CD8+ T cells, as well as IFN-γ, TNF-α and other cytokines, are necessary to protect against disease. The challenge is to determine which responses are sufficient for protection. It is unclear to what extent small animal models for TB reflect the human response to vaccine candidates. It is hoped that non-human primates will be the most informative model for human protection. Vaccine trials in humans that show at least partial protection may be the only way to fulfill these conditions. The first new candidate, MVA85A, which expresses a major Mtb antigen, 85A, in a modified vaccinia Ankara vector, was tested in a well-conducted Phase IIb trial in more than 3,000 infants in South Africa. The candidate, which was reported to induce IFN-γ and produce some protection in four animal species, failed to protect the infants from either infection or disease.

BCG is known to induce Th1 T cells and a number of cytokines — for example, IFN-γ, TNF-α, IL-12—that appear to be necessary for protection against TB in animal models and in human Mendelian gene defect studies. However, the immunological factors that are sufficient to generate protection are not yet known. It is very unlikely that large-scale studies will be conducted soon for new vaccine candidates, such as the study in southern India, which followed 360,000 people for 15 years and failed to show protection in any age group. Therefore, there is an urgent scientific need for the development of molecular "correlates of protection" that can be measured in a small number of recipients, that can predict which new vaccine candidates are likely to protect against infection and disease, and that can identify which individuals are likely to remain susceptible or relapse after treatment. In the absence of molecular markers of protection — either protecting against infection or preventing latent TB from progressing to active disease — the development of a safe, attenuated but live genetically engineered Mtb agent needs to be seriously considered. This development could be as valuable for the development of TB vaccines as live vaccines have been for malaria and enteritis vaccines.

Modeling the impact of potential new TB vaccines has been enormously valuable. They have shown that administering a more effective vaccine than BCG only to infants and children would have little impact on the epidemic, as children contribute little to transmission (Portevin et al., 2005). Modeling suggests that vaccination of adolescents, who had a high degree of protection (about 80%) in the original trials of BCG and *M. microti* in the United Kingdom, would be more effective than vaccination of infants in countries with high infection pressure. Vaccinating or boosting adolescents shortly before they reach the age of highest risk would probably have the greatest impact on the burden of disease.

Since many people in the general population need to be vaccinated to obtain sufficient statistical power for vaccine efficacy, the approach in practice is to test a smaller number of people in countries with a high disease burden to learn more about immunological parameters that may correlate with protection. For example, an experimental study with a small target population could determine whether immunization can prevent reinfection and relapse (after completion of treatment). Targeted immunization of a group of treated patients would shorten the time to find out if there is an effect on relapse and reduce the cost and time required for prevention trials in large populations. It is remarkable how little research has been devoted to the combination of chemotherapy and immunotherapy for TB.

7.8.4. Understanding the Immune Mechanisms Necessary and Sufficient for Protection

It is currently believed that a single vaccine administered at birth is unlikely to provide sufficient protection to prevent disease in adults who are at highest risk of disease. As the duration and cost of vaccine efficacy studies are very high, various strategies are being developed to gain insights into the key immune mechanisms required for protection in humans. Testing vaccine candidates in TST-negative individuals and evaluating their ability to prevent infection (as measured by IGRAs) could be accomplished in less time than disease prevention studies. As mentioned earlier, vaccinating patients after completion of drug treatment to prevent relapse or reinfection in areas of high disease burden could provide information in as little as one to two years. In all of these studies, it is important to examine multiple molecular and immunologic markers to develop correlates of protection. Finally, the most promising candidates need to be tested in small groups of volunteers to understand which of the different mechanisms each candidate triggers, which are likely to correlate with protection and which can be used as biomarkers for protection. This is where innovative study designs, such as randomized matched-pair studies, with far fewer subjects could provide meaningful information (Peyron et al., 2008).

Of importance are the older studies indicating that latent TB appears to induce sustained immune responses that provide substantial protection against the disease when compared with the risks of reinfection in TB patients who have been cured. This raises the concern that if chemotherapy kills most Mtb organisms, the susceptibility of people who have been successfully cured of TB will revert to that of naïve individuals. This suggests that the immunological value of latency may lie in the persistence of the pathogen and microbial antigens.

The duration of protective immune responses elicited by new vaccines could therefore be critical in protecting against reinfection and relapse. These results reinforce the approach of vaccinating or re-vaccinating people who have been "cured" by treatment to test whether vaccination reduces the incidence of relapse or reinfection.

Since BCG is the most widely used vaccine worldwide, especially in countries with high TB burden, the most likely vaccination strategy will be to vaccinate in early childhood with BCG or another whole-cell candidate and boost with a live attenuated TB vaccine, a vaccine with Mtb antigens expressed in a viral vector (such as an adenovirus or CMV), or a subunit vaccine containing multiple epitopes and an adjuvant. Particularly exciting are new vaccine platforms that offer the possibility of generating long-lasting immune responses to Mtb antigens. These include recombinant BCG vaccines designed to generate both CD4 and CD8 T cells (Kawate et al., 2013), attenuated TB vaccines, attenuated recombinant CMV vectors and mRNA vaccines.

It is clear that vaccine trials comparing multiple vaccine candidates in phases II and III are enormously expensive and time-consuming (in the order of 50 million US dollars per trial over a period of three to five years). Therefore, there is an urgent need to define molecular or immunological correlates of protection that would allow pre-selection of the most promising candidates from small human trials.

An alternative is to develop a safe, genetically engineered live Mtb vaccine strain that can survive long enough to allow the rapid evaluation of the efficacy of a vaccine that kills the strain but does not have the potential to cause disease. The ability of a vaccine candidate to kill the challenge strain would allow a small number of Phase II and III clinical trials to be conducted to test the efficacy of a particularly effective vaccine candidate against TB infection and disease, with Phase I trials conducted with a small number of people. Historically, all vaccines are iterative processes with continuous learning and improvement.

The development of biomarkers of protection, which would allow the identification of the most promising candidates for large clinical trials, would greatly accelerate the development of TB vaccines.

Effective new vaccines are essential for TB control, but their development, testing, and licensure require many years and significant investment.

The slow decline in TB incidence worldwide, particularly in high-burden countries, forces us to recognize that TB may not be controlled without a protective vaccine.

7.9. Financing for TB Programs

The WHO estimates that funding for the prevention, diagnosis, and treatment of TB amounts to USD 6.6 billion, of which USD 5.3 billion is for the diagnosis and treatment of drug-resistant TB and USD 1.8 billion for MDR TB. Of these funds, 84% come from domestic sources, which vary from country to country.

In 2014, 1.4 billion US dollars were provided for TB as part of development aid, a decrease of 9% compared to 2013, two-thirds of which came from the Global Fund. The WHO estimates the shortfall in funds required for the expansion of TB programs at around 2 billion US dollars. The Global Fund is the largest donor of TB aid worldwide and provides around 55% of its funding for HIV/AIDS, 27% for malaria and 18% for TB. Nevertheless, funding from the Global Fund accounts for about 50% of all current development assistance for health dedicated to TB. The United States does not have a dedicated entity for TB funding as it does for HIV/AIDS and malaria, but channels half of its $500 million in TB aid through the Global Fund; the remainder is provided bilaterally. In 2014, the Bill & Melinda Gates Foundation provided around 12.6% of total development aid for the health sector for TB. Other government donors were the United Kingdom (7.7%), France (7.0%), Germany (5.1%), Japan (3.4%), Canada (4.7%) and Australia (2.2%), and around 78% of these funds were provided by the Global Fund.

The WHO estimates that the funds required for a comprehensive approach to combating TB would be in the region of USD 8.8 billion, of which two-thirds would have to be spent on the diagnosis and treatment of drug-resistant TB and 20% on drug-resistant TB. This figure does not include the cost of research to develop new drugs, vaccines, and diagnostics, which the WHO estimates would require an additional 2.0 billion US dollars.

Given the scale of the TB epidemic, the emergence of MDR- and XDR-TB, and the need to strengthen health systems for TB, higher levels of funding will be required to scale up current efforts and enable the new approaches recommended here to dramatically reduce the incidence and transmission of the disease (Figures 7.8 and 7.9). A 2015 summary of recent recommendations from the Copenhagen Consensus Center, a consortium of international economists, suggests that additional investment in TB would be a good investment. For every US$1 invested, the return was estimated at US$43. If US$2 billion were invested to close the gap, the potential economic savings could be in the order of US$300 billion (Hariguchi et al., 2020). However, despite the increase in national and international funding, the WHO estimates the current funding gap at US$ 2.0 billion for the expansion of current measures and a further US$ 1.3 billion for research and new technologies. This leaves a funding gap of 2.7 billion US dollars per year to ensure a comprehensive response to the TB epidemic.

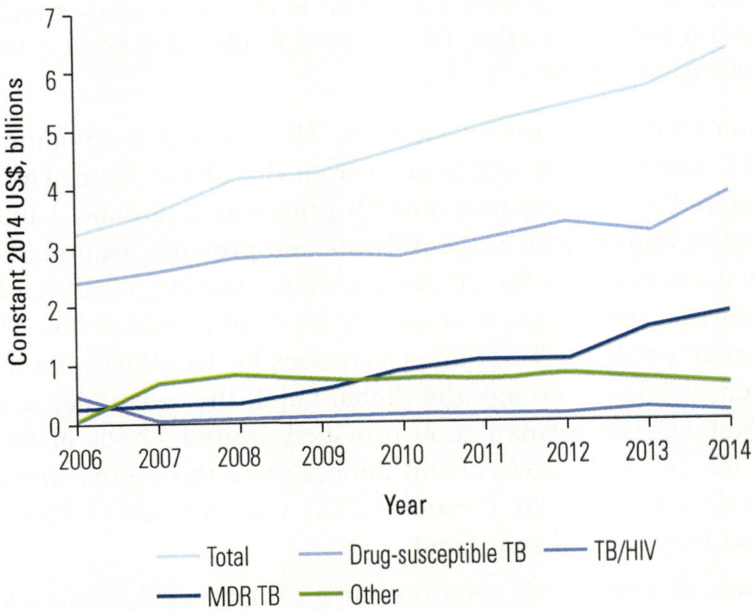

Figure 7.8. *Funding for TB prevention, diagnosis, and treatment, by intervention area, 2006–2014.*

Source: https://www.ncbi.nlm.nih.gov/books/NBK525174/figure/ch11.sec9.fig9/.

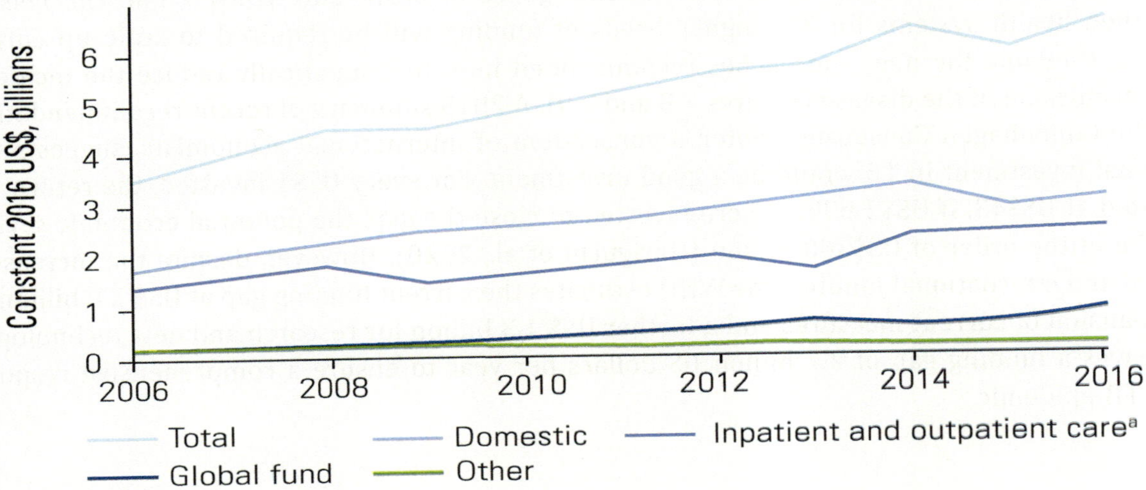

Figure 7.9. *Funding for TB prevention, diagnosis, and treatment by funding source, 2006–2016.*

Source: https://www.ncbi.nlm.nih.gov/books/NBK525174/figure/ch11.sec9.fig9/.

7.10. Economic Analyses and Cost-Effectiveness

As the pipeline for new TB diagnostic technologies expands, health, and economic evaluations are needed to inform decisions about the most promising options for different settings and patient populations. The economic evaluation of new diagnostic approaches can appear deceptively simple, but several factors should be considered if these evaluations are to provide credible and useful guidance for policy. These factors relate to both the quantification of potential impact and the estimation of costs (Grosset, 2003).

First, it is important to consider the pathway(s) through which new diagnostics are expected to lead to improved health outcomes. For example, efforts for new POC diagnostics point to the benefits of returning rapid test results, which can reduce the loss to follow-up by eliminating the need for a repeat visit. Faster diagnosis can increase the rate of treatment initiated, improve patient outcomes and reduce the risk of infection by shortening the time of contagiousness. However, shortcomings in implementation may mean that application in practice falls short of its maximum theoretical potential.

Furthermore, assessing the impact and cost-effectiveness of a new approach requires a comparison of the new approach with the status quo that it will replace. For example, a comparative evaluation of a new diagnostic approach should specify (1) where the diagnosis will be used (or example, only in centralized facilities such as district hospitals or also in peripheral health centers), (2) the sequence of tests and associated responses that will guide decision making in different groups of people or based on specific population-related factors (for example, in persons with HIV/AIDS), and (3) how the new approach will be used in different settings, for example, the current diagnostic approach in current settings, which represents the status quo comparison (that is, the extent to which bacterial cultures or drug susceptibility testing are currently used).

It is also critical to estimate the costs associated with scale-up and implementation, which are often much higher than the cost of the goods themselves or even the costs including other healthcare services utilized at the patient level (for example, the opportunity cost of the provider's time). At the simplest level, scaling new technologies is often associated with economies of scale (or costs) that relate to the shape of the average cost function relative to volume, and reflecting different mixes of fixed and variable costs at different levels. At a more complex level, achieving universal coverage of the population requires consideration of health system capacity, which constrains not only budget but also infrastructure and human and other resources. The validity of cost-effectiveness estimates depends on quantifying the costs of implementing an intervention or strategy in a way that is consistent with the benefits attributed to that intervention or strategy. Many published studies do not meet this requirement.

For diagnostic approaches, important questions should be asked about patients' pathways to treatment, the impact of a new diagnostic technology or strategy on these pathways, and potential delays or losses to follow-up, particularly as these may attenuate the expected benefits of a diagnosis. In HIV/AIDS, much attention has recently been paid to the so-called "cascade of care," and similar considerations are important in TB control interventions, including with regard to diagnosis (Ginsberg & Spigelman, 2007).

- Ø **Cost-Effectiveness of Using Xpert MTB/RIF:** Xpert MTB/RIF represents a significant technological advance in accelerating the diagnosis of TB and MDR diseases in many settings, however, it also has significant limitations. Several studies have examined the cost-effectiveness of Xpert MTB/RIF in different LMICs. A cost-effectiveness study published in 2011, which focused on India, South Africa and Uganda, estimated that Xpert devices in combination with swabs would have an incremental cost-effectiveness ratio of between US$41 and US$110 compared to the conventional use of swabs plus clinical diagnosis. A 2012 modeling study estimated the cost-effectiveness of Xpert at the regional level in sub-Saharan Africa and concluded that Xpert would reduce mortality and lower overall costs. Another 2012 study that focused on screening with Xpert before initiating ART in HIV/AIDS patients found much less favorable results, noting that the use of Xpert would cost US$5,100 per life-year saved compared to the next most attractive strategy, which included a smear and culture. A fourth study from 2012 examined the cost-effectiveness of Xpert in five southern African countries and found a cost-benefit ratio of approximately US$1,000 per DALY averted. Other studies have shown that the benefits of Xpert are lower than assumed.

The widely differing results reflect the many challenges in evaluating new diagnostic technologies and point to several areas that need further investigation. These include the extent to which frequent empiric treatment would reduce the potential benefit of Xpert technology compared to counterfactual diagnosis based on smear microscopy results. In the course of the dramatic expansion of Xpert in South Africa and other countries, further implementation challenges have come to light. These include the high overall costs associated with high coverage of Xpert, the feasibility of using Xpert at the POC, the inability to link Xpert results to health information systems, and the limitation of the potential benefits of faster diagnosis resulting from a failure to translate diagnostic improvements into faster initiation of treatment.

New technologies are needed that can be used at the point of care. Portable devices (for example, GeneXpert Omni) are currently being developed that can be used as POC diagnostic tests, however, it remains a major challenge to expand their capacity for sensitivity testing against the numerous drugs used in secondary and tertiary therapy.

7.10.1. Cost-Effectiveness of Developing New Drugs and Regimens

It is evident that investing in new TB drugs is a sound public health strategy (Zumla et al., 2015), but the substantial cost of drug development remains a major barrier to progress. Even if the efficiency of new drug development can be improved, the development of new TB drugs is likely to remain a difficult investment decision for many years to come.

The cost-effectiveness and affordability of first-line treatment for TB has long been recognized (World Bank, 1993), and there has been a focus on exploring the most cost-effective way to treat it. For countries that provide TB treatment in hospitals, studies have demonstrated the relative cost-effectiveness of outpatient treatment. Economic analyzes in other areas have focused on the provision of care through community structures and ensuring effective collaboration with the private sector. Although these studies show that the treatment of TB is feasible and cost-effective, the high cost of relatively prolonged antibiotic therapy in poorly resourced health systems is a concern, as are the high failure rates in some areas. These concerns are compounded by evidence of the significant economic and poverty-related impact of TB treatment on patients (and households). Numerous studies have found that multiple health service utilization can severely affect the economic well-being of TB patients.

The current approach to MDR-TB treatment is particularly challenging from an economic perspective, while several studies suggest that its treatment is cost-effective. A recent systematic review found that the cost per DALY prevented was lower than the gross domestic product per capita in all 14 WHO subregions studied. However, the absolute price of second-line drugs can run into the thousands of dollars even in LIC countries, increasing the total cost of the health system by three to four times. In South Africa, for example, the treatment of multidrug-resistant tuberculosis (MDR-TB) consumes more than half of the national budget allocated for TB control, with hospital treatment costs exceeding US$15,000 per patient. However, these costs can be significantly reduced by decentralizing MDR-TB treatment and care. Another potentially cost-effective approach is the use of drug susceptibility testing (DST) to confirm MDR-TB diagnoses. As highlighted earlier, culture-based DST presents a considerable challenge, particularly in facilities with limited laboratory capacity. Moreover, the economic burden of MDR-TB on households is often substantially higher than that of first-line treatment, and the financial impact can be catastrophic.

In light of these challenges, there is growing focus on developing cost-effective models for diagnosing and treating MDR-TB to expand access to treatment — for example, new outpatient models of care. In short, although current approaches to treating both drug-susceptible TB and MDR-TB are widely considered cost-effective, the relatively high cost of treatment for patients and health systems, the cost of DST, the high failure rates and the limited effectiveness of MDR-TB treatment in low- and middle-income health systems argue for investment in new TB drugs from an economic and public health perspective.

In recent years, considerable investment has been made in clinical trials of new TB drugs and therapies. The drugs under consideration impact treatment efficacy or effectiveness and cost in different ways, but the overall aim is to improve one or more of the following three dimensions:

- Reducing treatment duration; proven examples of first-line treatments include four-month moxifloxacin-based regimens and the Bangladesh regimen and bedaquiline-based regimens for MDR-TB.
- Increase treatment efficacy, particularly for MDR-TB; examples tested include delamanid and bedaquiline.
- Develop therapies that are effective for both drug-susceptible and MDR-TB. This will require new drugs to which resistance does not currently exist in most populations.

To justify and support investment, various economic and modeling efforts have explored the potential benefits of improving these dimensions of TB care in terms of cost-effectiveness, direct impact on treatment success, broader impact on transmission, and cost to patients and providers. In recent years, academic interest in both new drug investment and these analyzes has increased. At the time of writing, considerable work is already underway and much new work can be expected.

7.10.1.1. Shortening Treatment Regimens to Reduce Incidence

To date, modeling analyzes of TB treatment have focused on the population-level health benefits of investing in shortening the duration of treatment. For example, in examining first-line treatment, both Salomon and others (2006); and Abu-Raddad and others (2009) used a transmission model calibrated to the Southeast Asia region and found that the introduction of shortened regimens had a significant impact on incidence. Salomon and others (2006) concluded that non-inferior first-line two-month therapy would prevent approximately 13–21% of all new TB cases and 19–25% of TB deaths, depending on assumptions regarding the extension of current therapies over an 18-year period. The study suggests that a two- or three-fold reduction in incidence would be possible if the cost savings achieved by shortening treatment were invested in TB case detection. Abu-Raddad et al. (2009) concluded that a four-month treatment with similar efficacy to standard treatment would reduce incidence by up to 10% over a 35-year period and a two-month treatment with increased efficacy would reduce incidence by 23% over the same period. A more recent study by Fofana and others (2014) suggests a more modest but still positive effect, estimating that a four-month treatment would reduce incidence by 3% and a two-month treatment by 7% over a 10-year period.

The analysis of the economic benefits of shortened treatment is primarily based on decision analytic models of patient cohorts. A study examined a hypothetical non-inferior first-line regimen and investigated the trade-offs between drug price, treatment duration and healthcare system treatment costs for a cohort of new TB patients. This study found that a novel regimen with a four-month treatment duration costing US$1 per day would be highly cost-effective at worst and cost-saving at best, depending on the current level of treatment costs.

Ongoing work using an individual cohort model is examining these trade-offs in specific countries using primary cost data from Bangladesh, Brazil, South Africa and Tanzania (Gavalda et al., 2009). This study found that at a cost of US$1 per day, a four-month non-inferior first-line TB drug regimen would be cost-saving in South Africa (cost reduction of about 10%) and Brazil (cost reduction of 20%), highly cost-effective in Tanzania (savings of about US$120 per DALY prevented), but not cost-effective in Bangladesh. Even if the new first-line drugs cost up to US$10 and US$58 in South Africa and Brazil, respectively, while using a threshold analysis it was observed that the new TB regimen would be a cost-effective option compared to the standard regimen. This threshold price is USD 0.97 in Bangladesh and USD 1.13 in Tanzania. In all areas, the impact on health would be modest and dependent on current default rates; in areas with higher costs to the health system and the provision of TB treatment, the gains would be greatest. Unfortunately, the first first-line therapies with potentially treatment-shortening effects to emerge from trials in 2014 (moxifloxacin-based therapies) have not achieved sufficient cure rates, so these gains remain hypothetical at the time of writing.

Some also pointed to the importance of patient costs, with the greatest savings being achieved by reducing the economic burden of TB treatment on households. Savings in patient costs ranged from USD 175 (South Africa) to USD 45 (Bangladesh) depending on the setting.

7.10.1.2. Improving Therapeutic Efficacy in Patients with MDR TB

Compared to drug-resistant TB treatment regimens, there has been much less research into the potential cost-effectiveness and impact of new MDR-TB treatment regimens. In recent years, two new MDR-TB drugs (bedaquiline and delamanid) have been submitted for registration and programmatically approved by the WHO. As part of this process, an exploratory cost-effectiveness analysis was conducted using a decision analytic model for a cohort of new MDR-TB cases (Gavalda et al., 2014). These analyzes indicated that both drugs were potentially cost-effective given their impact on efficacy. However, the uncertainty about the impact of bedaquiline on mortality and, in the case of delamanid, the lack of randomization in the evaluation of long-term outcomes associated with the potential cardiotoxic effects have raised concerns. DALYs avoided varied by country, with countries that had already achieved good results benefiting less. However, the increased efficacy, even without shortening treatment, also led to a reduction in costs in some cases by reducing the need for re-treatment of MDR-TB and treatment of chronic cases. The results for LIC countries were less certain, as the potential benefits of increased efficiency for transmission were not considered, no definitive conclusion could be drawn for these countries.

In the case of bedaquiline, the impact of shortening MDR-TB treatment on cost-effectiveness was also investigated, as the study results indicated that the time to sustained sputum conversion could be shortened. When investigating shortening treatment by two months, the cost-effectiveness analysis showed cost savings at current drug prices. However, the extent of the cost savings depended on the length of hospitalization during treatment. The benefit in terms of avoided DALYS was less clear due to the trade-off between reducing the failure rate and the cure rate. Further studies with an integrated economic analysis are underway testing the use of bedaquiline as part of a nine-month MDR-TB regimen, the STREAM (Standardized Treatment Regimen of Anti-TB Drugs for Patients with Multi-Drug-Resistant TB) Trial. In 2016, the WHO recommended the new shortened regimen, which promises both lower drug prices and lower costs for the healthcare system while being just as effective as longer-term treatment.

7.10.1.3. Developing New Drugs for Treating Drug-Susceptible and MDR TB as First-Line Therapies

In the case of the drugs discussed here, the economic and health benefits of shortening the duration of treatment and improving efficacy have primarily been investigated to date. However, new drugs or regimens that are suitable for the treatment of both drug-susceptible and rifampicin-resistant TB could also be of great benefit. One example is PaMZ, a trial that is currently on hold. This new treatment regimen was hypothesized to have dual benefits: a shortened first-line treatment for drug-susceptible patients (four months) with efficacy non-inferior to the current standard treatment, and a shortened second-line treatment for patients with rifampicin-resistant TB (six months) with efficacy non-inferior to the first-line treatment for drug-susceptible TB patients. In this case, the introduction of the new regimen could lead to significant cost savings (at least 35%) from a societal perspective. The average cost per presumptive TB patient in South Africa was reduced by US$23 (28%) for treatment-related healthcare costs and US$42 (42%) for treatment-related patient costs. When the introduction of PaMZ was modeled in a cohort of only rifampicin-resistant patients, both the cost reduction and impact gains were greater. The clinical safety and efficacy of this new regimen remains to be determined, but the economic modeling can be applied to any new regimen that is effective for the treatment of both drug-resistant and drug-susceptible TB.

This model can be extended to explore the gains from a drug with the following optimal characteristics in all dimensions:

- Short duration (two weeks maximum shortening);
- High efficacy (95% cure rate for drug-susceptible TB, 85% for rifampicin-resistant TB);

- Ability to treat all forms of TB (that is, with no circulating resistance and no need for initial DST);
- Drug prices are set at US$5 per day.

Using the same model, some found that such a drug would be cost saving in an environment such as South Africa. Even with comparatively high daily costs compared to current treatment, these authors estimated a potential 51% reduction in overall TB diagnosis and treatment costs from a societal perspective when modeling a cohort of 10,000 presumptive TB patients. This is primarily a gain on the patient's side, including a reduction in direct treatment costs and a faster return to full productivity. In this high HIV/AIDS prevalence environment, there is a slight increase in ART-related costs (from a health care perspective) of 4% and an increase in DALYs avoided of 6.5%, primarily due to a reduction in treatment failures and an increase in cure rates among individuals with MDR-TB.

In summary, while much of the evidence on the potential economic and health benefits of investing in new TB drugs is based on models, emerging evidence suggests that reducing treatment duration, improving efficacy and expanding the scope of TB drugs has the potential for significant economic and health benefits in most situations (Table 7.7). In a field where there have been no new drugs in all but the last half century, the challenges in biomedicine and drug development cannot be underestimated, but new drugs are now being tested and much work is expected in the coming years to refine and validate these emerging predictions.

Table 7.7. *Population Impact, Patient Impact, Cost, and Cost-Effectiveness of New TB Drugs*

Study and Goal	Regimen	Setting	Time Horizon	Impact (Reduction)	Cost	Cost-Effectiveness
Shortening Treatment Duration						
Salomon et al. (2006)	First-line, 2 month	South-East Asia	2012–30: 18 years	13–21% incidence; 19–25% mortality	–	–
Abu-Raddad et al. (2009)	First-line, 4 month, noninferior to standard	South-East Asia	2015–50: 35 years	10% incidence	–	–
–	First-line, 2 month, 90% efficacy in drug-resistant cases.	–	–	23% incidence	–	–
–	First-line, 10 days, 90% efficacy in drug-resistant cases.	–	–	27% incidence	–	–

Fofana et al. (2014)	First-line, 4 month, noninferior to standard First-line, 2 month, noninferior to standard First-line, 2 weeks, noninferior to standard.	Global, nonspecific	10 years	1.9% incidence; 3.5% mortality 4.3% incidence; 7.5% mortality 6.7% incidence; 13.1% mortality.	–	–
Owens, Fofana, & Dowdy (2013)	First-line, 4 month, noninferior to standard, US$1 per day.	Global, nonspecific	Cohort lifetime	7.9 DALYs averted (100 cohort).	Health service cost: cost saving to US$5,900 (2012).	Highly cost-effective to cost saving, depending on current treatment costs.
–	First-line, 2 month, noninferior to standard, US$5 per day.	–	–	14.6 DALYs averted (100 cohort).	Health service cost: cost saving to US$20,200 (2012).	Cost saving
Trajman et al. (2016).	First-line, 4 month, noninferior to standard, US$1 per day.	South Africa	Cohort lifetime	Equivalent effect	10% societal cost reduction.	Cost saving
–	–	Brazil	–	–	20% societal cost reduction	Cost saving
–	–	Bangladesh	–	–	3.5% cost increase	Not cost-effective (ICER: 997)
–	–	Tanzania	–	–	Cost neutral	Cost-effective (ICER: 120)
Increasing Efficacy for MDR-TB Treatment						

Vassall (2013)	Bedaquiline	China, Estonia, Nepal, Russian Federation, Peru, Philippines.	Cohort lifetime	Varied by setting from 0.94 to 5.27 incremental DALYs, depending on current treatment success.	Varied by setting from US$823 to US$2,930, depending on ability to reduce retreatment costs.	Varied from US$202 to US$2,042 per DALY averted; likely to be cost-effective in all settings except low income, but ICER highly uncertain, depending on assumptions regarding trial results.
Vassall (2013)	Delamanid	China, Estonia, Nepal, Russian Federation, Peru, the Philippines.	Cohort lifetime	Varied by setting from 0.94 to 1.65 incremental DALYs depending on current treatment success.	Varied by setting from US$757 to US$2,548	Varied from US$501 to US$1,654 per DALY averted; likely to be cost-effective in all settings except low income, but ICER highly uncertain, depending on assumptions regarding trial results.
Developing Regimens that are Effective in Both Drug-Susceptible and MDR-TB						
Gomez et al. (2016)	First- (4 month) and second-line (6 month), PaMZ, noninferior to standard for first-line and equivalent to first-line treatment of drug-sensitive TB for MDR patients, less than US$1 per day.	South Africa	Cohort lifetime	Equivalent effect estimated, presumptive TB cohort 16% increase in DALYs averted, MDR cohort.	35% societal cost reduction 60% societal cost reduction.	Cost saving Cost saving
Future Developments						

Gomez et al. (2016)	Optimal: first- and second-line, 2 weeks, high efficacy, US$5 per day, no extra DST.	South Africa	Cohort lifetime	6.5% increase in DALYs averted	51% societal cost reduction; 58.1% patient costs reduction; 56.5% treatment costs reduction; no change in diagnosis costs.	Cost saving

Note: DALY: Disability-adjusted life year; ICER: incremental cost-effectiveness ratio; MDR: multidrug resistant; TB: Tuberculosis; PaMZ: pretomanid/moxifloxacin/pyrazinamide; DST: drug-sensitivity testing; and – = not available.

7.10.1.4. Costs to Patients of TB Treatment

The cost of diagnosis and several months of treatment for TB can be catastrophic for patients and their families. Data on patient costs in LMICs are limited and incomplete. In a systematic analysis of 11 publications on patient costs in eight African countries, it was estimated that patients' average prediagnostic costs ranged from US$36 to US$196, equivalent to 10.4% and 35.0% of their annual income, respectively. Patients' average treatment costs ranged from US$3 to US$662, equivalent to 0.2–30.0% of their annual income. Pre-diagnosis household costs accounted for 13–18.8% of patients' annual household income, while total household treatment costs ranged from US$26 to US$662, representing 2.9–9.3% of annual household income. Consequently, 18 to 61 of patients received financial support from outside their household to cope with TB treatment costs. In South Africa, patient costs for MDR-TB diagnosis and treatment were even more expensive: only 3 patients were still employed, and disability grants were the main source of income for 44 of patients (Philips & Ernst, 2012). Many of the patients reported having no source of income before (56%) and during (47%) treatment. These costs were likely to be catastrophic for many patients.

7.10.2. Modeling the Impact of New Vaccines

In the last 10 years, investment in the development of TB vaccines has increased significantly: More than 14 TB vaccine candidates have been tested in 50 human trials and funded with more than 600 million US dollars. Despite the significant cost of vaccine development, the complex task of selecting vaccine candidates must now be addressed. Therefore, efforts are underway to determine globally acceptable criteria for distinguishing and subsequently retaining the most promising candidates in the vaccine pipeline (Pawlowski et al., 2012).

Mathematical modeling can be used to differentiate candidates based on the potential impact that different vaccine characteristics targeting different populations could have on future TB burden. For example, modeling of the impact of vaccines targeting uninfected young children in Southeast Asia found that a novel vaccine introduced in 2015 could prevent more than 40% of the TB burden by 2050 and that such a vaccine would need to be effective in both uninfected and latently infected individuals to most rapidly reduce the TB burden. Linking this work to the economics of TB vaccines has shown that different TB vaccine profiles can also be cost-effective. However, it remains unclear how different vaccine characteristics (efficacy, duration of protection) and target group strategies (age, HIV/AIDS status) can be combined to maximize impact in countries with the highest TB burden.

The economic aspects of TB vaccines are also unclear, for example, depending on the vaccine profile, the likely price of administration and the dose of the vaccine is uncertain. Infant TB vaccines could be integrated into the standard infant vaccination program (DTP3 = diphtheria-tetanus-pertussis), and cost estimates are readily available. However, the economics of vaccinating adolescents and the elderly are largely unknown, and only recently have these populations been considered as a new platform for other vaccines such as human papillomavirus or measles booster. With these and other potential vaccines (for example, against measles, human papillomavirus or a future HIV/AIDS vaccine), increasing numbers of adolescents are likely to be vaccinated through schools in the future, which could reduce costs. Due to the widespread prevalence of TB infection in high-burden areas, adult TB vaccines can be used in mass prevention campaigns. There are few precedents for such campaigns, and there is controversy about what the coverage might be. Similarly, the lack of uptake of frequent mass campaigns could limit the potential impact of an adult TB vaccine. Finally, it is possible that vaccines could be targeted at patients being treated with TB or MDR-TB to either shorten treatment time or prevent relapse after drug treatment.

Some examined a wide range of vaccine profiles to understand which type of vaccine profile, targeting which age group, would have the greatest impact on TB incidence in LMICs. Vaccine profiles were defined by both efficacy and duration of protection, ranging from 40% to 80% and from five years to lifelong, respectively. It was assumed that the vaccine would be introduced in 2024. A comparison was then made between the targeted vaccination of infants and the targeted vaccination of adolescents or adults in mass campaigns. A new TB vaccine would likely be used as a booster for BCG due to the widespread use of BCG and its effectiveness in infants. The vaccine has been hypothesized to prevent active disease in both uninfected and latently infected individuals, with 40% less efficacy in individuals with HIV/AIDS. The "uptake" of the vaccine was modeled with an exact duration of protection. Each country was modeled separately, using calibration methods to capture uncertainty in both natural history parameters and TB burden data. Vaccination coverage was taken from similar mass campaigns in each country, for example for rubella, and was assumed to be at a frequency of 10 years or the duration of protection (whichever is shorter) from 2024. The cost-effectiveness was defined as cost per DALY prevented compared to gross national income per capita from a health sector perspective, with vaccine prices scaled by income group.

By estimating the TB burden in all LMICs for which data were available, the model was able to predict that a vaccine targeting adolescents or adults would have a much greater impact on TB burden before 2050 than a vaccine targeting young children (Figure 7.10) (Nahid et al., 2019). This is due to the difference in disease burden between these two age groups, with infants suffering higher levels of extrapulmonary TB and therefore contributing less to transmission. This conclusion also holds for the period 2024–2050, even considering the lifetime duration of protection.

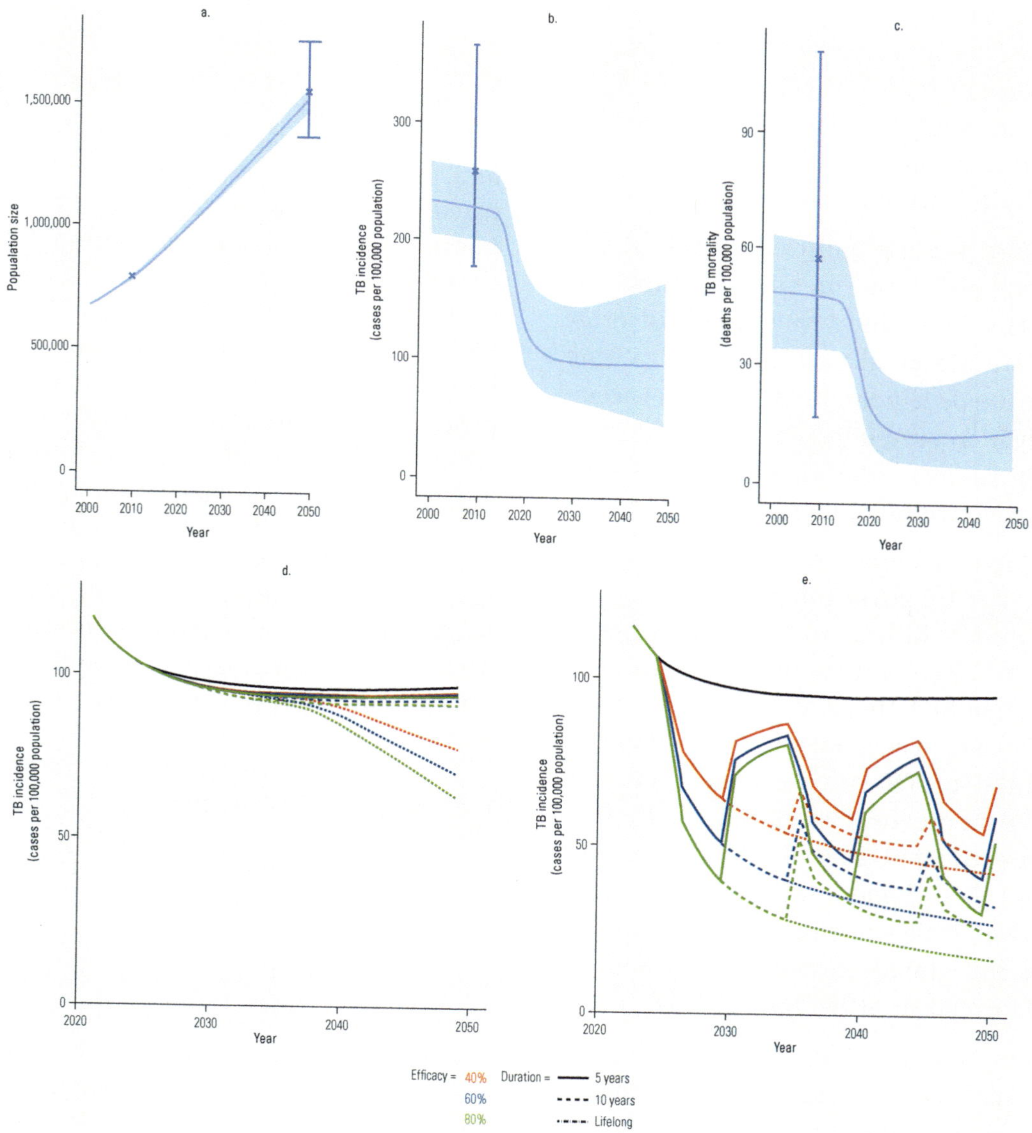

Figure 7.10. *Model calibration and vaccine impact in low-income countries.*

Source: https://www.ncbi.nlm.nih.gov/books/NBK525174/figure/ch11.sec1.fig10/.

Many reported that vaccines targeting adolescents or adults could be cost-effective at $149 (95% cost savings from $387) per DALY prevented at a cost of $1 per dose for a 10-year duration of protection and 60% efficacy in LICs. The same profile targeting infants would prevent only 0.89 (0.42–1.58) million TB cases, while 17 (11–24) million TB cases could be prevented in adolescents or adults and would not be considered cost-effective at a cost of US $1,692 (US $634–US $4,603) per DALY prevented. The threshold analysis determined the price per dose at which the vaccine profile would be cost-effective. Thus, a vaccine with a 10-year duration of protection and 60% efficacy targeting adolescents or adults could cost up to US $20 in middle-income countries and still be considered cost-effective. This reflects the large number of cases that could be prevented by targeting the age group where most cases of the disease occur and where most sources of transmission are found. Vaccines with a short duration of action (five years) and low efficacy (40%) were also found to be cost-effective when targeted at adolescents and adults.

A recent review pointed out that the development of TB vaccines is not funded to the same extent as the development of other vaccines (Mudde et al., 2022). For example, funding for the development of an Ebola vaccine was quickly increased following the 2013–2014 epidemic in Guinea, Liberia, and Sierra Leone, which claimed around 11,310 lives.

The global response to the outbreak was enormous. The US government alone allocated more than $5.4 billion to Ebola emergency response in 2015, much of which went to research, including the development of Ebola vaccines. In comparison, only US$ 85–90 million was allocated to TB vaccine development in 2015 (based on previous years' funding figures), despite an estimated 29,000 people per week dying from TB (based on 2014 mortality estimates) and little evidence of any meaningful decline in the global spread of Mtb and the continued spread of MDR- and XDR-TB.

In summary, vaccines have tremendous potential to reduce the incidence and prevalence of TB when targeting adolescents or adults, suggesting that increased investment in vaccine candidates targeting this group is warranted. Vaccines are also likely to be highly cost-effective, even if they have relatively modest clinical efficacy. Given the age-dependent risk period, special consideration should be given to the development of vaccine candidates that offer long-term protection.

7.11. Extended Cost-Effectiveness Analysis of Universal Public Financing of TB Treatment

TB causes around 28 million active infections and 480,000 deaths in India every year. The disease burden is largely concentrated in the poorer sections of the population: TB is four times more common in people from lower socioeconomic groups, and the incidence is higher in rural areas than in urban areas. Private health expenditure also accounts for a large proportion of India's total health expenditure, and most TB patients see a private physician at their first visit, resulting in significant OOP expenditure on TB. In India, as in many other countries, OOP costs for medical services are a major cause of impoverishment. For example, Kruk, Goldmann, & Galeo (2009) and Sengupta & Nundy (2005) found that about 40% of Indian households borrowed money or sold assets to pay for health care. In light of these findings, the government is increasingly taking responsibility for financing TB treatment.

Universal public financing (UPF) is when the government finances an intervention regardless of who uses it. For any given health intervention, UPF has consequences in several areas. Firstly, UPF increases the acceptance of the intervention, secondly, it removes the need for private expenditure, and finally, it provides financial risk protection (insurance) by covering catastrophic expenses that would otherwise drive households into poverty. This section examines these three consequences of UPF using the results of the Extended Cost-Effectiveness Analysis (ECEA) on the expansion of DOTs in India (Marrakchi et al., 2014).

Given the importance of OOP costs, international organizations have supported the use of health sector interventions to mitigate health-related financial risks. Despite the attention given to its significant potential as part of broader social insurance, in practice

UPF covers few interventions in most LMICs, with little consensus on what should be covered in a severely resource-constrained environment. In India, UPF has typically funded disease-specific programs (for example leprosy, HIV/AIDS, and cataract blindness) or, more recently, secondary, and tertiary care insurance schemes such as the Rashtriya Swasthya Bima Yojana and the Arogyasri program (in Andhra Pradesh). These insurance schemes are believed to provide significant financial protection as they cover the high OOP costs associated with hospitalization.

Currently, about 70% of TB cases receive DOTS treatment, with only about half of these services being free in the public sector. For various reasons, including transportation costs and waiting times, people do not always receive TB treatment in a public hospital. Most low-income people would rather go to a private doctor after working hours than take a day off without pay to go to a public hospital. Nevertheless, privately purchased TB treatment is often ineffective because private doctors do not necessarily provide standard treatment with proven efficacy. A potential benefit of the UPF is that it eliminates substandard treatments in the private sector, enabling the introduction of higher quality treatments and increasing technical efficiency. However, this requires a well-managed public sector program, which is only largely achieved in parts of India.

We have estimated the results of expanding DOTS through UPF to 90% for an Indian population of 1 million (Table 7.8). The total number of lives saved would be about 80 per 1 million per year, and the health benefits would be concentrated in the lowest two income quintiles (80%) because TB is more prevalent in these socioeconomic groups. The total amount of private spending averted by the program would be about $30,000 per 1 million population per year, and the lowest two quintiles would benefit from about 40% of the averted private spending. The total financial protection for this population sample (measured as the monetary value of insurance) would amount to around 10,000 US dollars, of which 80% would be attributable to the two lowest quintiles. The total (additional) treatment costs of the UPF for the sample would amount to around USD 65,000.

Table 7.8. *Public Financing of TB Treatment up to 90% coverage in India, by Income Quintile (Per Million Population)*

Outcome	Total	Income Quintile				
		I	II	III	IV	V
TB deaths averted	80	40	25	12	3	0
Private expenditures crowded out[a]	29	6	6	7	6	4
Insurance value[a]	9	5	2	1	1	0

This analysis illustrates how UPF can be used to improve financial protection and technical efficiency by avoiding the purchase of substandard treatments. It is only a limited view of the wider opportunities, for example, a detailed assessment could provide more comprehensive estimates of TB costs (assessing household transportation costs, income, and impact on productivity). The focus here is on the OOP costs of treatment and excludes the costs of reduced income due to the disease. To illustrate, the number of working days lost due to TB in southern India can range from 30 to 90, and the indirect costs of lost earnings can be substantial (Tahlan et al., 2012), which, in the absence of other forms of social insurance, would increase UPF insurance benefits.

A limitation of focusing on the financial cost of treatment is that people also do not seek treatment for other reasons, such as lack of information about TB and its treatment. Primary health centers in India can be difficult to reach due to poor travel conditions, overcrowding, and lack of respect for patients' dignity. Health services may not always be available, even when information and financial barriers have been removed: expanding coverage may therefore not be feasible, and the extent of subsequent health benefits of UPF may be substantially reduced without supply-side interventions. If demand for TB treatment does not match disease incidence for any of these reasons, the achievable level of coverage will be limited.

Researchers used ECEA to demonstrate that the potential health and financial risk protection benefits of UPF would primarily accrue to the low-socioeconomic populations. The reduction in OOP spending would prove beneficial as UPF displaces private financing of substandard treatments often purchased by low-income individuals. Reducing the cost of credit for this population could potentially achieve some of the health benefits of UPF, but at the cost of increasing the indebtedness (Table 7.9).

Table 7.9. *Borrowing to Finance TB Treatment in India, by Income Quintile (per million population)*

Outcome	Total	Income Quintile				
		I	II	III	IV	V
TB deaths averted	29	13	10	5	1	0
Private expenditures crowded out[a]	−25	−12	−8	−4	−1	0
Insurance value[a]	0	0	0	0	0	0

A Closer Look

Chemotherapy

Chemotherapy remains a cornerstone in the treatment of various cancers, employing cytotoxic agents to inhibit the proliferation of cancer cells. This systemic therapy is designed to target rapidly dividing cells, which is a hallmark of malignant growth. The mechanism of action typically involves disrupting DNA replication or damaging the cellular structure of cancer cells, ultimately leading to cell death. A significant advantage of chemotherapy is its ability to reach cancer cells throughout the body, making it effective for treating metastatic disease. Research conducted by the American Society of Clinical Oncology (ASCO) emphasizes the importance of tailoring chemotherapy regimens based on the specific cancer type and patient characteristics, which enhances treatment efficacy while minimizing adverse effects (Burstein et al., 2018).

The efficacy of chemotherapy can vary significantly depending on several factors, including tumor type, stage, and patient health. Recent studies, such as the meta-analysis conducted by Haller et al. (2018), revealed that while chemotherapy can prolong survival in certain cancer types, its effectiveness is notably influenced by the individual's genetic makeup. Pharmacogenomics, the study of how genes affect a person's response to drugs, is emerging as a crucial factor in personalizing chemotherapy. For instance, variations in the gene TPMT can affect a patient's response to thiopurine drugs, leading to either toxicity or inadequate treatment (Wang et al., 2019).

Despite its effectiveness, chemotherapy is often associated with a range of side effects due to its impact on normal, healthy cells, particularly those that also divide rapidly, such as those in the bone marrow, gastrointestinal tract, and hair follicles. Common side effects include nausea, vomiting, hair loss, and increased susceptibility to infections. A study by Norrie et al. (2020) highlighted the psychological impact of these side effects on patients, revealing that emotional well-being significantly influences treatment adherence. Supportive care strategies, including antiemetic therapies and counseling, have been shown to improve the overall treatment experience and quality of life for patients undergoing chemotherapy.

In recent years, there has been a growing interest in combining chemotherapy with other treatment modalities, such as immunotherapy and targeted therapy, to enhance treatment outcomes. Research by Choueiri et al. (2021) showed that the combination of chemotherapy with immune checkpoint inhibitors could lead to improved survival rates in patients with advanced melanoma and non-small cell lung cancer. This integrated approach not only targets cancer cells more effectively but also helps in overcoming resistance mechanisms that tumors often develop against single-agent therapies. As research in oncology continues to evolve, the future of chemotherapy will likely focus on personalized and combination strategies that maximize efficacy while reducing toxicity.

Summary

- Despite significant progress in recent decades, TB remains a serious global health challenge, exacerbated by the rise of MDR-TB, extensively XDR-TB, and co-infection with HIV/AIDS. While mortality rates have decreased, TB still poses a significant threat, requiring early detection, prompt treatment, and prevention strategies.
- Efforts to combat TB must focus on improving case detection, ensuring rapid initiation of effective treatment, and promoting adherence to treatment regimens. A major obstacle is the identification and treatment of asymptomatic individuals, those unaware of their TB status, or those without access to treatment, as they contribute to ongoing transmission.
- Addressing TB effectively requires a revision of global control strategies, particularly in high-burden countries, and substantial investments in health systems and research. These investments should aim to strengthen healthcare infrastructure, improve diagnostic capabilities, and enhance access to treatment and prevention services.
- Therefore, combating TB requires a multifaceted approach that addresses not only medical aspects but also social determinants of health. The prioritizing of early detection, effective treatment, and prevention strategies, can lead to the significant reduction of the global burden of TB and improve health outcomes for affected individuals.

References

1. Acharya, B., Acharya, A., Gautam, S., Ghimire, S. P., Mishra, G., Parajuli, N., & Sapkota, B. (2020). Advances in diagnosis of tuberculosis: An update into molecular diagnosis of *Mycobacterium tuberculosis*. *Molecular Biology Reports, 47*(5), 4065–4075.
2. Aggarwal, A., Parai, M. K., Shetty, N., Wallis, D., Woolhiser, L., Hastings, C., Dutta, N. K., Galaviz, S., Dhakal, R. C., Shrestha, R., et al. (2017). Development of a novel lead that targets *M. tuberculosis* polyketide synthase 13. *Cell, 170*(2), 249–259.e25.
3. Bhatt, A., Molle, V., Besra, G. S., Jacobs, W. R., Jr., & Kremer, L. (2007). The *Mycobacterium tuberculosis* FAS-II condensing enzymes: Their role in mycolic acid biosynthesis, acid-fastness, pathogenesis and in future drug development. *Molecular Microbiology, 64*(6), 1442–1454.
4. Brecik, M., Centárová, I., Mukherjee, R., Kolly, G. S., Huszár, S., Bobovská, A., Kilacsková, E., Mokošová, V., Svetlíková, Z., Šarkan, M., et al. (2015). DprE1 is a vulnerable tuberculosis drug target due to its cell wall localization. *ACS Chemical Biology, 10*(7), 1631–1636.
5. Brown, J. R., North, E. J., Hurdle, J. G., Morisseau, C., Scarborough, J. S., Sun, D., Korduláková, J., Scherman, M. S., Jones, V., Grzegorzewicz, A., et al. (2011). The structure–activity relationship of urea derivatives as anti-tuberculosis agents. *Bioorganic & Medicinal Chemistry, 19*(18), 5585–5595.
6. Campbell, E. A., Korzheva, N., Mustaev, A., Murakami, K., Nair, S., Goldfarb, A., & Darst, S. A. (2001). Structural mechanism for rifampicin inhibition of bacterial RNA polymerase. *Cell, 104*(6), 901–912.
7. Carroll, P., Faray-Kele, M. C., & Parish, T. (2011). Identifying vulnerable pathways in *Mycobacterium tuberculosis* by using a knockdown approach. *Applied and Environmental Microbiology, 77*(15), 5040–5043.

8. Chahine, E. B., Karaoui, L. R., & Mansour, H. (2014). Bedaquiline: A novel diarylquinoline for multidrug-resistant tuberculosis. *Annals of Pharmacotherapy, 48*(1), 107–115.

9. Chai, Q., Zhang, Y., & Liu, C. H. (2018). *Mycobacterium tuberculosis*: An adaptable pathogen associated with multiple human diseases. *Frontiers in Cellular and Infection Microbiology, 8*, 158.

10. Chatterji, M., Shandil, R., Manjunatha, M. R., Solapure, S., Ramachandran, V., Kumar, N., Saralaya, R., Panduga, V., Reddy, J., Kr, P., et al. (2014). 1,4-Azaindole, a potential drug candidate for treatment of tuberculosis. *Antimicrobial Agents and Chemotherapy, 58*(10), 5325–5331.

11. Chiang, C. Y., Centis, R., & Migliori, G. B. (2010). Drug-resistant tuberculosis: Past, present, future. *Respirology, 15*(3), 413–432.

12. Chikhale, R. V., Barmade, M. A., Murumkar, P. R., & Yadav, M. R. (2018). Overview of the development of DprE1 inhibitors for combating the menace of tuberculosis. *Journal of Medicinal Chemistry, 61*(20), 8563–8593.

13. Cole, S. T., Brosch, R., Parkhill, J., Garnier, T., Churcher, C., Harris, D., Gordon, S. V., Eiglmeier, K., Gas, S., Barry, C. E., 3rd, et al. (1998). Deciphering the biology of *Mycobacterium tuberculosis* from the complete genome sequence. *Nature, 393*(6685), 537–544.

14. Degiacomi, G., Benjak, A., Madacki, J., Boldrin, F., Provvedi, R., Palù, G., Kordulakova, J., Cole, S. T., & Manganelli, R. (2017). Essentiality of mmpL3 and impact of its silencing on *Mycobacterium tuberculosis* gene expression. *Scientific Reports, 7*, 43495.

15. Deidda, D., Lampis, G., Fioravanti, R., Biava, M., Porretta, G. C., Zanetti, S., & Pompei, R. (1998). Bactericidal activities of the pyrrole derivative BM212 against multidrug-resistant and intramacrophagic *Mycobacterium tuberculosis* strains. *Antimicrobial Agents and Chemotherapy, 42*(12), 3035–3037.

16. Dorhoi, A., & Kaufmann, S. H. (2015). Pathology and immune reactivity: Understanding multidimensionality in pulmonary tuberculosis. *Seminars in Immunopathology, 38*(2), 153–166.

17. Flynn, J. L., & Chan, J. (2001). Tuberculosis: Latency and reactivation. *Infection and Immunity, 69*(7), 4195–4201.

18. Gande, R., Gibson, K. J. C., Brown, A. K., Krumbach, K., Dover, L., Sahm, H., Shioyama, S., Oikawa, T., Besra, G., & Eggeling, L. (2004). Acyl-CoA carboxylases (accD2 and accD3), together with a unique polyketide synthase (Cg-pks), are key to mycolic acid biosynthesis in *Corynebacterianeae* such as *Corynebacterium glutamicum* and *Mycobacterium tuberculosis*. *Journal of Biological Chemistry, 279*(43), 44847–44857.

19. Gavalda, S., Bardou, F., Laval, F., Bon, C., Malaga, W., Chalut, C., Guilhot, C., Mourey, L., Daffé, M., & Quémard, A. (2014). The polyketide synthase Pks13 catalyzes a novel mechanism of lipid transfer in mycobacteria. *Chemical Biology, 21*(12), 1660–1669.

20. Gavalda, S., Leger, M., van der Rest, B., Stella, A., Bardou, F., Montrozier, H., Chalut, C., Burlet-Schiltz, O., Marrakchi, H., Daffe, M., et al. (2009). The Pks13/FadD32 crosstalk for the biosynthesis of mycolic acids in *Mycobacterium tuberculosis*. *Journal of Biological Chemistry, 284*(29), 19255–19264.

21. Gengenbacher, M., & Kaufmann, S. H. (2012). *Mycobacterium tuberculosis*: Success through dormancy. *FEMS Microbiology Reviews, 36*(3), 514–532.

22. Ginsberg, A. M., & Spigelman, M. (2007). Challenges in tuberculosis drug research and development. *Nature Medicine, 13*(3), 290–294.

23. Goude, R., Amin, A. G., Chatterjee, D., & Parish, T. (2009). The arabinosyltransferase EmbC is inhibited by ethambutol in *Mycobacterium tuberculosis. Antimicrobial Agents and Chemotherapy, 53*(10), 4138–4146.

24. Grosset, J. (2003). *Mycobacterium tuberculosis* in the extracellular compartment: An underestimated adversary. *Antimicrobial Agents and Chemotherapy, 47*(3), 833–836.

25. Grzegorzewicz, A. E., Pham, H., Gundi, V. A., Scherman, M. S., North, E. J., Hess, T., Jones, V., Gruppo, V., Born, S. E., Kordulakova, J., et al. (2012). Inhibition of mycolic acid transport across the *Mycobacterium tuberculosis* plasma membrane. *Nature Chemical Biology, 8*(4), 334–341.

26. Hariguchi, N., Chen, X., Hayashi, Y., Kawano, Y., Fujiwara, M., Matsuba, M., Shimizu, H., Ohba, Y., Nakamura, I., Kitamoto, R., et al. (2020). OPC-167832, a novel carbostyril derivative with potent antituberculosis activity as a DprE1 inhibitor. *Antimicrobial Agents and Chemotherapy, 64*(1), e02020-19.

27. Hunter, R. L. (2011). Pathology of post-primary tuberculosis of the lung: An illustrated critical review. *Tuberculosis, 91*(6), 497–509.

28. Huszár, S., Chibale, K., & Singh, V. (2020). The quest for the holy grail: New antitubercular chemical entities, targets and strategies. *Drug Discovery Today, 25*(5), 772–780.

29. Ioerger, T. R., O'Malley, T., Liao, R., Guinn, K. M., Hickey, M. J., Mohaideen, N., Murphy, K. C., Boshoff, H. I., Mizrahi, V., Rubin, E. J., et al. (2013). Identification of new drug targets and resistance mechanisms in *Mycobacterium tuberculosis. PLoS ONE, 8*(11), e75245.

30. Kaufmann, S. H., & Schaible, U. E. (2005). 100th anniversary of Robert Koch's Nobel Prize for the discovery of the tubercle bacillus. *Trends in Microbiology, 13*(9), 469–475.

31. Kawate, T., Iwase, N., Shimizu, M., Stanley, S. A., Wellington, S., Kazyanskaya, E., & Hung, D. T. (2013). Synthesis and structure–activity relationships of phenyl-substituted coumarins with anti-tubercular activity that target FadD32. *Bioorganic & Medicinal Chemistry Letters, 23*(21), 6052–6059.

32. Kolly, G. S., Boldrin, F., Sala, C., Dhar, N., Hartkoorn, R. C., Ventura, M., Serafini, A., McKinney, J. D., Manganelli, R., & Cole, S. T. (2014). Assessing the essentiality of the decaprenyl-phospho-D-arabinofuranose pathway in *Mycobacterium tuberculosis* using conditional mutants. *Molecular Microbiology, 92*(1), 194–211.

33. Koul, A., Arnoult, E., Lounis, N., Guillemont, J., & Andries, K. (2011). The challenge of new drug discovery for tuberculosis. *Nature, 469*(7331), 483–490.

34. Koul, A., Dendouga, N., Vergauwen, K., Molenberghs, B., Vranckx, L., Willebrords, R., Ristic, Z., Lill, H., Dorange, I., Guillemont, J., et al. (2007). Diarylquinolines target subunit c of mycobacterial ATP synthase. *Nature Chemical Biology, 3*(6), 323–324.

35. Kuhn, M. L., Alexander, E., Minasov, G., Page, H. J., Warwrzak, Z., Shuvalova, L., Flores, K. J., Wilson, D. J., Shi, C., Aldrich, C. C., et al. (2016). Structure of the essential Mtb FadD32 enzyme: A promising drug target for treating tuberculosis. *ACS Infectious Diseases, 2*(8), 579–591.

36. La Rosa, V., Poce, G., Canseco, J. O., Buroni, S., Pasca, M. R., Biava, M., Raju, R. M., Porretta, G. C., Alfonso, S., Battilocchio, C., et al. (2012). MmpL3 is the cellular target of the antitubercular pyrrole derivative BM212. *Antimicrobial Agents and Chemotherapy, 56*(1), 324–331.

37. Leung, A. N. (1999). Pulmonary tuberculosis: The essentials. *Radiology, 210*(2), 307–322.

38. Li, W., Gu, S., Fleming, J., & Bi, L. (2015). Crystal structure of FadD32, an enzyme essential for mycolic acid biosynthesis in mycobacteria. *Scientific Reports, 5*, 15493.

39. Li, W., Obregón-Henao, A., Wallach, J. B., North, E. J., Lee, R. E., Gonzalez-Juarrero, M., Schnappinger, D., & Jackson, M. (2016). Therapeutic potential of the *Mycobacterium tuberculosis* mycolic acid transporter, MmpL3. *Antimicrobial Agents and Chemotherapy, 60*(8), 5198–5207.

40. Li, W., Stevens, C. M., Pandya, A. N., Darzynkiewicz, Z. M., Bhattarai, P., Tong, W., Gonzalez-Juarrero, M., North, E. J., Zgurskaya, H. I., & Jackson, M. C. (2019). Direct inhibition of MmpL3 by novel antitubercular compounds. *ACS Infectious Diseases, 5*(8), 1001–1012.

41. Locher, C. P., Jones, S. M., Hanzelka, B. L., Perola, E., Shoen, C. M., Cynamon, M. H., Ngwane, A. H., Wiid, I. J., van Helden, P. D., Betoudji, F., et al. (2015). A novel inhibitor of gyrase B is a potent drug candidate for treatment of tuberculosis and nontuberculosis mycobacterial infections. *Antimicrobial Agents and Chemotherapy, 59*(3), 1455–1465.

42. Louw, G. E., Warren, R. M., van Pittius, N. C. G., Leon, R., Jimenez, A., Hernandez-Pando, R., McEvoy, C. R. E., Grobbelaar, M., Murray, M., van Helden, P. D., et al. (2011). Rifampicin reduces susceptibility to ofloxacin in rifampicin-resistant *Mycobacterium tuberculosis* through efflux. *American Journal of Respiratory and Critical Care Medicine, 184*(3), 269–276.

43. Lu, P., Lill, H., & Bald, D. (2014). ATP synthase in mycobacteria: Special features and implications for a function as drug target. *Biochimica et Biophysica Acta, 1837*(8), 1208–1218.

44. Lu, X., Williams, Z., Hards, K., Tang, J., Cheung, C. Y., Aung, H. L., Wang, B., Liu, Z., Hu, X., Lenaerts, A., et al. (2019). Pyrazolo[1,5-a]pyridine inhibitor of the respiratory cytochrome bcc complex for the treatment of drug-resistant tuberculosis. *ACS Infectious Diseases, 5*(2), 239–249.

45. Luies, L., & du Preez, I. (2020). The echo of pulmonary tuberculosis: Mechanisms of clinical symptoms and other disease-induced systemic complications. *Clinical Microbiology Reviews, 33*(2), e00036–20.

46. Lun, S., Guo, H., Onajole, O. K., Pieroni, M., Gunosewoyo, H., Chen, G., Tipparaju, S. K., Ammerman, N. C., Kozikowski, A. P., & Bishai, W. R. (2013). Indoleamides are active against drug-resistant *Mycobacterium tuberculosis. Nature Communications, 4*, 2907.

47. Lun, S., Xiao, S., Zhang, W., Wang, S., Gunosewoyo, H., Yu, L. F., & Bishai, W. R. (2021). Therapeutic potential of coumestan Pks13 inhibitors for tuberculosis. *Antimicrobial Agents and Chemotherapy, 65*(10), e01887–20.

48. Makarov, V., Lechartier, B., Zhang, M., Neres, J., Van Der Sar, A. M., Raadsen, S. A., Hartkoorn, R., Ryabova, O. B., Vocat, A., Decosterd, L., et al. (2014). Towards a new combination therapy for tuberculosis with next generation benzothiazinones. *EMBO Molecular Medicine, 6*(3), 372–383.

49. Makarov, V., Manina, G., Mikusova, K., Möllmann, U., Ryabova, O., Saint-Joanis, B., Dhar, N., Pasca, M. R., Buroni, S., Lucarelli, A. P., et al. (2009). Benzothiazinones kill *Mycobacterium tuberculosis* by blocking arabinan synthesis. *Science, 324*(5928), 801–804.

50. Makarov, V., Neres, J., Hartkoorn, R. C., Ryabova, O. B., Kazakova, E., Šarkan, M., Huszár, S., Piton, J., Kolly, G. S., Vocat, A., et al. (2015). The 8-pyrrole-benzothiazinones are noncovalent inhibitors of DprE1 from *Mycobacterium tuberculosis. Antimicrobial Agents and Chemotherapy, 59*(7), 4446–4452.

51. Manjunatha, U. H., & Smith, P. W. (2015). Perspective: Challenges and opportunities in TB drug discovery from phenotypic screening. *Bioorganic & Medicinal Chemistry, 23*(17), 5087–5097.

52. Marrakchi, H., Laneelle, M. A., & Daffe, M. (2014). Mycolic acids: Structures, biosynthesis, and beyond. *Chemical Biology, 21*(1), 67–85.

53. Mdluli, K., & Ma, Z. (2007). *Mycobacterium tuberculosis* DNA gyrase as a target for drug discovery. *Infectious Disorders Drug Targets, 7*(2), 159–168.

54. Mdluli, K., Kaneko, T., & Upton, A. (2015). The tuberculosis drug discovery and development pipeline and emerging drug targets. *Cold Spring Harbor Perspectives in Medicine, 5*(11), a021154.

55. Migliori, G. B., Tiberi, S., Zumla, A., Petersen, E., Chakaya, J. M., Wejse, C., Muñoz Torrico, M., Duarte, R., Alffenaar, J. W., Schaaf, H. S., et al. (2020). MDR/XDR-TB management of patients and contacts: Challenges facing the new decade. The 2020 clinical update by the Global Tuberculosis Network. *International Journal of Infectious Diseases, 92*(S1), S15–S25.

56. Mudde, S. E., Upton, A. M., Lenaerts, A., Bax, H. I., & De Steenwinkel, J. E. M. (2022). Delamanid or pretomanid? A Solomonic judgement! *Journal of Antimicrobial Chemotherapy, 77*(4), 880–902.

57. Nahid, P., Mase, S. R., Migliori, G. B., Sotgiu, G., Bothamley, G. H., Brozek, J. L., Cattamanchi, A., Cegielski, J. P., Chen, L., Daley, C. L., et al. (2019). Treatment of drug-resistant tuberculosis. An official ATS/CDC/ERS/IDSA clinical practice guideline. *American Journal of Respiratory and Critical Care Medicine, 200*(5), e93–e142.

58. Pawlowski, A., Jansson, M., Skold, M., Rottenberg, M. E., & Kallenius, G. (2012). Tuberculosis and HIV co-infection. *PLoS Pathogens, 8*(2), e1002464.

59. Pethe, K., Bifani, P., Jang, J., Kang, S., Park, S., Ahn, S., Jiricek, J., Jung, J., Jeon, H. K., Cechetto, J., et al. (2013). Discovery of Q203, a potent clinical candidate for the treatment of tuberculosis. *Nature Medicine, 19*(10), 1157–1160.

60. Peyron, P., Vaubourgeix, J., Poquet, Y., Levillain, F., Botanch, C., Bardou, F., Daffe, M., Emile, J. F., Marchou, B., Cardona, P. J., et al. (2008). Foamy macrophages from tuberculous patients' granulomas constitute a nutrient-rich reservoir for *M. tuberculosis* persistence. *PLoS Pathogens, 4*(11), e1000204.

61. Philips, J. A., & Ernst, J. D. (2012). Tuberculosis pathogenesis and immunity. *Annual Review of Pathology: Mechanisms of Disease, 7*, 353–384.

62. Portevin, D., De Sousa-D'Auria, C., Houssin, C., Grimaldi, C., Chami, M., Daffe, M., & Guilhot, C. (2004). A polyketide synthase catalyzes the last condensation step of mycolic acid biosynthesis in mycobacteria and related organisms. *Proceedings of the National Academy of Sciences USA, 101*(2), 314–319.

63. Portevin, D., de Sousa-D'Auria, C., Montrozier, H., Houssin, C., Stella, A., Laneelle, M. A., Bardou, F., Guilhot, C., & Daffe, M. (2005). The acyl-AMP ligase FadD32 and AccD4-containing acyl-CoA carboxylase are required for the synthesis of mycolic acids and essential for mycobacterial growth: Identification of the carboxylation product and determination of the acyl-CoA carboxylase components. *Journal of Biological Chemistry, 280*(10), 8862–8874.

64. Rao, S. P. S., Lakshminarayana, S. B., Kondreddi, R. R., Herve, M., Camacho, L. R., Bifani, P., Kalapala, S. K., Jiricek, J., Ma, N. L., Tan, B. H., et al. (2013). Indolcarboxamide is a preclinical candidate for treating multidrug-resistant tuberculosis. *Science Translational Medicine, 5*(214), 214ra168.

65. Rawat, R., Whitty, A., & Tonge, P. J. (2003). The isoniazid-NAD adduct is a slow, tight-binding inhibitor of InhA, the *Mycobacterium tuberculosis* enoyl reductase: Adduct affinity and drug resistance. *Proceedings of the National Academy of Sciences USA*, *100*(24), 13881–13886.

66. Reece, S. T., & Kaufmann, S. H. (2012). Floating between the poles of pathology and protection: Can we pin down the granuloma in tuberculosis? *Current Opinion in Microbiology*, *15*(1), 63–70.

67. Remuiñán, M. J., Pérez-Herrán, E., Rullás, J., Alemparte, C., Martínez-Hoyos, M., Dow, D. J., Afari, J., Mehta, N., Esquivias, J., Jiménez, E., et al. (2013). Tetrahydropyrazolo[1,5-a]pyrimidine-3-carboxamide and N-benzyl-6′,7′-dihydrospiro[piperidine-4,4′-thieno[3,2-c]pyran] analogues with bactericidal efficacy against *Mycobacterium tuberculosis* targeting MmpL3. *PLoS ONE*, *8*(7), e60933.

68. Russell, D. G., Cardona, P. J., Kim, M. J., Allain, S., & Altare, F. (2009). Foamy macrophages and the progression of the human tuberculosis granuloma. *Nature Immunology*, *10*(9), 943–948.

69. Sacksteder, K. A., Protopopova, M., Barry, C. E. III, Andries, K., & Nacy, C. A. (2012). Discovery and development of SQ109: A new antitubercular drug with a novel mechanism of action. *Future Microbiology*, *7*(7), 823–837.

70. Schluger, N. W. (2005). The pathogenesis of tuberculosis: The first 100 (and 23) years. *American Journal of Respiratory Cell and Molecular Biology*, *32*(3), 251–256.

71. Sensi, P. (1983). History of the development of rifampin. *Clinical Infectious Diseases*, *5*(Suppl. S3), S402–S406.

72. Shirude, P. S., Shandil, R. K., Manjunatha, M. R., Sadler, C., Panda, M., Panduga, V., Reddy, J., Saralaya, R., Nanduri, R., Ambady, A., et al. (2014). Lead optimization of 1,4-azaindoles as antimycobacterial agents. *Journal of Medicinal Chemistry*, *57*(14), 5728–5737.

73. Shirude, P. S., Shandil, R., Sadler, C., Naik, M., Hosagrahara, V., Hameed, S., Shinde, V., Bathula, C., Humnabadkar, V., Kumar, N., et al. (2013). Azaindoles: Noncovalent DprE1 inhibitors from scaffold morphing efforts, kill *Mycobacterium tuberculosis* and are efficacious *in vivo*. *Journal of Medicinal Chemistry*, *56*(24), 9701–9708.

74. Sotgiu, G., Centis, R., D'Ambrosio, L., & Migliori, G. B. (2015). Tuberculosis treatment and drug regimens. *Cold Spring Harbor Perspectives in Medicine*, *5*(5), a017822.

75. Stanley, S. A., Kawate, T., Iwase, N., Shimizu, M., Clatworthy, A. E., Kazyanskaya, E., Sacchettini, J. C., Ioerger, T. R., Siddiqi, N. A., Minami, S., et al. (2013). Diarylcoumarins inhibit mycolic acid biosynthesis and kill *Mycobacterium tuberculosis* by targeting FadD32. *Proceedings of the National Academy of Sciences USA*, *110*(28), 11565–11570.

76. Stec, J., Onajole, O. K., Lun, S., Guo, H., Merenbloom, B., Vistoli, G., Bishai, W. R., & Kozikowski, A. P. (2016). Indole-2-carboxamide-based MmpL3 inhibitors show exceptional antitubercular activity in an animal model of tuberculosis infection. *Journal of Medicinal Chemistry*, *59*(13), 6232–6247.

77. Stout, J. E., Koh, W. J., & Yew, W. W. (2016). Update on pulmonary disease due to non-tuberculous mycobacteria. *International Journal of Infectious Diseases*, *45*, 123–134.

78. Su, C. C., Klenotic, P. A., Bolla, J. R., Purdy, G. E., Robinson, C. V., & Yu, E. W. (2019). MmpL3 is a lipid transporter that binds trehalose monomycolate and phosphatidylethanolamine. *Proceedings of the National Academy of Sciences USA*, *116*(22), 11241–11246.

79. Sutherland, H. S., Tong, A. S., Choi, P. J., Blaser, A., Conole, D., Franzblau, S. G., Lotlikar, M.

U., Cooper, C. B., Upton, A. M., Denny, W. A., et al. (2019). 3,5-Dialkoxypyridine analogues of bedaquiline are potent antituberculosis agents with minimal inhibition of the hERG channel. *Bioorganic & Medicinal Chemistry, 27*(6), 1292–1307.

80. Tahlan, K., Wilson, R., Kastrinsky, D. B., Arora, K., Nair, V., Fischer, E., Barnes, S. W., Walker, J. R., Alland, D., Barry, C. E. III, et al. (2012). SQ109 targets MmpL3, a membrane transporter of trehalose monomycolate involved in mycolic acid donation to the cell wall core of *Mycobacterium tuberculosis. Antimicrobial Agents and Chemotherapy, 56*(4), 1797–1809.

81. Tima, H. G., Al Dulayymi, J. R., Denis, O., Lehebel, P., Baols, K. S., Mohammed, M. O., L'Homme, L., Sahb, M. M., Potemberg, G., Legrand, S., et al. (2016). Inflammatory properties and adjuvant potential of synthetic glycolipids homologous to mycolate esters of the cell wall of *Mycobacterium tuberculosis. Journal of Innate Immunity, 9*(2), 162–180.

82. Trefzer, C., Skovierova, H., Buroni, S., Bobovska, A., Nenci, S., Molteni, E., Pojer, F., Pasca, M. R., Makarov, V., Cole, S. T., et al. (2012). Benzothiazinones are suicide inhibitors of mycobacterial decaprenylphosphoryl-beta-D-ribofuranose 2'-oxidase DprE1. *Journal of the American Chemical Society, 134*(2), 912–915.

83. Varela, C., Rittmann, D., Singh, A., Krumbach, K., Bhatt, K., Eggeling, L., Besra, G. S., & Bhatt, A. (2012). MmpL genes are associated with mycolic acid metabolism in mycobacteria and corynebacteria. *Chemistry & Biology, 19*(5), 498–506.

84. Xu, Z., Meshcheryakov, V. A., Poce, G., & Chng, S. S. (2017). MmpL3 is the flippase for mycolic acids in mycobacteria. *Proceedings of the National Academy of Sciences USA, 114*(30), 7993–7998.

85. Yee, D., Valiquette, C., Pelletier, M., Parisien, I., Rocher, I., & Menzies, D. (2003). Incidence of serious side effects from first-line antituberculosis drugs among patients treated for active tuberculosis. *American Journal of Respiratory and Critical Care Medicine, 167*(11), 1472–1477.

86. Zhang, B., Li, J., Yang, X., Wu, L., Zhang, J., Yang, Y., Zhao, Y., Zhang, L., Yang, X., Yang, X., et al. (2019). Crystal structures of membrane transporter MmpL3, an anti-TB drug target. *Cell, 176*(3), 636–648.e13.

87. Zhang, W., Lun, S., Liu, L. L., Xiao, S., Duan, G., Gunosewoyo, H., Yang, F., Tang, J., Bishai, W. R., & Yu, L. F. (2019). Identification of novel coumestan derivatives as polyketide synthase 13 inhibitors against *Mycobacterium tuberculosis*. Part II. *Journal of Medicinal Chemistry, 62*(7), 3575–3589.

88. Zhang, W., Lun, S., Wang, S. H., Jiang, X. W., Yang, F., Tang, J., Manson, A. L., Earl, A. M., Gunosewoyo, H., Bishai, W. R., et al. (2018). Identification of novel coumestan derivatives as polyketide synthase 13 inhibitors against *Mycobacterium tuberculosis. Journal of Medicinal Chemistry, 61*(2), 791–803.

89. Zhang, Y., & Mitchison, D. (2003). The curious characteristics of pyrazinamide: A review. *International Journal of Tuberculosis and Lung Disease, 7*(1), 6–21.

90. Zumla, A., Chakaya, J., Centis, R., D'Ambrosio, L., Mwaba, P., Bates, M., Kapata, N., Nyirenda, T., Chanda, D., Mfinanga, S., et al. (2015). Tuberculosis treatment and management—an update on treatment regimens, trials, new drugs, and adjunct therapies. *Lancet Respiratory Medicine, 3*(3), 220–234.

91. Zumla, A., Nahid, P., & Cole, S. T. (2013). Advances in the development of new tuberculosis drugs and treatment regimens. *Nature Reviews Drug Discovery, 12*(5), 388–404.

Chapter 8

HUMAN IMMUNODEFICIENCY VIRUS INFECTION

Contents

Introduction

Human Immunodeficiency Virus (HIV) infection, despite its global impact, can be considered a rare disease in many contexts. HIV attacks the immune system, specifically targeting CD4 cells (T cells), which are crucial for the body's defense against infections. This progressive destruction of the immune system can lead to acquired immunodeficiency syndrome (AIDS), a life-threatening condition.

While HIV/AIDS has had a profound impact worldwide, its prevalence varies significantly between regions. According to the World Health Organization (WHO), approximately 37.7 million people worldwide were living with HIV/AIDS in 2020. In many high-income countries, effective prevention strategies and access to antiretroviral therapy (ART) have reduced the number of new HIV infections and AIDS-related deaths, leading to HIV/AIDS being considered a rare disease by some definitions.

In low- and middle-income countries, however, HIV/AIDS remains a significant public health challenge. Sub-Saharan Africa is the most affected region, with nearly two-thirds of all people living with HIV globally. Despite progress in expanding access to ART, many people in these regions still lack access to HIV testing, prevention, and treatment services. In addition to regional disparities, certain populations are disproportionately affected by HIV/AIDS, including homosexuality among men, people who inject drugs, sex workers, transgender people, and prisoners. Stigma, discrimination, and lack of access to healthcare are among the barriers that contribute to the continued spread of HIV in these populations (Alvarado et al., 2020).

New information has emerged from ongoing clinical observation, surveillance systems, and epidemiologic studies. In this chapter, we focus on some important aspects of the disease and the epidemic in areas where new data have either confirmed or changed initial impressions, or alternatively where a deeper understanding of the disease has emerged. These areas include the causative agent of AIDS, the proportion of seropositive persons who will develop AIDS, HIV infection as a continuum of conditions, the modalities and efficiency of HIV transmission, and the prevalence and incidence of HIV infection and dimensions of the epidemic in the United States (global epidemiology is discussed in this chapter.

Orientation and Directional Terms

Term	Definition	Illustration
T cells	A type of white blood cell that plays a central role in the immune response by directly attacking infected cells, coordinating other immune cells, or regulating the immune response.	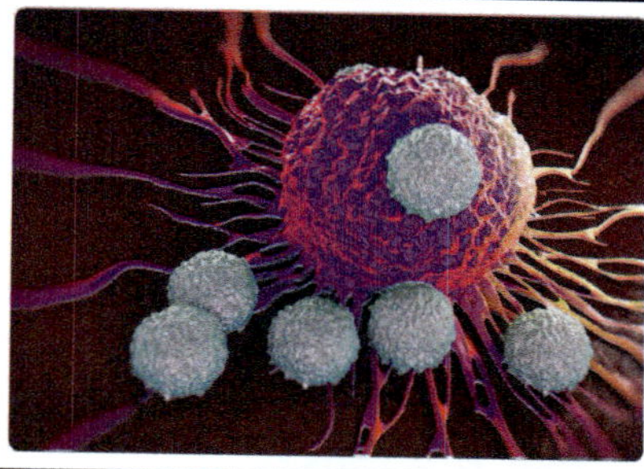
Intravenous (IV) drug abusers	Individuals who inject drugs directly into the veins, often using syringes, which increases the risk of infections, diseases, and other health complications.	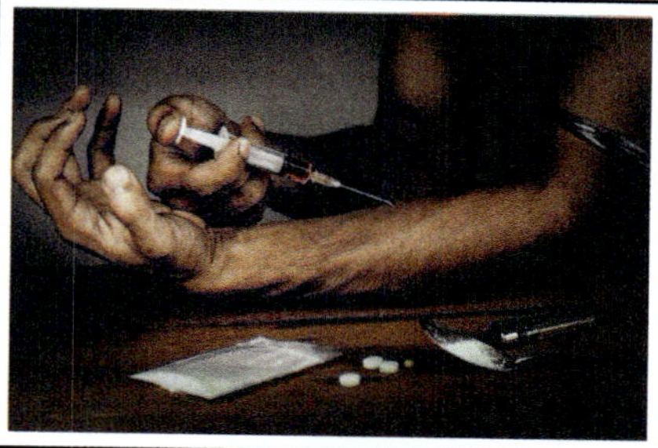
T lymphocytes	Another name for T cells; these are a subtype of lymphocytes (a type of white blood cell) involved in the immune system's response to pathogens.	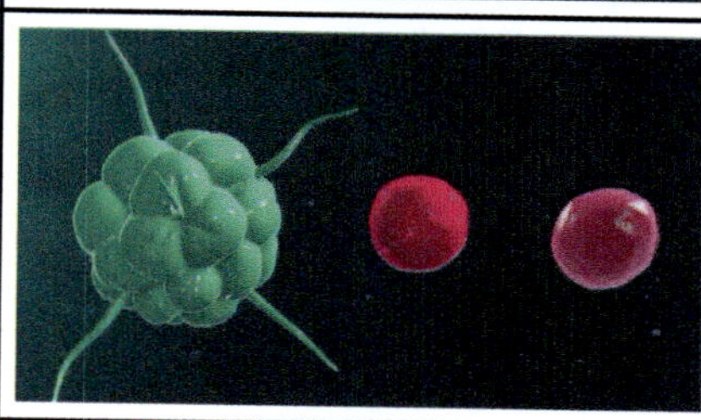
Chronic diarrhea	Diarrhea that lasts for more than four weeks, often caused by infections, gastrointestinal disorders, or conditions like irritable bowel syndrome or Crohn's disease.	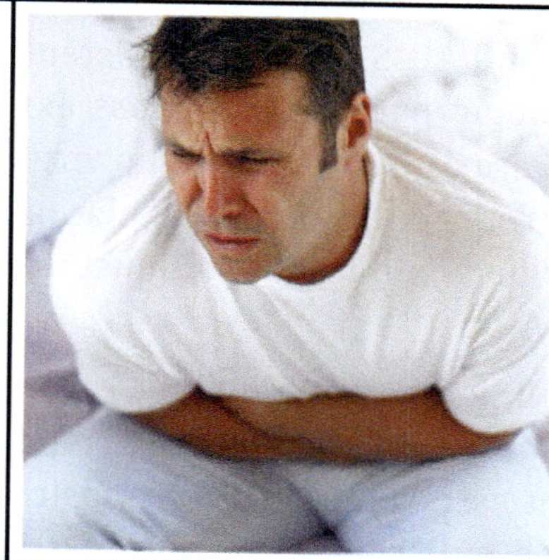
Sexually transmitted disease (STD)	Infections that are primarily spread through sexual contact, caused by bacteria, viruses, or parasites, and can lead to various health issues if untreated.	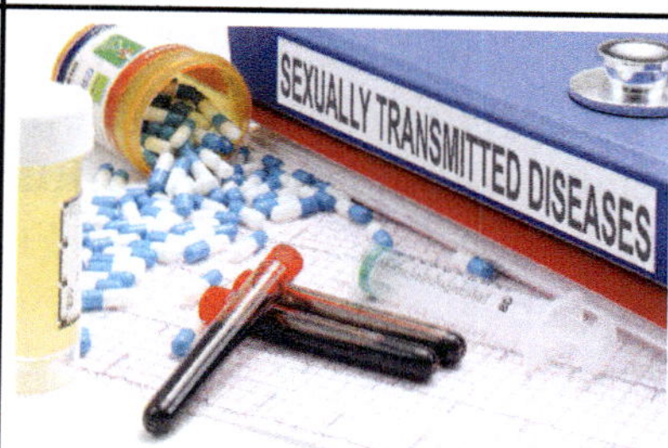

8.1. HIV: The Etiologic Agent of Aids

At the beginning of the epidemic, epidemiologic analysis of the pattern of spread of AIDS showed that it was reminiscent of that of the hepatitis B virus, an observation that pointed scientists in the right direction in their search for an etiologic agent. In 1983 and 1984, several researchers identified a retrovirus, now known as HIV, as the cause of AIDS. The Committee believes that the evidence that HIV causes AIDS is scientifically conclusive.

That a particular organism causes a disease is proven by a confluence of evidence linking the two: HIV and AIDS are linked in time, place, and population. In San Francisco, for example, antibodies against HIV were detected in frozen blood samples from a cohort of homosexual men as early as 1978. At that time, the prevalence of HIV infection in the population of male homosexuals in San Francisco was probably less than 5%, and the first cases of AIDS in homosexual men in San Francisco were detected in 1981 (Babel et al., 2021). This association between the cumulative incidence of HIV infection and AIDS cases is consistent with the epidemiologic pattern that must exist if HIV and AIDS are causally linked: the virus must be newly introduced into the population, it must spread widely, and its spread must precede the onset of AIDS.

The link heralded by the co-occurrence of HIV and AIDS has been confirmed by their persistent association. HIV seropositivity rates in defined subgroups of homosexual men in San Francisco and New York City and among intravenous (IV) drug abusers in New York City are associated with subsequent AIDS cases in the same groups (Balaji et al., 2011). In San Francisco, these subgroups can be further disaggregated by neighborhood, where the association between HIV seropositivity and AIDS is also high. Conversely, AIDS is unknown in populations that are free of HIV antibodies.

The virus has been isolated from persons with AIDS. As testing techniques have improved, the virus can be detected in nearly 100% of affected individuals. The virus is not found in people who are not at risk of infection. These points are supported by epidemiologic data from the ongoing San Francisco Men's Health Study, which began in 1984, where results showed among 374 homosexual men who were not infected with HIV during the first 30 months of follow-up, no case of AIDS occurred. Among 36 homosexual men who became infected with HIV during this period, however, 3 cases of AIDS (8%) occurred, and of the 399 study participants who were infected with HIV when they entered the study, 52 (13%) developed AIDS. None of the heterosexual men in the study acquired HIV infection, and none developed AIDS. The probability that this distribution occurred by chance is less than one in a million.

Perhaps the clearest evidence of the link between HIV and AIDS is the tragic consequences of blood transfusions in the United States and around the world. Transmission of HIV through contaminated blood and blood products has been clearly linked to AIDS; in the United States, over 1,500 reported AIDS cases have been linked to blood transfusions. Since routine screening of the blood supply for HIV antibodies began in 1985, HIV transmission by this route has virtually disappeared. Nevertheless, 13 recipients from 7 donors who originally tested negative for HIV antibodies are known to have acquired HIV infection between March 1985 and October 1987. The 7 donors who were tested at the time of donation probably had negative test results because the test was performed shortly after infection and before the development of detectable antibodies. However, in a later repeat test, all 7 donors were found to have detectable HIV antibodies in their blood.

Results demonstrate that of the 13 recipients, 1 developed AIDS and 3 developed HIV-related illnesses, and of the 3 who became ill, 1 was a set of twins who had received transfusions shortly after birth, and their fraternal twin, who had not received transfusions, remained healthy. Thus, 13 people without other risk factors were infected, and 4 of them became ill after receiving transfusions from donors who were initially thought not to be infected. After careful investigation, it turned out that the donors were indeed infected with HIV.

The causal role of HIV in AIDS is also supported by the high risk (30–50%) of perinatal HIV transmission from an infected mother to her child and the subsequent diagnosis of AIDS in the infected children.

The pathogenesis of HIV infection, that is the way in which the organism causes disease, is still not fully understood. Several mechanisms have been proposed for the profound immunodeficiency that results from HIV infection, including aggregation of uninfected and infected T lymphocytes into multinucleated syncytia that subsequently die, infection of stem cells, and inhibition of lymphocyte function by viral products. However, a complete understanding of the pathogenesis of a disease is not a prerequisite for knowledge of its etiology (Bautista-Arredondo et al., 2013).

8.1.1. Proportion of Infected Individuals Who Will Develop Aids

The observation of epidemiologic cohorts of HIV-infected persons over time has shown that an increasing proportion of seropositive persons develop AIDS. The available data indicate that the vast majority of HIV-infected individuals will eventually develop AIDS if there is no effective therapy to slow or halt the progression of the infection.

The group of people who have been studied the longest in relation to AIDS is a group of homosexual men in San Francisco who took part in a trial of a vaccine against the hepatitis B virus in the late 1970s. As part of the study, blood samples were taken and the serum was stored and frozen. As it later emerged that this group of men were at high risk of AIDS, samples of the frozen serum were tested for HIV infection and the infected individuals were examined for clinical and laboratory signs of AIDS. In the first 2 years after the infection was discovered, almost no cases of AIDS occurred, however, after 8 1/2 years, more than 40% of the infected cohort have developed AIDS and a similar proportion have developed symptoms of HIV infection, and are expected to progress to AIDS. The statistical modeling of the incidence of AIDS in this cohort predicts the possibility that 100% will develop AIDS within 13 years of initial infection (Chow et al., 2015).

The analysis of another cohort of 288 seropositive homosexual men in San Francisco who were seropositive at baseline showed that 22% developed AIDS after 3 years of observation. Another 19% have clinical symptoms of infection, and another 24% show laboratory evidence of immunologic impairment. Projections for this cohort suggest that 50% of the men will develop AIDS within 6 years of observation (or probably 9 years after infection) and that many more will develop the disease in subsequent years.

Data from individuals who have contracted HIV through blood transfusion and data from individuals with hemophilia suggest that the rate of progression from HIV infection to AIDS increases with age. The exception to this pattern is newborns, who have the highest rate of progression of all age groups, while the rate of progression in adults with hemophilia appears to be similar to that in male homosexuals.

8.2. The Spectrum of HIV Infection

When dealing with a new disease, especially one that is rapidly reaching epidemic proportions, terminology, and definitions become essential for clinical management of patients, data collection and research, and decisions about coverage and reimbursement. In 1982, the CDC developed a definition of AIDS for surveillance purposes based on the presence of opportunistic infections and malignancies. In August 1987, the definition was revised to include two additional syndromes indicative of AIDS: Dementia and wasting syndrome (see Appendix B). However, quite early in the epidemic, it became clear that many infected persons who suffered from clinical symptoms and laboratory abnormalities suggestive of HIV infection did not meet the CDC criteria for the disease. For example, persistent generalized lymphadenopathy (PGL) was thought to be associated with an increased risk of AIDS, especially when combined with oral candidiasis and certain laboratory abnormalities. Another group of patients had other chronic AIDS symptoms — fever, weight loss, night sweats, chronic diarrhea and fatigue — and a high proportion of this group also had laboratory abnormalities. Nevertheless, these patients did not meet the standard definition of the disease, although some of them appeared to develop AIDS at a rapid pace. They were labeled AIDS-related complex (ARC), and the clinical ARC syndrome was eventually incorporated into a CDC definition (although it was never used as a basis for reporting cases). Clinicians, however, realized that even this definition did not capture some patients who were at high risk for developing AIDS, and thus a third, more broadly defined syndrome was labeled an AIDS-related condition (Chuang et al., 2021).

Today, as we better understand the natural history of HIV infection and can more accurately assess disease progression in the laboratory, the Committee believes that the term ARC is not useful from either a clinical or public health perspective and that HIV infection itself should be considered a disease. It is more accurate to describe HIV infection as a continuum of conditions ranging from the acute, transient, mononucleosis-like syndrome associated with seroconversion, to asymptomatic HIV infection, to symptomatic HIV infection, and finally to AIDS, a spectrum that includes a wide variety of clinical symptoms. The terms ARC and PGL no longer have the precise prognostic meaning they were once thought to have, for example, it is now known that the presence of persistent, generalized lymphadenopathy does not in itself mean a worse prognosis than HIV seropositivity. For clinical (treatment or research) purposes, a patient can be more accurately described by a combination of a description of symptoms and laboratory evidence of immune dysfunction than by terms such as ARC or PGL.

Experience with cohorts of infected individuals shows that the majority of HIV-infected individuals show signs of progressive immunodeficiency and are likely to develop AIDS without effective therapy. AIDS, a dramatic and devastating syndrome, attracted the attention of physicians and public health authorities earlier than the milder manifestations of HIV infection, but it is now clear that AIDS is the final stage of HIV infection. Like many other progressive disease processes, both infectious and non-infectious, HIV has an asymptomatic phase that varies in length (Coelho et al., 2021).

It is important to consider HIV infection as a disease because it may be amenable to treatment. The drug zidovudine (AZT) has been shown to prolong the lives of AIDS patients, and along with other drugs, they are currently being tested to determine whether they can halt or slow the progression of the disease in infected asymptomatic individuals. If an effective therapy is found,

HIV infection must be treated early, similarly with diseases such as gonorrhea where they are often diagnosed and treated in asymptomatic infected patients. Even if no treatment is available, diagnosis of HIV infection is still important now so that opportunistic infections and malignancies can be detected as early as possible. Many treatments for these complications are more effective and less toxic if initiated early (Di Ciaccio et al., 2020).

Viewing HIV infection as a disease is important for other aspects of the AIDS crisis. From a public health perspective, the population infected with the virus is of greatest concern because these individuals are capable of infecting others. Medical care should be based on the symptoms associated with HIV infection and not on arbitrary definitions of the onset of "disease." The terminology that reflects the progression of the disease from the initial, acute stage of infection through asymptomatic HIV infection to symptomatic HIV infection and AIDS (Figure 8.1) would be useful for clinical care and community management of the disease. The CDC has developed a classification system (see Appendix B) that could form the basis for such terminology.

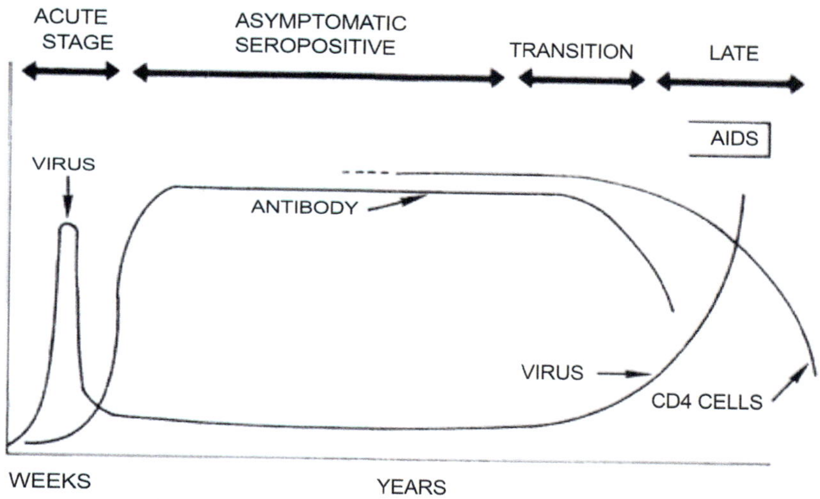

Figure 8.1. *The course of disease from HIV infection to AIDS.*

Source: Courtesy of David Baltimore, Whitehead Institute for Biomedical Research, Cambridge, Massachusetts; https://www.ncbi.nlm.nih.gov/books/NBK218872/.

8.3. Modes and Efficiencies of HIV Transmission

Epidemiologic data further support the observation that HIV transmission is limited to sexual contact, sharing of contaminated needles and syringes, contact with infected blood or blood products, transplantation of infected organs or tissues, and transmission from mother to child either via the placenta or during delivery. A recent follow-up of more than 1,100 AIDS cases initially reported to the CDC without identified risk factors has shown that transmission in these individuals was also limited to the known routes. Finally, additional data from studies of health care workers, nonsexual household contacts (Dyer et al., 2012), and insect bites support the conclusion that HIV is not transmitted by casual contact or insect bites. A change in the mode of transmission of HIV would be biologically unprecedented for a virus, and there is no evidence that HIV is capable of such a change.

8.3.1. Heterosexual Transmission

There is clear evidence that HIV infection can be transmitted from men to women and from women to men through vaginal and anal intercourse. To date, however, heterosexual spread of the virus in the United States has been limited primarily to individuals whose sexual partners have contracted HIV in other ways — for example, by sharing contaminated needles and syringes or through blood transfusions.

The evidence to date shows that the spread of infection among heterosexuals tends to be slow in cases where neither partner can be assigned to a known risk category. In nine seroprevalence surveys of heterosexual men and women attending sexually transmitted disease (STD) clinics in six cities, the prevalence of HIV infection ranged from 0 to 2.6% (CDC, 1987b). STD clinics treat people who are most likely to be infected with HIV based on their sexual behavior. In studies conducted in clinics where data were collected through face-to-face interviews rather than self-reported questionnaires, and where seropositive individuals were re-interviewed to obtain better information about their risk status, the prevalence of HIV infection in individuals with no known risk factors ranged from 0 to 1.2%. The results of large-scale studies of over 36 million blood donors and 1.5 million military personnel (where there is evidence of self-exclusion of high-risk individuals) show that the overall prevalence of HIV in these populations was less than 1% between 1985 and 1987. This low prevalence among heterosexuals (compared to the 20 to 50% prevalence among male homosexuals) seems to indicate that the virus is not spreading rapidly in populations that are primarily considered low-risk (Earnshaw & Chaudoir, 2009).

However, it would be a mistake to become complacent in the face of this obvious trend, and heterosexual transmission of the virus is a proven fact. Although the numbers are small, cases acquired through heterosexual transmission represent the fastest growing group of AIDS cases in the United States. In parts of Africa, heterosexual transmission of HIV is even large enough to keep AIDS in epidemic status. It is useful to look at the African experience with AIDS and try to identify conditions that might predict changes in the patterns of spread of the disease in the United States.

It is believed that HIV infection in Africa first appeared in large numbers in the heterosexual community and that prostitution has played an important role in its spread. Prostitution is not uncommon in some urban areas in Central and East Africa, and the prevalence of HIV infection is quite high (25–88%) among prostitutes tested in some of these areas (Gayet et al., 2007). Case-control studies have also shown that sexual activity with female prostitutes is more common among men with AIDS than among control subjects; African AIDS patients also report contact with more heterosexual partners than control subjects. On the other hand, homosexuality, and intravenous drug abuse do not play a major role in HIV transmission in Africa. In addition, STDs, particularly genital ulcers, are quite common in some sexually active populations in Africa and are associated with an increased risk of infection, perhaps because they provide a more direct portal of entry into the bloodstream. Contamination of the African blood supply and frequent contact with non-sterile needles and syringes, both in medical settings and during ritual practices, may also be important factors in the spread of AIDS in the African heterosexual population. In addition, African heterosexual adults are more likely than American heterosexual men to have chronically activated immune systems, which may be a factor that increases their susceptibility to HIV infection.

The pattern of spread of the disease in the United States was quite different, where the epidemic began in a few cities and within a closed community, male homosexuals, and high-risk behaviors were practiced (multiple partners and receptive anal intercourse). These behaviors promoted the rapid spread of HIV infection within this community, which also had high STD rates — another factor that may have increased the risk of HIV infection. The observation that HIV infection spreads much more slowly in the heterosexual community suggests that one or more of the following may be true: (1) there was relatively little sexual contact between this pool of infected men and heterosexuals; (2) heterosexuals probably change partners less frequently than homosexual men; and (3) vaginal intercourse may not transmit the virus as easily as anal intercourse. Therefore, HIV infection has been somewhat contained in the heterosexual population in the United States.

Similar to the incidence of the disease among homosexual men, HIV infection was also pronounced in communities of IV drug users who practiced high-risk behaviors — in this case, frequent drug injections and sharing contaminated injection equipment. These behaviors are the functional equivalent of frequent receptive anal intercourse and multiple sexual partners among homosexual men. Again, the spread of infection was rapid but limited (Goffman & Estigma, 1963). The potential for spread of infection beyond the IV drug-using population is discussed below.

Will HIV infection reach epidemic proportions in the "general" heterosexual population in the United States, and are the conditions necessary for such an epidemic already present? To sustain the spread of the disease, a "chain of transmission" is needed from individuals who engage in high-risk behaviors with their partners and from them to individuals who have no known risks. This chain of transmission would need to include a sufficient number of infected women interacting with men who are not otherwise at high risk. Such a reservoir of infected women can arise in various ways: one mechanism is bisexuality, and another, probably more significant, route is IV drug abuse. Of all IV drug users, 90% are heterosexual, and 30% are women. In addition, between 30 and 50% of female IV drug abusers have engaged in prostitution. There is therefore the possibility of a pool of infected prostitutes, whose source of infection is the sharing of contaminated needles and syringes. The HIV infection could then enter the heterosexual community via male clients of female prostitutes.

To date, most AIDS cases among heterosexuals are due to IV drug abuse, and the number of infected addicts is growing. Additionally, seroprevalence among heterosexuals without known risk factors is higher in areas of the country where seroprevalence among IV drug abusers is high. This consistency implies that IV drug users play a central role in the spread of HIV to adults through heterosexual transmission (and to infants through perinatal transmission).

A 30% increase in syphilis was reported for 1987 in the United States, primarily among heterosexuals, where higher rates were reported for blacks and Hispanics than for whites populations. Moreover, the areas that reported the largest absolute increases in syphilis cases (that is, Florida, New York City, and California) were also areas with high rates of HIV infection. The increase in syphilis cases suggests that behaviors that increase the likelihood of HIV infection among heterosexuals are not being effectively curbed.

In summary, heterosexual HIV transmission occurs from men to women and from women to men through vaginal and anal intercourse.

The virus is capable of spreading among heterosexuals, but so far the prevalence of infection in the heterosexual population with no known risk of infection is low. However, the extent of future spread among heterosexuals is uncertain. There appears to be a "window of opportunity" to prevent further spread of the infection in the heterosexual population.

8.3.2. Efficiencies of Transmission

The modalities of HIV transmission are well documented. What is less clear, however, is how easily or how "efficiently" HIV is transmitted by a particular route when a person is exposed. Specially designed epidemiologic studies provide information to help estimate the likelihood of HIV transmission by the various known routes, such as blood transfusions. The efficiency of this route of transmission can be estimated from studies of recipients of blood from donors who were subsequently found to have AIDS or HIV antibodies. Between 66% and 100% of blood transfusion recipients were infected if the donors either tested positive for HIV antibodies or later developed antibodies or AIDS themselves (Hess et al., 2017). In addition, recipients were more likely to be infected if the transfusion took place close to the time when the donor developed symptoms. All recipients of blood transfusions were infected if the donors developed AIDS within 23 months of the donation. The high dose of virus that a blood transfusion represents therefore appears to be quite efficient in conjunction with this particular route of transmission.

Another route includes through perinatal transmission, where the risk of transmission can be estimated from studies that assess the risk of an HIV-infected pregnant woman giving birth to an HIV-infected child. The results of such studies indicate that the probability of HIV transmission from mother to infant is between 30 and 50%, while some studies suggest that the risk of transmission is higher in infants born to mothers who have symptoms of HIV infection or show signs of immunosuppression during pregnancy (Hessou et al., 2019).

IV drug abuse is another route of HIV transmission, as mentioned previously, however due to the illicit nature of IV drug abuse, it is difficult to collect information on the sharing of contaminated needles and syringes. However, several studies have shown that once HIV is introduced into a community, it spreads rapidly among IV drug users and most of them soon become infected. In New York City, where there are large numbers of infected IV drug users, used needles and other drug paraphernalia are rented in "shooting galleries" where the users congregate. Studies among IV drug users have shown an association between HIV seropositivity and the frequency of drug injections and the sharing of drug injection equipment.

Homosexual transmission is another route mentioned previously, and while the risk of HIV transmission through receptive anal intercourse between homosexual men has been estimated, partner tracing among homosexuals may be difficult in situations where there have been multiple sexual partners. Cohort and case-control studies of homosexual men show that the risk of HIV infection is greatest among those who have receptive anal intercourse. The risk of infection is lower in partners who have insertive anal intercourse, and the risk appears to be even lower with oral receptive intercourse.

Heterosexual transmission is another route of HIV transmission, and estimates of its risk has been derived from studies of the sexual partners of infected individuals. In this particular study design, an index case (the infected person) is identified and the antibody status of his or her sexual partner is determined at baseline and monitored over time. In several other studies on female partners of IV drug addicts, the risk of infection was reported to be around 50% (Hoff et al., 2012). Studies on the male sexual partners of female IV drug addicts showed a similarly high risk of infection, although the number of male partners tested was low. In these studies, HIV transmission through the shared use of contaminated needles and syringes cannot be ruled out.

The risk of transmission is lower in female partners of hemophiliacs and bisexual men and in partners of transfusion-infected persons than in male or female partners of IV drug abusers. In studies on the wives or partners of hemophiliacs, the risk of infection was about 10%, while studies on female partners with bisexual men reported a transmission risk of around 25%. A similarly high risk was found in studies with the spouses of transfusion-infected persons, and in a more recent study, of the 55 wives who had sexual contact with their infected partners, 10 (18%) were seropositive. In the later study, the risk of infection was not related to the number of sexual contacts a woman had with her infected spouse, but rather, seropositive wives reported fewer sexual contacts and were slightly older than seronegative wives. This finding suggests that in addition to behavioral factors, biological factors probably play a role in how easily HIV is transmitted. There may be differences in transmissibility due to changes in the infectiousness of the infected person over time. For example, heterosexual contact during periods of high risk of infection is more likely to transmit the virus than contact during periods of low risk of infection. A similar result was reported in a cohort study with partners of infected hemophiliacs. In this study, the best predictor of HIV transmission was the absolute number of T helper lymphocytes of hemophiliacs, suggesting that as their immune systems became more suppressed, they were more likely to infect their sexual partners, regardless of the frequency of sexual contact or the duration of their infection (Huebner et al., 2015).

Another result of the study of spouses of transfusion-infected persons was a higher transmission rate from men to women than from women to men. While 10 out of 55 wives (18%) became seropositive through sexual contact with their infected husbands, only 2 out of 25 husbands (8%) became seropositive through sexual contact with their infected wives. Although this difference was not statistically significant, the finding that HIV transmission from men to women may be more efficient than from women to men has been reported in other studies.

Needlestick injuries are a recognized route of HIV transmission, particularly among healthcare workers. Studies on accidental needlestick injuries or cuts with sharp objects provide crucial data on the risk of HIV infection through this route. One notable collaborative surveillance study conducted by the CDC followed 489 healthcare workers who had been exposed to HIV-infected blood. Both acute and convalescent serum samples were collected from these individuals. By December 31, 1987, three of the 489 healthcare workers (0.6%) had seroconverted within six months of exposure. Additionally, two other prospective studies in the United States assessed the risk of HIV transmission from accidental needlestick exposure among healthcare workers. These studies contribute valuable insight into understanding the risks of HIV transmission in healthcare settings.

As of April 15, 1988, a similarly designed study at the College of California at San Francisco had reported that 1 of 180 health care workers (0.5%) had seroconverted after a follow-up period of at least 6 months. By April 30, 1988, the National Institutes of Health had collected both acute and convalescent serum samples from 108 health care workers with needlestick injuries at least 6 months after exposure; none were seroconverted. The results of these studies, as well as those conducted in England and Canada, suggest that the risk of transmission through needlestick injuries is less than 1% and probably closer to 0.5%. In most cases, these risks are associated with a single exposure, in contrast to the studies on sexual partners, which involve multiple exposures over time.

8.3.3. Relative Efficiencies of HIV Transmission

Several researchers have estimated the probability of HIV transmission for different transmission routes (for example, per episode of heterosexual intercourse or per controlled blood transfusion), but these estimates are uncertain because the calculations are based on very limited information (Liu et al., 2012). It is also not possible to rank the transmission routes from most to least efficient with absolute certainty. In addition to the route of transmission, other factors also appear to be decisive in determining whether the virus is transmitted. These factors include the dose (size of the inoculum) of the transmitted virus, the frequency of exposure, differences in host susceptibility, variations in the infectivity of an infected person over time, possible differences in the virulence of HIV isolates, and the presence of other sexually transmitted diseases or other co-factors. While the study designs differ, making it difficult to compare the results, nevertheless, some preliminary conclusions can be drawn. Recipients of infected blood transfusions are at very high risk of infection, as are children born to infected mothers. Studies on infected IV drug users also report high infection rates in this group, suggesting that sharing contaminated needles and syringes in combination with frequent injections carries a high risk of infection. The sexual partners of IV drug users have a higher risk of becoming infected than the sexual partners of people who have become infected by other means, suggesting that the route of transmission could be either heterosexual transmission or unacknowledged sharing of contaminated needles and syringes. Studies of the sexual partners of individuals infected by means other than IV drug abuse show a much lower risk of infection, as do studies of the risk of infection from accidental contact with needle sticks. It is important to point out that while the risk of infection from an episode of heterosexual sex and a needlestick injury is about the same, studies of sexual transmission involve repeated exposures over years, whereas studies of needlestick injuries usually involve one or a few episodes. Although it seems intuitively correct that the risk increases with increasing exposure, other factor, for example, the apparent inability of a particular infected person to transmit the virus, may play a role.

In the case of sexual transmission, the risk of infection is greater for the receptive partner during anal intercourse than for the insertive partner. Vaginal intercourse is probably less efficient as a transmission route than receptive anal intercourse, while initial indications also suggest that the infectiousness of vaginal intercourse is somewhat greater from men to women than from women to men.

8.4. Prevalence and Incidence of HIV Infection in the United States

The importance of accurate descriptions of the prevalence and incidence of HIV infection, both now and in the future, cannot be overestimated. Defined AIDS cases are only the clinical end-stage of the devastating effects of HIV infection. Describing HIV infection by demographic characteristics and other distinguishing features helps to determine target groups for intervention strategies to prevent the further spread of infection.

8.4.1. HIV Prevalence in Groups at Recognized Risk

In November 1987, the CDC summarized the current state of knowledge about the prevalence and incidence of HIV infection for various population groups in the United States by age, sex, racial or ethnic group, and geographic area. The report analyzed data from various sources (including federal agencies, health departments, and medical centers) on the prevalence of HIV infection as measured by the presence of HIV antibodies in the blood (that is, seroprevalence).

The observed prevalence of HIV infection is highest in the risk groups responsible for most AIDS cases reported to the CDC. Nevertheless, caution is required when interpreting the prevalence data. For example, the prevalence of HIV infection in STD clinics may differ in different geographic areas because background prevalence may be different in two communities. Other problems in comparing data arise from differences in questionnaire design, the inclusion or exclusion of symptomatic individuals in seroprevalence reports, and differences in the demographic characteristics of those tested. In addition, the reported prevalence may be higher or lower than the actual prevalence for a given group depending on who "walked in the door" (that is, most of these surveys are based on self-selected samples).

Estimates of the prevalence of HIV infection among gay and bisexual men based on data from 23 cities range from 10–70%, with most estimates between 20 and 50%. Prevalence is highest in cohorts of homosexual men in San Francisco. However, the data probably overestimate the true prevalence of HIV infection in this group because most participants in these surveys either sought medical attention for STDs or were concerned that their past or current sexual behavior had put them at risk (Mak & Cheung, 2010).

The population of IV drug abusers appears to be less mobile than the population of homosexual men, as greater differences in HIV prevalence are reported by geographic area. Surveys consistently show very high prevalence (50–60%) in large East Coast cities with geographic or close cultural ties to New York City and northern New Jersey; prevalence is much lower (less than 5%) in other areas of the country. Most surveys measuring prevalence among IV drug users are conducted in chronic heroin abuse treatment facilities. It is believed that only 10–20% of the estimated 1.2 million drug abusers in the United States are currently in treatment and that those who are not in treatment may be habitual users who are at even greater risk for HIV infection.

The prevalence of HIV infection in persons with hemophilia ranges from 15% to more than 90%, depending on the type and severity of hemophilia and thus the amount of clotting factor received (Martinez et al., 2020). Individuals with severe hemophilia A have the highest prevalence (approximately 70%), while individuals with hemophilia B or mild hemophilia A have a slightly lower prevalence (approximately 35%). Within these clinical categories, however, the prevalence is consistent across the country and reflects the distribution of clotting factor concentrates received prior to 1985. Only hemophiliacs undergoing treatment are tested. Therefore, the prevalence reported here may be an overestimate of the true prevalence for hemophiliacs as a group.

HIV prevalence among female sex workers in the United States varies from 0% to more than 50%, and seropositivity is observed to be higher among black and Hispanic prostitutes than among white prostitutes. The differences in prevalence appear to be related to the extent of IV drug abuse in the groups tested and the background prevalence of HIV among IV drug abusers in the region.

In studies of seroprevalence among persons who are heterosexual sexual partners of HIV-infected persons but have no other identifiable risk factors for HIV infection, prevalence ranged from less than 10% to 60%. As mentioned earlier in this chapter, STD clinic surveys of heterosexual men and women who do not belong to a risk group and do not have partners from a risk group show prevalence rates between 0 and 2.6%, depending on the population studied and the method of data collection. Seroprevalence is higher among heterosexuals in areas where seroprevalence is high among IV drug users. However, such studies may overstate the true HIV prevalence among heterosexuals, as those interviewed in STD clinics may be more sexually active than the "general" heterosexual population.

8.4.2. HIV Prevalence Among Selected Segments of the General Population

The prevalence of HIV infection in the general population has been estimated primarily from studies of various special populations: blood donors, civilian applicants to the military, Job Corps entrants, sentinel hospital patients, and newborns (whose antibody status at birth reflects the presence or absence of antibodies in their mothers) (Martinez et al., 2017). Since 1985, more than 36 million blood or plasma donations have been tested for HIV antibodies in the United States. HIV prevalence among first-time donors was 0.04% between 1985 and 1987. The prevalence was significantly higher among men than women and higher among blacks and Hispanics than whites. Since October 1985, the blood samples of over 1.5 million applicants for military service have also been tested for HIV antibodies. The prevalence of HIV infection increases with age in applicants between their late teens and late 20s. The prevalence by birth cohort also increased from the first screening period (1985–1986) to the second (1986–1987). As with blood donors, seropositivity was higher among men than women and higher among blacks and Hispanics than whites. The overall prevalence (for October 1985 through September 1987), adjusted for age, sex, and racial and ethnic composition of the U.S. adult population aged 17 to 59 years, was 0.14%. Since March 1987, HIV antibody screening has been conducted for new Job Corps members participating in a training program. This program recruits disadvantaged youth ages 16 to 21 from rural and inner-city areas, with Preliminary data from the first 25,000 participants showing a seroprevalence of 0.33%. The prevalence of infection across the nation is likely higher than that observed in blood donors, military applicants and Job Corps participants, as those at highest risk of infection are likely underrepresented.

To avoid the self-selection bias associated with volunteer programs, anonymous HIV antibody testing of selected hospital patients (excluding AIDS cases and other conditions associated with HIV infection) has also recently been implemented in sentinel hospitals. Based on the first 8,668 test results, the age- and sex-adjusted prevalence of infection was 0.32%, and this sample represents hospitalized patients who are at low risk of infection. In addition, the hospitals selected to participate in the program may serve specific segments of the community, and therefore, the data collected is not representative of all hospitalized patients.

Several states have initiated programs to determine the prevalence of HIV infection in women of childbearing age by testing for HIV antibodies in their newborns. Maternal antibodies to HIV cross the placenta and are therefore present in the baby's blood. A baby with HIV antibodies may or may not be infected, but the presence of antibodies in the baby's blood always indicates that the mother is infected. Hospitals routinely take blood samples from newborns to test for metabolic disorders, and testing for HIV antibodies has been included in this program. A recent study found that 1 in 476 women (0.2%) who gave birth in Massachusetts was antibody-positive from December 1986 through June 1987, and the prevalence of HIV infection varied by type and location of maternity hospital. Prevalence was highest in inner-city hospitals (0.8%), lower in mixed urban and suburban hospitals (0.25%), and lowest in suburban and rural hospitals (0.09%) (Mercer et al., 2016). In New York, the prevalence of HIV infection among women who gave birth in hospitals in the five New York City boroughs between November 1987 and February 1988 was 1.45%, and the prevalence of HIV infection among women who gave birth in hospitals outside the metropolitan area was 0.18%.

8.4.3. Incidence of New Infections

Data on the incidence (the number of new infections over time) of HIV infection are more difficult to obtain than prevalence data, but they are crucial for longer-term projections about the course of the epidemic. The results of eight cohort studies of homosexual men indicate that the HIV incidence rate in this population was lower in 1985–1987 than in the first half of the decade. This observed decline in the incidence of infection can be attributed to several factors but is consistent with reports of a decline in other sexually transmitted diseases in this group as well as changes in sexual behavior (Mimiaga et al., 2015). Serologic screening of blood and plasma donors and heat treatment of factor concentrates, as well as efforts to exclude high-risk donors, have also reduced the rate of new infections among transfusion recipients and hemophiliacs since 1985. In contrast, HIV incidence among IV drug abusers in New York City and San Francisco appears to be increasing. These data suggest that the epidemic of HIV infection in the United States can be viewed as a series of overlapping smaller epidemics, each with its own dynamics and time course.

8.4.4. National Estimates of HIV Infection

In 1986, the CDC estimated the size of various population groups known to be infected (that is, male homosexuals, IV drug abusers, hemophiliacs, and heterosexuals with no known risks) and the prevalence of HIV infection for each of these groups. From these estimates, she calculated that 1 to 1.5 million people in the United States are currently infected with HIV. In November 1987, the CDC reviewed these estimates and modified them slightly based on new information about the size of the various population groups and new data on seroprevalence for these groups. In retrospect, the estimates made by the CDC in 1986 appear to have been too high. The CDC estimates that between 945,000 and 1.4 million Americans are currently infected with HIV. The major limitation of both the original and revised estimates is the unknown size of the homosexual population that engages in risk behaviors (Mimiaga et al., 2019). The CDC will continue to update national estimates of the prevalence of HIV infection as more information becomes available. Other groups and researchers have also estimated the prevalence of HIV infection in the United States. These estimates have been both higher and lower than those of the CDC, ranging from 400,000 to 2.2 million for late 1987, and they give an overall picture of the scale of the epidemic. More important, however, are the data esimates on seroprevalence and incidence in specific risk groups, as they provide the necessary information to target prevention strategies and evaluate their effectiveness in containing the epidemic.

8.4.5. The Program of HIV Surveys and Studies

The CDC has responded to the urgent need to monitor the spread of HIV infection by introducing a series of seroprevalence studies and surveillance systems (Mimiaga et al., 2015). In approximately 30 major cities in the United States, blood samples are routinely collected from persons receiving treatment in STD clinics, substance abuse treatment centers, family planning and women's health clinics, and tuberculosis clinics, as well as from selected hospital admissions and newborns. These studies will provide local authorities with information on HIV prevalence so that measures can be developed to control HIV infection in specific areas. The neonatal surveys will provide some of the most valuable information as the sample selection is unbiased and will include the entire population of mothers of childbearing age. As mentioned earlier, HIV antibody testing, which is conducted in approximately 30 states, will be added to existing programs that routinely test newborns for metabolic disorders. These surveys will therefore be population-based and, by providing information on the antibody status of newborns, will reflect the prevalence of infection among mothers delivering in these hospitals.

In addition to these activities, studies of HIV infection among civilian applicants to the armed forces, active military personnel, blood donors, and Job Corps participants will continue. HIV prevalence surveys are also conducted in other populations of special interest, such as emergency room patients, patients receiving other hospital services, students on campus, and prisoners. The National Center for Health Statistics (NCHS) will also conduct a study to determine the feasibility of a nationwide seroprevalence survey in private households. In addition, the NCHS plans to conduct anonymous HIV antibody testing on an estimated 17,000 adult blood samples collected over a 6-year period as part of the National Health and Nutrition Examination Survey.

It is important to note that some of these surveys will be 'blinded' (that is, the HIV antibody test will be conducted on blood samples collected for other purposes, with personal information about the individual permanently removed) to avoid the uninterpretable effects of self-selection. However, other surveys will not be blinded, and in these cases, voluntary participants will be interviewed to identify risk factors for HIV transmission.

8.5. AIDS Cases in the United States

In October 1986, when Confronting AIDS was published, about 24,500 AIDS cases had been reported to the CDC. In May 1988, 62,200 AIDS cases had been reported since June 1981, and of which 35,051 had resulted in death (Mustanski et al., 2017). It is assumed that a further 10–20% of cases have been overlooked by the surveillance system. The number of cases reported annually continues to increase, although the rate of increase is less steep than at the beginning of the decade. Cases have been reported from all 50 states and the District of Columbia.

Since the publication of Confronting AIDS, the distribution of cases by risk group and by gender, race, age, and geographic area has not changed significantly: 63% of cases are homosexual or bisexual men who are not known to have abused IV drugs, 19% are heterosexual IV drug abusers, 7% are both male homosexuals and IV drug abusers, 1% are patients with hemophilia and related disorders, 4% are persons who acquired the disease through heterosexual contact, 3% are blood transfusion recipients, and 3% are cases where the risk information is undetermined because it is incomplete (the patients have died, refused to be interviewed, or have not been followed up) or the patients are still under investigation. The latter 3% also includes men who report contact with a prostitute and patients for whom no risk factor is identifiable. Of the 981 pediatric AIDS cases reported to CDC through May 1988, 77% are offspring of a parent with AIDS or at high risk for AIDS. Of the remaining pediatric cases, 6% are children with hemophilia, 14% are transfusion recipients, and 4% are children for whom no risk information can be determined.

In the last 2 years, the largest increases in new cases have been observed in two groups: heterosexual partners of HIV-infected persons and children whose mothers are IV drug abusers or sexual partners of high-risk men. While Blacks and Hispanics are overrepresented in both of these groups, the only group in which the incidence of AIDS has steadily declined over the past 2 years is children with transfusion-associated AIDS. This decline is attributed to the screening of blood and blood products, which began in early 1985, and the relatively short incubation period of 12 months or less observed in children with transfusion-associated AIDS. It is now believed that more than 80% of HIV infections in children can be directly linked to IV drug abuse by the mother or father (Oldenburg et al., 2015).

8.6. The Demographic Impact of AIDS

AIDS has already begun to change the demographics of New York City and San Francisco. A disease that was virtually unknown to Americans 8 years ago is now the leading cause of death in New York City among men ages 25 to 44 and women ages 25 to 34. In 1986, mortality from AIDS was the eighth leading cause of loss of potential years of life before age 65. Recent data from New York City has shown that one in 66 infants born between November 1987 and February 1988 tested positive for HIV antibodies, reflecting the prevalence of HIV infection among women of childbearing age in that city (Pachankis et al., 2015). In San Francisco, about 50% of the male homosexual population is infected with the virus, suggesting that a large proportion of the city's population may be affected in the future. In 1986, New York City and San Francisco accounted for about 40% of all AIDS cases, and by 1991, these two cities accounted for less than 20% of cases nationwide, suggesting that other metropolitan areas will soon face large economic and demographic losses (Passaro et al., 2019).

The proportion of AIDS cases is higher in the Black and Hispanic population than in the White population (on the West Coast, the proportion is three times higher in the Black and Hispanic population than in the white population and 12 times higher on the East Coast), largely due to higher HIV prevalence among Black and Hispanic IV drug abusers and their sexual partners as well as offspring. Recent data also suggest that the virus is spreading faster among vulnerable Blacks and Hispanics than among other populations, particularly in Northeast cities, suggesting that the future composition of AIDS cases will be primarily poor, urban minorities (Pettigrew et al., 2011).

8.7. Future Research Needs

Epidemiologic studies are the primary source of information on the prevalence and incidence of HIV infection and AIDS, the modalities and efficiency of HIV transmission, the proportion of infected persons who progress to AIDS, serologic markers of disease progression, and the distribution of behaviors associated with increased HIV exposure. Epidemiologic studies have also provided some of the strongest evidence for the link between HIV infection and AIDS. Whether these studies are prevalence or incidence surveys, cohort or case-control studies, they provide important data for understanding and controlling the epidemic (Pitpitan et al., 2016).

Although we have already learned much about the epidemiology of HIV infection, more research is needed to answer the many unanswered questions. The Committee therefore urges the continuation of epidemiologic research to support appropriate prevention and control measures. The CDC must be provided with the necessary resources to ensure that expertly trained staff, space, and technical resources are adequate for the task of continued epidemiologic research (Prati et al., 2014).

A Closer Look

T Lymphocytes

T lymphocytes, or T cells, are critical components of the adaptive immune system, playing essential roles in the body's defense against infections, tumors, and other pathologies. Derived from hematopoietic stem cells in the bone marrow, T cells undergo maturation in the thymus, where they differentiate into various subsets, including helper T cells (CD4+), cytotoxic T cells (CD8+), and regulatory T cells (Tregs). Each subset possesses unique functions; for example, CD4+ T cells orchestrate immune responses by producing cytokines that regulate other immune cells, while CD8+ T cells directly kill virus-infected cells and tumors. The understanding of T cell biology has advanced significantly, revealing their complex roles beyond direct pathogen elimination, such as their involvement in maintaining immune homeostasis and tolerance.

Recent research has highlighted the plasticity of T cells, enabling them to adapt to various immune challenges and environmental cues. A study by Wherry et al. (2015) emphasized the phenomenon of T cell exhaustion in chronic infections and cancer, where T cells lose their effector functions due to persistent antigen stimulation. This state is characterized by the upregulation of inhibitory receptors, such as PD-1, leading to diminished immune responses. Importantly, therapeutic strategies targeting these inhibitory pathways, such as immune checkpoint inhibitors, have shown promising results in revitalizing exhausted T cells in cancer patients, showcasing the potential of manipulating T cell responses for therapeutic benefit.

Another crucial aspect of T cell function is their memory formation. Research by Ramesh et al. (2018) illustrated that memory T cells provide long-lasting immunity by persisting in the body after the initial infection has resolved. These cells can rapidly respond upon re-exposure to the same pathogen, making them a key focus in vaccine development. The study identified mechanisms governing memory T cell differentiation, such as the role of transcription factors like T-bet and Eomesodermin, which dictate whether T cells become short-lived effector cells or long-lived memory cells. This knowledge has implications for designing effective vaccines against infectious diseases and for developing strategies to enhance memory T cell responses in immunotherapy.

Furthermore, Tregs, a specialized subset of CD4+ T cells, are crucial for maintaining immune tolerance and preventing autoimmune diseases. Research by Sakaguchi et al. (2008) demonstrated that Tregs play a vital role in suppressing unwanted immune responses, including those against self-antigens. Dysfunction or depletion of Tregs has been implicated in the pathogenesis of various autoimmune disorders, such as multiple sclerosis and type 1 diabetes. Consequently, therapeutic approaches aimed at enhancing Treg function or numbers are being explored as potential treatments for these conditions. The intricate balance of T lymphocyte subsets, including their activation, differentiation, and regulatory mechanisms, underscores their importance in health and disease, driving ongoing research to harness their potential for therapeutic interventions.

Summary

- HIV infection is a global health challenge characterized by the progressive destruction of the immune system, primarily targeting CD4 cells. This depletion of immune cells can lead to the development of AIDS, a life-threatening condition.
- Despite its widespread impact, the prevalence of HIV/AIDS varies significantly between regions, with sub-Saharan Africa being the most affected.
- Effective prevention strategies and access to antiretroviral therapy have reduced the number of new HIV infections and AIDS-related deaths in high-income countries, leading some to consider HIV/AIDS a rare disease in these contexts.
- However, in low- and middle-income countries, challenges remain in terms of access to HIV testing, prevention, and treatment services.
- Certain populations, such as men who have sex with men, people who inject drugs, and sex workers, are disproportionately affected by HIV/AIDS due to stigma, discrimination, and barriers to healthcare.
- Efforts to combat HIV/AIDS require a comprehensive approach that addresses prevention, testing, treatment, and social and structural barriers to care.

References

1. Alvarado, B., Mueses, H. F., Galindo, J., & Martínez-Cajas, J. L. (2020). Application of the "syndemics" theory to explain unprotected sex and transactional sex: A cross-sectional study in men who have sex with men (MSM), transgender women, and non-MSM in Colombia. *Biomedica, 40*, 391–403.
2. Babel, R. A., Wang, P., Alessi, E. J., Raymond, H. F., & Wei, C. (2021). Stigma, HIV risk, and access to HIV prevention and treatment services among men who have sex with men (MSM) in the United States: A scoping review. *AIDS Behavior, 25*(12), 3574–3604.
3. Balaji, A. B., Bowles, K. E., Hess, K. L., Smith, J. C., & Paz-Bailey, G. (2017). Association between enacted stigma and HIV-related risk behavior among MSM, National HIV Behavioral Surveillance System, 2011. *AIDS Behavior, 21*(1), 227–237.
4. Bautista-Arredondo, S., Colchero, M. A., Romero, M., Conde-Glez, C. J., & Sosa-Rubí, S. G. (2013). Is the HIV epidemic stable among MSM in Mexico? HIV prevalence and risk behavior results from a nationally representative survey among men who have sex with men. *PLoS ONE, 8*(12), e72616.
5. Chow, E. P., Chen, X., Zhao, J., Zhuang, X., Jing, J., & Zhang, L. (2015). Factors associated with self-reported unprotected anal intercourse among men who have sex with men in Changsha City of Hunan Province, China. *AIDS Care, 27*(10), 1332–1342.
6. Chuang, D. M., Newman, P. A., Fang, L., & Lai, M. C. (2021). Syndemic conditions, sexual risk behavior, and HIV infection among men who have sex with men in Taiwan. *AIDS Behavior, 25*(11), 3503–3518.
7. Coelho, L. E., Torres, T. S., Veloso, V. G., Grinsztejn, B., Jalil, E. M., Wilson, E. C., & McFarland, W. (2021). The prevalence of HIV among men who have sex with men (MSM) and young MSM in Latin America and the Caribbean: A systematic review. *AIDS Behavior, 25*(9), 3223–3237.

8. Di Ciaccio, M., Sagaon-Teyssier, L., Mimi, M., Suzan-Monti, M., Protiere, C., Castro, D. R., Meyer, L., Tremblay, C., Chidiac, C., Capitant, C., et al. (2020). What are the situational and behavioral factors associated with condomless anal sex without pre-exposure prophylaxis in MSM? *AIDS, 34*(9), 1367–1375.

9. Dyer, T. P., Shoptaw, S., Guadamuz, T. E., Plankey, M., Kao, U., Ostrow, D., Chmiel, J. S., Herrick, A., & Stall, R. (2012). Application of syndemic theory to black men who have sex with men in the Multicenter AIDS Cohort Study. *Journal of Urban Health, 89*(4), 697–708.

10. Earnshaw, V. A., & Chaudoir, S. R. (2009). From conceptualizing to measuring HIV stigma: A review of HIV stigma mechanism measures. *AIDS Behavior, 13*(6), 1160–1177.

11. Gayet, C., Magis, C., Sacknoff, D., & Guli, L. (2007). *Prácticas sexuales de las poblaciones vulnerables a la epidemia de VIH/SIDA en México*. CE SIDA: Mexico City, Mexico.

12. Goffman, E. (1963). *Estigma. La Identidad Deteriorada*. Amorrortu Editores: Buenos Aires, Argentina.

13. Hess, K. L., Hu, X., Lansky, A., Mermin, J., & Hall, H. I. (2017). Lifetime risk of a diagnosis of HIV infection in the United States. *Annals of Epidemiology, 27*(4), 238–243.

14. Hessou, P. H. S., Glele-Ahanhanzo, Y., Adekpedjou, R., Ahouada, C., Johnson, R. C., Boko, M., Zomahoun, H. T. V., & Alary, M. (2019). Comparison of the prevalence rates of HIV infection between men who have sex with men (MSM) and men in the general population in sub-Saharan Africa: A systematic review and meta-analysis. *BMC Public Health, 19*(1), 1634.

15. Hoff, C. C., Chakravarty, D., Beougher, S. C., Neilands, T. B., & Darbes, L. A. (2012). Relationship characteristics associated with sexual risk behavior among MSM in committed relationships. *AIDS Patient Care and STDs, 26*(12), 738–745.

16. Huebner, D. M., & Perry, N. S. (2015). Do behavioral scientists really understand HIV-related sexual risk behavior? A systematic review of longitudinal and experimental studies predicting sexual behavior. *Archives of Sexual Behavior, 44*(7), 1915–1936.

17. Liu, J., Qu, B., Ezeakile, M. C., & Zhang, Y. (2012). Factors associated with unprotected anal intercourse among men who have sex with men in Liaoning Province, China. *PLoS ONE, 7*(12), e50493.

18. Mak, W. W., & Cheung, R. Y. (2010). Self-stigma among concealable minorities in Hong Kong: Conceptualization and unified measurement. *American Journal of Orthopsychiatry, 80*(2), 267–281.

19. Martinez, O., Brady, K. A., Levine, E., Page, K. R., Zea, M. C., Yamanis, T. J., Grieb, S., Shinefeld, J., Ortiz, K., Davis, W. W., et al. (2020). Using syndemics theory to examine HIV sexual risk among Latinx men who have sex with men in Philadelphia, PA: Findings from the National HIV Behavioral Surveillance. *Equidad, 13*, 217–236.

20. Martinez, O., Muñoz-Laboy, M., Levine, E. C., Starks, T., Dolezal, C., Dodge, B., Icard, L., Moya, E., Chavez-Baray, S., Rhodes, S. D., et al. (2017). Relationship factors associated with sexual risk behavior and high-risk alcohol consumption among Latino men who have sex with men: Challenges and opportunities to intervene on HIV risk. *Archives of Sexual Behavior, 46*(4), 987–999.

21. Mercer, C. H., Prah, P., Field, N., Tanton, C., Macdowall, W., Clifton, S., Hughes, G., Nardone, A., Wellings, K., Johnson, A. M., et al. (2016). The health and well-being of men who have sex with men (MSM) in Britain: Evidence from the third National Survey of Sexual Attitudes and Lifestyles (Natsal-3). *BMC Public Health, 16*, 525.

22. Mimiaga, M. J., Biello, K. B., Robertson, A. M., Oldenburg, C. E., Rosenberger, J. G., O'Cleirigh, C., Novak, D. S., Mayer, K. H., & Safren, S. A. (2015). High prevalence of multiple syndemic conditions associated with sexual risk behavior and HIV infection among a large sample of Spanish- and Portuguese-speaking men who have sex with men in Latin America. *Archives of Sexual Behavior, 44*(7), 1869–1878.

23. Mimiaga, M. J., Hughto, J. M. W., Biello, K. B., Santostefano, C. M., Kuhns, L. M., Reisner, S. L., & Garofalo, R. (2019). Longitudinal analysis of syndemic psychosocial problems predicting HIV risk behavior among a multicity prospective cohort of sexually active young transgender women in the United States. *Journal of Acquired Immune Deficiency Syndromes, 81*(2), 184–192.

24. Mimiaga, M. J., O'Cleirigh, C., Biello, K. B., Robertson, A. M., Safren, S. A., Coates, T. J., Koblin, B. A., Chesney, M. A., Donnell, D. J., Stall, R. D., et al. (2015). The effect of psychosocial syndemic production on 4-year HIV incidence and risk behavior in a large cohort of sexually active men who have sex with men. *Journal of Acquired Immune Deficiency Syndromes, 68*(3), 329–336.

25. Mustanski, B., Phillips, G., Ryan, D. T., Swann, G., Kuhns, L., & Garofalo, R. (2017). Prospective effects of a syndemic on HIV and STI incidence and risk behaviors in a cohort of young men who have sex with men. *AIDS and Behavior, 21*(3), 845–857.

26. Oldenburg, C. E., Perez-Brumer, A. G., Hatzenbuehler, M. L., Krakower, D., Novak, D. S., Mimiaga, M. J., & Mayer, K. H. (2015). State-level structural sexual stigma and HIV prevention in a national online sample of HIV-uninfected MSM in the United States. *AIDS, 29*(7), 837–845.

27. Pachankis, J. E., Hatzenbuehler, M. L., Hickson, F., Weatherburn, P., Berg, R. C., Marcus, U., & Schmidt, A. J. (2015). Hidden from health: Structural stigma, sexual orientation concealment, and HIV across 38 countries in the European MSM Internet Survey. *AIDS, 29*(10), 1239–1246.

28. Passaro, R. C., Castañeda-Huaripata, A., Gonzales-Saavedra, W., Chavez-Gomez, S., Segura, E. R., Lake, J. E., Cabello, R., & Clark, J. L. (2019). Contextualizing condoms: A cross-sectional study mapping intersections of locations of sexual contact, partner type, and substance use as contexts for sexual risk behavior among MSM in Peru. *BMC Infectious Diseases, 19*, 958.

29. Pettigrew, T. F., Tropp, L. R., Wagner, U., & Christ, O. (2011). Recent advances in intergroup contact theory. *International Journal of Intercultural Relations, 35*(3), 271–280.

30. Pitpitan, E. V., Smith, L. R., Goodman-Meza, D., Torres, K., Semple, S. J., Strathdee, S. A., & Patterson, T. L. (2016). "Outness" as a moderator of the association between syndemic conditions and HIV risk-taking behavior among men who have sex with men in Tijuana, Mexico. *AIDS and Behavior, 20*(3), 431–438.

31. Prati, G., Mazzoni, D., & Zani, B. (2014). The influence of knowing someone with HIV/AIDS on preventive behaviors in Italy. *AIDS Care, 26*(3), 292–296.

32. Prati, G., Zani, B., Pietrantoni, L., Scudiero, D., Perone, P., Cosmaro, L., Cerioli, A., & Oldrini, M. (2016). The role of knowing someone living with HIV/AIDS and HIV disclosure in the HIV stigma framework: A Bayesian mediation analysis. *Quality & Quantity, 50*(2), 637–651.

33. Ransome, Y., Kawachi, I., Braunstein, S., & Nash, D. (2016). Structural inequalities drive late HIV diagnosis: The role of black racial concentration, income inequality, socioeconomic deprivation, and HIV testing. *Health & Place, 42*, 148–158.

34. Rao, A., Stahlman, S., Hargreaves, J., Weir, S., Edwards, J., Rice, B., Kochelani, D., Mavimbela, M., & Baral, S. (2017). Sampling key populations for HIV surveillance: Results from eight cross-sectional studies using respondent-driven sampling and venue-based snowball sampling. *JMIR Public Health and Surveillance, 3*(3), e72.

35. Rodriguez-Hart, C., Nowak, R. G., Musci, R., German, D., Orazulike, I., Kayode, B., Gureje, O., Crowell, T. A., Baral, S., & Charurat, M. (2017). Pathways from sexual stigma to incident HIV and sexually transmitted infections among Nigerian MSM. *AIDS, 31*(16), 2415–2420.

36. Santos, G. M., Do, T., Beck, J., Makofane, K., Arreola, S., Pyun, T., Hebert, P., Wilson, P. A., & Ayala, G. (2014). Syndemic conditions associated with increased HIV risk in a global sample of men who have sex with men. *Sexually Transmitted Infections, 90*(4), 250–253.

37. Semple, S. J., Pitpitan, E. V., Goodman-Meza, D., Strathdee, S. A., Chavarin, C. V., Rangel, G., Torres, K., & Patterson, T. L. (2017). Correlates of condomless anal sex among men who have sex with men (MSM) in Tijuana, Mexico: The role of public sex venues. *PLoS ONE, 12*(8), e0186814.

38. Singer, M., Bulled, N., Ostrach, B., & Mendenhall, E. (2017). Syndemics and the biosocial conception of health. *The Lancet, 389*(10072), 941–950.

39. Skaathun, B., Pines, H. A., Patterson, T. L., Semple, S. J., Pekar, J., Harvey-Vera, A., Rangel, G., & Mehta, S. R. (2020). Recent HIV infection among men who have sex with men and transgender women in Tijuana. *Revista de Saúde Pública, 54*, 82.

40. Sun, S., Pachankis, J. E., Li, X., & Operario, D. (2020). Addressing minority stress and mental health among men who have sex with men (MSM) in China. *Current HIV/AIDS Reports, 17*(1), 35–62.

41. Tomori, C., McFall, A. M., Solomon, S. S., Srikrishnan, A. K., Anand, S., Balakrishnan, P., Mehta, S. H., & Celentano, D. D. (2018). Is there synergy in syndemics? Psychosocial conditions and sexual risk among men who have sex with men in India. *Social Science & Medicine, 206*, 110–116.

42. Tsai, A. C., & Burns, B. F. (2015). Syndemics of psychosocial problems and HIV risk: A systematic review of empirical tests of the disease interaction concept. *Social Science & Medicine, 139*, 26–35.

43. Verduzco, I. L. (2014). Barriers to sexual expression and safe sex among Mexican gay men: A qualitative approach. *American Journal of Men's Health, 10*(3), 270–284.

44. Wang, Y., Wang, Z., Jia, M., Liang, A., Yuan, D., Sun, Z., Gan, F., Wang, Y., Cai, Y., & Zhang, Z. (2017). Association between a syndemic of psychosocial problems and unprotected anal intercourse among men who have sex with men in Shanghai, China. *BMC Infectious Diseases, 17*, 46.

45. Zhu, Y., Liu, J., Chen, Y., Zhang, R., & Qu, B. (2018). The relation between mental health, homosexual stigma, childhood abuse, community engagement, and unprotected anal intercourse among MSM in China. *Scientific Reports, 8*(1), 3984.

INDEX

F

G

H

I

L

Printed and bound by CPI Group (UK) Ltd, Croydon, CR0 4YY
18/09/2026
14965062-0001